TRACE ELEMENTS,
HAIR ANALYSIS
AND NUTRITION

Other relevant Keats Publishing titles

Brain Allergies by William H. Philpott, M.D. and Dwight K. Kalita, Ph.D.

Diet and Disease by E. Cheraskin, M.D., D.M.D.; W. M. Ringsdorf, D.M.D.; and J. W. Clark, D.D.S.

Medical Applications of Clinical Nutrition edited by Jeffrey Bland, Ph.D.

Mental and Elemental Nutrients by Carl C. Pfeiffer, Ph.D., M.D.

Minerals and Your Health by Len Mervyn, Ph.D.

Nutrients to Age Without Senility by Abram Hoffer, Ph.D., M.D. and Morton Walker, D.P.M.

Orthomolecular Nutrition by Abram Hoffer, Ph.D., M.D., and Morton Walker, D.P.M.

Physician's Handbook on Orthomolecular Medicine, edited by Roger J. Williams, Ph.D. and Dwight K. Kalita, Ph.D.

The Poisons Around Us by Henry A. Schroeder, M.D.

Recipe for Survival by Doris Grant

The Saccharine Disease by T. L. Cleave, M.D.

Selenium as Food and Medicine by Richard A. Passwater, Ph.D.

Victory Over Diabetes by William H. Philpott, M.D. and Dwight K. Kalita, Ph.D.

TRACE ELEMENTS, HAIR ANALYSIS AND NUTRITION

Richard A. Passwater, Ph.D.
and Elmer M. Cranton, M.D.

Foreword by Jeffrey Bland, Ph.D.

KEATS PUBLISHING, INC. NEW CANAAN, CT

Neither the authors nor the publisher has authorized the use of their names or the use of any of the material contained in this book in connection with the sale, promotion or advertising of any product or apparatus. Any such use is strictly unauthorized and in violation of the rights of Richard A. Passwater, Elmer M. Cranton and Keats Publishing, Inc.

The information contained in this book is in no way to be considered as medical advice. It is advisable to seek professional advice or consult your physician in every case where you are in doubt about your health, or when you have continuing symptoms.

Library of Congress Cataloging in Publication Data

Passwater, Richard A.
  Trace elements, hair analysis, and nutrition.

  Includes bibliographical references and index.
  1. Trace elements in nutrition. 2. Trace elements in the body. 3. Hair—Analysis.
4. Health. I. Cranton, Elmer M. II. Title. [DNLM: 1. Hair—Analysis—Popular
works. 2. Trace elements—Deficiency—Popular works. 3. Trace elements—Poisoning—
Popular works. DU 130 P289t]
QP534.P37   1983   612'.3924   83-75
ISBN   0-87983-265-7
Library of Congress Catalog Card Number: 81-83892

Trace Elements, Hair Analysis and Nutrition

Printed in the United States of America
Keats Publishing, Inc., 27 Pine Street (Box 876) New Canaan, CT 06840
Design by Betty Binns Graphics/Madeleine Sanchez

ACKNOWLEDGMENT

The authors wish to thank the following for their help in reviewing the manuscript: Dr. Garry Gordon, MineraLab; Bob L. Smith, Doctor's Data; James Davenport, Parmae Laboratories; and Dr. Jeffrey Bland, University of Puget Sound. Chapter 31 is published with permission of the Hair Analysis Standardization Board of the American Holistic Medical Institute. Janet Ralston, MineraLab, did much of the work to compile the tables contained in Chapter 32.

We also thank Allison Turner and Barbara Passwater for typing the manuscript.

R.A.P. AND E.M.C.

CONTENTS

FOREWORD

INTRODUCTION

1 MINERALS AND TRACE ELEMENTS 1

2 CHELATION 14

3 THE PROCESS OF HAIR ANALYSIS 18

The macro-minerals

4 CALCIUM 31

5 PHOSPHORUS 60

6 MAGNESIUM 64

The electrolyte minerals

7 POTASSIUM 79

8 SODIUM AND CHLORIDE 92

Trace elements

9 IRON 105

10 ZINC 122

11 COPPER 147

12 MANGANESE 161

13 IODINE 170

Ultra-trace elements

14 CHROMIUM 179

15 SELENIUM 200

16 MOLYBDENUM 209

Research trace elements

17 SILICON 215

18 VANADIUM 222

19 NICKEL 227

20 TIN 230

21 LITHIUM 231

22 RUBIDIUM 234

23 STRONTIUM 239

24 SULFUR 240

25 COBALT 241

Toxic elements

26 LEAD 245

27 CADMIUM 262

28 MERCURY 272

29 ALUMINUM 281

30 ARSENIC 287

Hair analysis interpretation and application: the techniques

31 STANDARDIZATION AND INTERPRETATION OF
   HUMAN HAIR FOR ELEMENTAL CONCENTRATION 291

32 DOCUMENTATION OF THE UTILITY OF
   HAIR ELEMENT ANALYSIS 304

INDEX 368

FOREWORD

The field of trace element nutrition and its relationship to human health and disease is one of the most rapidly advancing fields within the health sciences area. There has been a considerable need over the past two or three years for a comprehensive book which would address the major implications of trace element nutrition in such a way that it would encompass: how to recognize trace element insufficiencies, what the health implications are of these insufficiencies and what the treatment for these problems is.

Such is the value of this excellent book by Dr. Richard Passwater and Dr. Elmer Cranton entitled *Trace Elements, Hair Analysis and Nutrition*. The authors have accomplished the herculean task of consolidating a vast body of clinical and research data into a concise summary which allows the nonspecialist to appreciate not only the large questions concerning mineral nutrition and health, but some of the more subtle and important relationships. The section of the use and misuse of hair mineral analysis in assessment is well written and is the first definitive survey of clinical implications of hair mineral analysis in the literature.

Although the field of mineral metabolism and assessment is still rapidly changing, this volume provides up-to-date and concise information which should be the measuring stick in the field for the next period of time.

This book represents a major contribution to the field and will considerably improve the understanding and knowledge about the important role that trace elements play in human health. I recommend this book as part of the library of all nutritionists who are concerned about the important role that trace elements play in human health and disease.

JEFFREY BLAND, PH.D.
Professor, Biochemistry
University of Puget Sound
Tacoma, Washington
September, 1982

INTRODUCTION

The majority of diseases begin when biochemical imbalances occur at the cellular level. "Deficiencies or excesses of metal ions cause most adverse biological effects," comments D. R. Williams.[1] Occasionally these imbalances actually cause illness; more often they simply hinder the body's efficiency, thereby weakening any number of chemically based immunity processes.

Imbalance of those elements essential to health or interference due to heavy metal accumulation will leave the door open to potential disease; yet more and more, research points out that modern health care has the potential to correct these imbalances before disease reaches the stage of physical symptoms.

This book discusses how nutrient minerals and toxic elemental pollutants affect your health and how a simple hair analysis for trace metals (those elements present in minute quantities) can uncover many mineral deficiencies and toxic accumulations. We want to make you aware that your health depends on what you eat, but just as important, your health depends on what is missing from or contaminating the food you select and how much of that nourishment is digested and assimilated by your body. It is not just a matter of what you put in your mouth, but what reaches every cell in your body.

We feel that this book will help many people overcome health problems that range from "not feeling well" or unexplained tiredness to forestalling the major killer diseases such as cancer and heart disease. We present documented evidence showing how proper mineral balance can achieve this.

This book is jointly written by a biochemist with more than twenty years in trace element research and a physician who has been a leader in incorporating nutrition into a holistic clinical practice and who is also the Chairman of the Hair Analysis Standardization Board, a committee of experts who have no commercial laboratory ties. This book is for you if you have a disease or health problem that has not responded to treatment. It is directed toward everyone; appendices are included in certain discussions to accommodate additional technical details.

This book is for you if you are concerned about the effects of air, water and food pollution on *you*.

Joggers, how much lead are you breathing from car exhausts? Seafood lovers, how much mercury have you accumulated? Ladies, are you developing frail and brittle bones as you pass menopause? Gentlemen, are you developing prostate trouble? Will you be able to respond well to surgery? Do you have increased risk of cancer or heart disease? Are *your* foods supplying the proper balance of minerals?

There is no need to worry about these things needlessly if *you* are not in danger. But how do you know? This book will answer that question by alerting you to the dangers, showing you *how* to protect yourself and how to determine your nutrient mineral levels and toxic element levels.

On the other hand, if you do have a mineral deficiency or toxic accumulation, this book may save your life!

Let's look at a few common examples. A housewife in her early forties had been troubled with that dragging, tired feeling. After running all the standard tests, her doctor said she was in "fine shape." But she was still tired. Finally, her doctor did an analysis for trace minerals in her hair. The hair analysis showed her body had high amounts of toxic lead that caused her tired feeling. Most of the lead came from auto exhaust (this will be explained in Chapter 26).

Once her problem was understood, the cure came easily. She was feeling better in two weeks and the tired feeling vanished within a month.

Undiagnosed lead poisoning had institutionalized a printer as a manic depressive before he discovered his real problem. Simple treatment "cured" him and he has had no symptoms for eight years.

We have seen many hyperactive children and children suffering personality changes that have been solely due to "mild" lead poisoning. One woman went to twenty-two doctors without proper diagnosis until she diagnosed herself as having lead poisoning. She was correct, but it proved to be too late to save her life.

Another example is an executive who suffered from "unexplained" headaches, backaches, weakness and tremors. Most doctors he consulted advised him it was "nerves" due to stress. One psychotherapist gave him antidepressant drugs and shock treatment; they did not work. Later he was found to have mercury poisoning, an increasingly common finding explained in Chapter 28.

That is the toxic pollutant side of the story, which is relatively easy to detect and correct. The nutritional deficiency side escapes detection more frequently, is more difficult to diagnose, and it is not always a simple matter to correct. Without proper guidance, improper attempts to correct a mineral deficiency by taking massive amounts of that one mineral may create deficiencies in other minerals, due to imbalance. This book will show you how to uncover mineral deficiencies, confirm that they do exist and restore mineral balance.

Mineral imbalance increases vulnerability to disease, aggravates existing diseases and shortens the lifespan. When mineral balance is restored, you'll begin to feel better and look better within weeks. Proper mineral balance can restore vigor, put luster back in your hair, a healthy glow in your skin, sparkle in your eye, and a spring to your step. We have records of improved sex life, prostates returning to normal health, and menopausal symptoms disappearing when mineral balance is restored.

Dieters who had been physical wrecks for months after taking diuretics while they dieted, athletes who had suddenly become weak, and heart patients on medication who had become tired and impotent have improved immediately when proper mineral balance was restored. This book contains many such case histories.

Our experience suggests that most people have mineral imbalances. We agree with Dr. Donald Oberleas, Chairman of the Department of Nutrition and Food Sciences at the University of Kentucky, who estimates that as many as 80 percent of Americans are deficient in mineral intake.[2] Dr. William Strain, Director of the Trace Elements Laboratory at Case Western Reserve University, has done trace mineral analysis on more than 16,000 people and has found virtually all of them to have mineral deficiencies.[3]

It is clear that Americans are becoming essential element-starved and toxic element-polluted due to improper diet, depleted and contaminated soils, food processing and environmental pollution. What can you do about it? Protect yourself by reading on!

REFERENCES

1 Williams, D. R., ed. 1976. *An Introduction to Bio-Inorganic Chemistry*. Springfield, Illinois: Charles C. Thomas, p. 315.

2 Vaisrub, S. May 31, 1976. *J. Amer. Med. Assoc.* 235(22): 2422.

3 Gibson, R. Nov. 29, 1977. *Nat. Eng.* 37.

TRACE ELEMENTS,
HAIR ANALYSIS
AND NUTRITION

This review covers the following elements:

CALCIUM

PHOSPHORUS

MAGNESIUM

POTASSIUM

SODIUM and CHLORIDE

IRON

ZINC

COPPER

MANGANESE

IODINE

CHROMIUM

SELENIUM

MOLYBDENUM

SILICON

VANADIUM

NICKEL

TIN

LITHIUM

RUBIDIUM

STRONTIUM

SULFUR

COBALT

LEAD

CADMIUM

MERCURY

ALUMINUM

ARSENIC

1

MINERALS AND TRACE ELEMENTS

In recent years there has been much concern about vitamin deficiencies in the American diet. Government surveys show that only 28 percent of American diets have vitamin A intakes providing 100 percent of the Recommended Dietary Allowance (RDA) and only 60 percent of the American diets have vitamin C intakes providing 100 percent of the RDA.[1]

However, the greatest deficiencies are the deficiencies of various elements in our diets commonly called minerals. There has not been much concern expressed over mineral deficiencies until now because only recently have the essential roles of many of these minerals been understood. The fact that these vital minerals are disappearing from modern diets has not been appreciated because few surveys ever include minerals and "trace elements." The Hanes survey (the U.S. Department of Health and the Health and Nutrition Examination Survey) includes only two minerals, calcium and iron. It found only 39 percent of Americans to be receiving 100 percent of the RDA for calcium and 64 percent receiving the RDA for iron (95 percent of females aged eighteen to forty-four had iron intakes below the RDA).[1]

The distinction between minerals and trace elements will be made shortly, but common usage groups them together as minerals.

Few physicians speak of trace elements because most physicians have not been exposed to studies showing the role of minerals and trace elements in protecting us against heart disease, cancer, arthritis and other ailments. Others believe that since the required quantities are so small they cannot be very important

Most physicians who do learn of the roles of minerals and trace elements also learn of the complicated interrelationships between the various elements and decide to await further clarification. We hope this book will offer clarification of the existing knowledge of this new science.

The quantities of minerals and trace elements in our diets and in our bodies are often in the "milligram" or "microgram" range, and are sometimes referred to as a "part per million" or "part per billion." These units are not in common usage and may not be familiar to everyone. We'll try to give you a feeling for these small quantities now and later show how such small quantities exert such large influence on health.

Most people can visualize either an ounce or gram of something. A gram is the metric unit of weight which is one-twenty eighth of an ounce. A milligram is a thousandth of a gram and a microgram is a millionth of a gram (or a thousandth of a milligram). A milligram of most substances is just a speck or two, while a microgram is difficult to see with the naked eye.

If a gram of material contains a microgram of another substance, then the material is said to contain one-part-per-million of the other substance. If only a nanogram (a billionth of a gram or a thousandth of a microgram) of another substance is present in each gram of a material, then the substance is said to contain one part-per-billion of that material.

These are very small quantities indeed. A favorite device of scientists describing these quantities is to imagine that it was necessary to put one drop of an additive into 14,000 gallons of jet fuel. The drop represents one-part-per-billion concentration. Yet that drop makes the difference in whether a jet plane gets to its destination or not when flying from New York to Greece.

Our bodies consist of molecules made up of atoms of the basic elements. The vast majority of atoms in our bodies are of the elements hydrogen, carbon, nitrogen, oxygen and sulfur. These atoms are combined into molecules of protein, carbohydrates, fats, vitamins and water. Our bodies do not need elemental hydrogen, nitrogen or sulfur as such, but we do need to ingest certain essential groupings of these elements. The groupings, called molecules, are obtained from food, and we each have specific requirements for certain amino acids (portions of proteins), fatty acids (portions of fats) and vitamins. (Carbohydrates are not considered essential dietary components, but we all experience better health when adequate amounts are in the diet.)

An exception is oxygen, which we need as the pure element, as the diatomic molecule, O_2, and also as a component of proteins, carbohydrates, fats, vitamins and water.

Other elements in the body play major roles, even though their concentrations are low. Some of these elements are present in appreciable quantities, while others are present only in hard-to-measure "traces." Those elements of the former type—such as calcium, which typically totals 1200 grams in the adult—have structural functions as well as enzymatic functions. In common usage these elements have been called "minerals." The elements of the latter type—such as selenium, which typically totals less than a milligram in an adult—do not usually contribute to the structure of the body, but only to enzymatic reactions. These elements are called "trace elements." How so few atoms of specific elements can be so important has to do with their role in enzymes and this will be explained later.

The body processes minerals as elements: therefore, the term "mineral" (an inorganic compound—a mixture of elements) is inappropriate. We can digest and absorb some of the elements in some minerals, but most of our "mineral" intake is a part of organic living tissue (plant or animal) and not inorganic. Some of the "mineral" is still in the elemental form, but much is incorporated into tissue or enzymes, just as it will eventually become in our bodies.

However, we are stuck with the common usage term for the most part. Today general usage in nutrition confines the term "mineral" to those elements that are largely incorporated into bone tissue, which contains compounds identical to true inorganic minerals found in the ground.

The Food and Nutrition Board of the National Academy of Sciences makes the following classifications:

MACRO-MINERALS calcium, phosphorus, magnesium, sodium, potassium and chlorine (The latter three are sub-classified as electrolytes)

TRACE ELEMENTS iron, zinc, copper, manganese, iodine, chromium, selenium, molybdenum

The Food and Nutrition Board also includes fluorine. Generally, fluorine is listed as a trace element. We do not consider the existing evidence sufficient to establish fluorine or fluoride as an essential element. We are aware of the many studies claiming improved resistance to tooth decay for fluoride, but these studies are not conclusive. We are also aware of studies showing that excesses are toxic.

Since fluoride deficiencies do not exist (by definition) and hair analysis for fluorine as a toxicant does not exist (due to instrumental limitation), we offer no further discussion of this element.

We also acknowledge the research indicating silicon, vanadium, nickel, tin, strontium, and arsenic as very likely to be essential, with lithium and rubidium as being probably essential.

When we discuss hair analysis, we refer to elements contained in the hair, not to "mineral" compounds. The elements incorporated into hair are usually attached to proteins, and are never present as inorganic minerals.

Our knowledge of trace elements is expanding, and at the present time, it is felt that we probably have not identified all of the elements that are necessary for life. Some elements have been proven essential, others have shown evidence of being essential but need more research, and still others may have escaped our suspicion of being essential but may eventually enter that category.

Dr. Walter Mertz of the U.S. Department of Agriculture explains: "By the simplest definition, an essential element is one required for maintenance of life; its absence results in death of the organism. Severe deficiencies of an element that results in death are difficult to produce, particularly if the element is required in very low concentrations. A broader definition of essential elements has therefore been proposed and is widely accepted: an element is essential when a deficient intake consistently results in an impairment of a function from optimal to suboptimal and when supplementation with physiological levels of this element, but not of others, prevents or cures this impairment."[2]

FIGURE 1.1

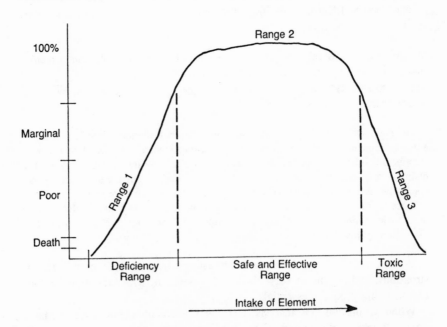

The "Supernutrition Curve" showing the three ranges of intake versus health benefits described in the text. *Source:* Based on Passwater, R. 1975. *Supernutrition.* New York: Dial Press.

How much?

Deficiencies in essential elements are those that produce death or impaired function. This implies that increasing quantities brings about increasing function and health. Actually there are three ranges to consider with dietary intake of elements—*and two of these are bad!*

Range one is where the intake is insufficient and causes death or poor health. Range two is a safe and adequate range which includes the ideal intake for optimal health. Range three is where the intake is excessive and brings about toxicity directly, or causes poor health by interfering with the utilization of other elements. Figure 1.1 illustrates the range concept, and Figure 1.2 illustrates that some minerals may interfere with certain others. These ranges may differ significantly from one person to another.

In other words, there is one optimal range of intake for each element for each person; less is bad and more is bad.

Unknowledgeable tinkering with the diet—either stripping trace elements away in food processing or improper supplementation—can lead to serious disease. We hope this book will point out the dangers of both without causing undue alarm, and we hope it will guide you in optimizing *your* diet to achieve the fullest health possible.

FIGURE 1.2A HOW TO INTERPRET THE MINERAL WHEEL:

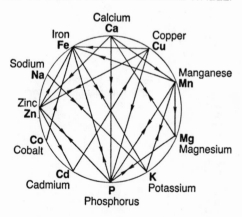

If a mineral has an arrow pointing to another mineral, it means a deficiency of that mineral or interference with its metabolism may be caused by excesses of the mineral from whence the arrow *originates.*

Source: Based on research of several investigators in animal testing, the above mineral interrelationships appear to be established.

FIGURE 1.2 MINERAL INTERFERENCES

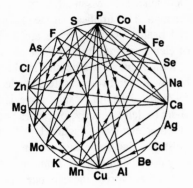

If a mineral has an arrow pointing to another mineral, it means a deficiency of that mineral or interference with its metabolism may be caused by excesses of the mineral from whence the arrow *originates*.

Source: Ashmead, H. 1970. *J. Applied Nutrition* 22(1&2) 44.

FIGURE 1.2B

METAL
$V+^3$
$Fe+^3$
$In+^3$
$Th+^4$
$Hg+^2$
$Ti+^3$
$Ga+^3$
$Cu+^2$
$VO+^2$
$Ni+^2$
$Pd+^2$
$Y+^3$
$Pb+^2$
$TiO+^2$
$Zn+^2$
$Cd+^2$
$Co+^2$
$Al+^3$
$Fe+^2$
$Mn+^2$
$V+^2$
$Ca+^2$
$Sc+^3$
$Mg+^2$
$Sr+^2$
$Ba+^2$
Rare Earths

Excessive levels of any one mineral depress other minerals that are lower in the electromotive series.

While we are discussing mineral and trace element toxicity, it is interesting to note that recent research has demonstrated essential functions for at least three trace elements—selenium, chromium and arsenic—which previously had been known only as toxic.[2]

Why minerals are so vital to health

Minerals and trace elements do not supply fuel or energy to the body; they assist in the production of energy and in the other chemical reactions of life.

The vast majority of chemical reactions that make up the life process are governed by certain proteins in the body called enzymes. There are thousands and thousands of different enzymes, each type controlling one specific chemical reaction. Enzymes are catalysts—that is, they control the rate of the reaction without being consumed by the reaction themselves. Thus they are reusable.

Minerals and trace elements are constituents of or interact with enzymes. Magnesium is known to be part of many different enzymes, and thus controls many different functions in the body. Sometimes elements are constituents of enzymes that govern other body components such as hormones, which in turn regulate other reactions. This biological amplification explains how a hundred nanograms of a mineral or trace element such as cobalt (which is a constituent of vitamin B12) can be a life or death factor to an adult weighing a trillion times more.

This phenomenon is illustrated in Figure 1.3. You can see that a little does a lot, but keep in mind that a small difference in intake—a few micrograms—can make a large difference in health. It reminds one of the story of the famous biologist who once pointed out that there is really very little difference between the male and the female; to which the classic rejoinder was, "Vive la difference!"

Today's problems

Mineral intakes may not have been widespread problems in the past, with a few classic exceptions such as iodine deficiency in the goiter belt. Today there are several serious problems that should concern us all.

■ We are eating less food, but still need the same amount of minerals and trace elements.

■ We are eating more empty calories and highly processed foods stripped of most of their minerals and trace elements.

■ Modern farming practices have decreased the mineral content of soil and some fertilizers have made some minerals unavailable to plants.

■ Other elements, such as sodium and phosphorus, have been overabundantly added to the diet and can disturb the natural mineral ratios.

Today, most people are less active, so they eat fewer calories in an effort to maintain their desired weight. The fewer calories consumed means less food eaten. Although the energy content of the diet is decreased, essentially the same amounts of minerals and trace elements are needed to "fire" the various reactions of the life process.

Yet, there is also a trend towards eating more processed foods that have lost their natural mineral and trace element supply, and more food "substitutes" such as artificial orange juice or artificial eggs.

FIGURE 1:3 BIOLOGICAL AMPLIFICATION OF TRACE ELEMENT ACTION (Source)

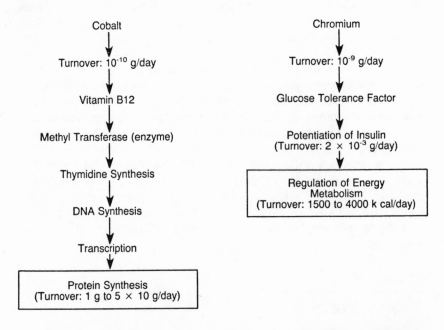

As Dr. Walter Mertz told Congress in 1977, "A continuation of the present trend toward consumption of more partitioned, refined and fabricated foods must eventually lead to a point where the rest of the diet cannot meet the requirements for all essential nutrients any more. In the future, we will not be able to rely any more on our premise that the consumption of a varied, balanced diet will provide all of the essential trace elements, because such a diet will be very difficult to obtain for millions of people."[3]

In the same year, Dr. Carole Christopher of Pennsylvania State University warned newspaper food editors that "the consumption of refined foods is inappropriately and excessively replacing conventional foods and they are not the nutritional counterparts of the foods they replace. . . . Trace minerals are of particular concern because there are only a very few about which we know enough to include them in foods without risking toxicity or creating imbalances with other essential nutrients."[3]

One comment regarding "balanced" diets. We are not sure what is normally meant by balanced. In this book we report several so-called "balanced" diets that are almost completely devoid of chromium or greatly lacking in iron or zinc. To us a "balanced" diet implies a balance of all essential nutrients, not just the macronutrients (protein, carbohydrates, fats).

If the minerals aren't in the soil, the elements won't be in the food. In October 1981, the Associated Press carried the following story warning about the loss of topsoil.

The loss of topsoil in the United States and other countries is so severe that it could trigger food shortages in the 1980s surpassing the impact of oil shortages during the 1970s, a new study concluded yesterday.

The study, done by Lester Brown, head of the Worldwatch Institute, said a doubling in world food output since 1950 was achieved at the expense of severe land abuse.

"Perhaps the most serious single threat humanity now faces is the widespread loss of topsoil," Brown, an agricultural specialist, said in the study, which is being published as a book titled *Building a Sustainable Society*.

"Civilization cannot survive this continuing loss of topsoil," Brown said. "If not arrested, this loss of soil could cause the food problem to unfold during the '80s as the energy problem did during the '70s.

"The productivity of 34 percent of American cropland is declining because of an excessive loss of topsoil each year," Brown said.

A detailed survey by the Agriculture Department last year discovered "alarmingly high" erosion in several states. It estimated soil losses of 14.1 tons an acre in Tennessee, 11.4 tons an acre in Missouri and 10.9 tons in Mississippi.

The yearly loss of 5.5 billion tons of topsoil has been expressed in another way by the U. S. Department of Agriculture: "Enough soil goes into the Mississippi River in one year to build an island a mile long and 1¼-mile wide and 2000 feet high. It contains the equivalent of 808 rail carloads of phosphorus, 21,121 carloads of potassium, 291,511 carloads of calcium and 67 carloads of magnesium. Iowa, the latest terrible reminder of our neglect of a primary resource, has already lost half of its original topsoil in one century."

However, the concern expressed is for the loss of topsoil and its minerals needed for crops—not for human nutrition. If a soil is too low in minerals such as magnesium, iron or manganese, plants will not grow in it. Plants do *not* need some trace minerals which are of vital importance to humans—as examples, iodine, selenium and chromium. Soils deficient in one or more of these nutrients can yield bountiful, healthy crops. Yet humans or other animals that consume these crops may develop severe deficiency diseases.

Many trace elements are removed from the soil by weather and years of cultivation. Of the forty-four minerals and trace elements now found in the sea, twenty are no longer in the land. They are not replaced by the fertilizers which usually contain only nitrates, phosphates, potassium, and occasionally sulfates, or lime which contains calcium.

Mineral forms

There are several forms of minerals and trace elements. That is, the required elements may be present in the diet as metals, inorganic salts, organic salts (called esters), chelates or incorporated into protein.

Iron is an essential element, but we will absorb little iron by swallowing metallic iron pellets. In order for our body to absorb the iron, it must first be "ionized" (dissolved) and then "chelated" (surrounded or insulated) by amino acids in the intestine so that the dissolved iron—which is an electrically charged ion—can be carried through the intestinal walls which are also charged. Chelated minerals are discussed in fuller detail in an appendix to this chapter, for those interested.

Stomach acid dissolves iron metal very poorly. However, if we take iron salts, such as ferrous sulfate (ferrous and ferric are the chemists' names for iron compounds), which dissolves very efficiently in stomach acid, iron ions are readily formed. The ions can then be chelated and carried through the intestinal walls.

However, ferrous sulfate sometimes is rough on the digestive system and can cause constipation or abdominal discomfort. Organic iron complexes, such as ferrous gluconate or ferrous fumerate are also efficiently dissolved (ionized), but they are milder and usually do not produce gastric upset or constipation.

Still, the organic iron complex must be chelated to pass efficiently through the electrically charged intestinal walls. One way to increase the probability of having the iron chelated is to take the iron as iron chelate. This is merely iron complexed in a very specific fashion with amino acids so that it can be more readily absorbed. This does not mean that other forms of iron cannot be very effective for most people. Chelated elements are reported to be more efficiently absorbed than other forms of the element, although the degree of increased efficiency varies from element to element.

Typical inorganic salts are oxides, carbonates, sulfates and chlorides. Typical organic complexes are lactates, fumarates and gluconates. Chelates are designated as chelates. All chelates are organic complexes, but not all organic complexes are chelates. Some mineral organic complexes such as gluconates have been called "weak chelates." This usage is accepted by some scientists but not by others.

Toxic elements

Not all elements are essential to life. Some elements sneak into our bodies that are not only useless as nutrients, but also toxic. And to compound the issue, most essential nutrients have toxic effects when taken in excessive amounts.

Therefore, we cannot truly divide elements into "nutrients" and "poisons." In this book, we have made a distinction between those elements known to be essential nutrients, those elements under active research to establish if they are essential or not, and those elements that frequently have been associated with toxicity problems, even though some may be essential nutrients at lower levels while others in this group have no known nutrition value. This group includes lead, cadmium, mercury and aluminum.

TABLE 1.1 ESSENTIALITY OR TOXICITY OF MINERAL ELEMENTS FOR HUMANS

Elements	Importance	Reference
Calcium	Essentiality well-documented	1
Magnesium	Essentiality well-documented	1
Phosphorus	Essentiality well-documented	1
Sodium	Essentiality well-documented	1
Potassium	Essentiality well-documented	1
Iron	Essentiality well-documented	1
Zinc	Essentiality well-documented	1
Copper	Essentiality well-documented	1
Manganese	Essentiality well-documented	1
Chromium	Essentiality well-documented	1
Selenium	Essentiality well-documented	1
Molybdenum	Deficiency states in humans not known but negative balances seen in subjects consuming 0.1 mg, thus estimated adequate RDA intake provided. Excess Mo intake may relate to gout and urinary loss of Cu.	1
Cobalt	Essential as part of B12 molecule; no utility in measuring cobalt directly as indicator of Co-B12 status. Toxicity low but has been observed in man.	2
Nickel	Evidence for Ni deficiency in human has not been found but restricted intakes of Ni may occur and there may be an increased need for Ni in certain disorders. Orally ingested Ni relatively non-toxic; inhaled Ni more toxic and some forms carcinogenic.	3
Lithium	No known essential function. Toxicity can occur at pharmacological dose levels.	4

MINERALS AND TRACE ELEMENTS

ESSENTIALITY OR TOXICITY OF MINERAL ELEMENTS FOR HUMANS (*cont.*)

Elements	Importance	Reference
Vanadium	Presumed essential for man; borderline deficiency more of concern than toxicity. Occasional cases of industrial toxicity have been reported.	5
Lead	Toxicity well-established	1
Mercury	Toxicity well-established	1
Cadmium	Toxicity well-established	1
Arsenic	Toxicity well-established	1
Aluminum	No known essential function; can be toxic to some persons under certain conditions.	6, 7
Strontium	No known essential function; no evidence that stable Sr exerts deleterious effects at usual dietary levels; radioactive Sr more hazardous.	8
Iodine	Essentiality well-established	1
Silicon	Si deficiency has not been described in man; Si has important functions in human growth and maintenance of connective tissues. Adequate Si nutrition should not be taken for granted.	9
Tin	Deficiencies or toxicities of tin are unknown in man.	10
Silver	No evidence that silver is essential, nor is it considered very toxic.	2
Fluorine	Essentiality debated and toxicity recognized.	1
Antimony	No essential function. Potential exposure from food, therapeutic or occupational use; low toxicity.	2, 11
Beryllium	Toxic to humans; potential occupational exposure hazard.	11

In today's world elemental toxicity is becoming a serious, but usually undetected, health problem. Hair analysis provides a convenient screening procedure to detect elemental toxicity as well as nutritional deficiency. The advantages of this beneficial technique are discussed in the following chapter.

REFERENCES FOR ESSENTIALITY OR TOXICITY OF MINERAL ELEMENTS

1 *Recommended Dietary Allowances*. National Research Council. 1980.

2 Underwood, E.J. 1977. *Trace Elements in Human and Animal Nutrition*. Fourth Edition. New York: Academic Press.

3 Nielsen, F. *et al*. 1977. In: *Geochemistry and the Environment, vol. II—The Relation of Other Selected Trace Elements to Health and Disease*. Washington, D.C.: National Academy of Sciences, p. 40–53.

4 Mertz, N. *et al*. 1974. In: *Geochemistry and the Environment, vol. I—The Relation of Selected Trace Elements to Health and Disease*, Washington, D.C.: National Academy of Sciences, p. 36–42.

5 Hopkins, L. *et al*. 1977. In: *Geochemistry and the Environment, vol. II*. Washington, D.C.: National Academy of Sciences, p. 93–107.

6 Schenk, R., Bjorksten, J., Lipert, R., and Mortell, M. March 1981. *Rejuvenation* 9(1).

7 Bowdler, N. *et al*. 1979. *Pharm. Biochem. Behavior* 10: 505–512.

8 Wasserman, R., *et al*. 1977. In: *Geochemistry and the Environment, vol. II*. Washington, D.C.: National Academy of Sciences, p. 73–87.

9 Nielsen, F. 1976. In: *Trace Elements in Human Health and Disease, vol. II*. Ananda Prasad, ed. New York: Academic Press, p. 379–399.

10 Beeson, K. *et al*. 1977. In: *Geochemistry and the Environment, vol. II*. Washington, D.C.: National Academy of Sciences, p. 88–92.

11 Jenkins, D. 1981. *Biological Monitoring of Toxic Trace Elements*. Las Vegas, Nevada: EPA Project Summary.

REFERENCES FOR CHAPTER ONE

1 U.S. Dept. of Health. 1971–72. First Health and Nutrition Examination Survey (HANES), United States, Preliminary Findings, Pub. Health Service, HRA.

2 Mertz, W. 1981. *Science* 213:1332–1338.

3 Burros, M. Jan. 19, 1978. *The Washington Post*, El.

2

CHELATION

"Chelated" minerals are often confused with a medical technique called "chelation therapy." This chapter discusses both the degree of improved assimilation of mineral "chelates" and the medical procedure called "chelation therapy" that removes toxic elements from the body.

Mineral chelates

A chelate (pronounced key-late) is a special complex involving a particular type of attraction between an organic complex and a mineral or trace element. The element (mineral, metal or trace element) is surrounded by the organic complex which has formed a ring-like arrangement of its atoms. This "ring" arrangement also holds the element in place within the ring by a special type of loose chemical bond. This special type of attraction of the element to the organic complex is likened to the pincer action of the claws of a crab. In fact, the term "chelate" originates from the Greek word "chele" which means "crab claw."

A chelate consists of a metal ion held in place by a special attraction which chemists refer to as a "coordinate covalent bond" which is formed by five or

14

six atoms in a ring. The atoms usually include carbon, oxygen, hydrogen and nitrogen.

Chelates can have various stabilities. A "strong" chelate is useless as a nutrient because it will never release its metal ion for use by the body. On the other hand, a strong chelate is excellent for removing unwanted metals from the body. The synthetic amino acid, EDTA, is a strong chelating agent and is widely used to sequester metallic pollutants and carry them out of the body. EDTA is used in intravenous chelation therapy.

A weak chelate offers little advantage over an inorganic salt or organic complex if it dissociates prematurely. If the metal ion is released in the digestive tract it can then combine with another ion to form an insoluble complex or be trapped on the intestinal wall due to electronic attraction.

Most dissolved minerals and trace elements are ions having positive charges, while the intestinal mucosa is negatively charged. Minerals and trace elements in inorganic form cannot pass through the electrical barrier of the intestinal wall. They adhere to the intestinal wall until the muscular contractions of the digestive system push them into the colon from where they are excreted intact. If the intestinal wall becomes heavily plugged with metal ions, then a fluid is released which washes the trapped elements away in diarrhea.

Some organic complexes such as gluconates contain carbon, oxygen and hydrogen, but do not contain nitrogen. Gluconate forms a weaker chelate than nitrogen compounds. Such complexes may dissociate in the stomach. The metal ion can become trapped as discussed above for the case of weak chelates, and the gluconate is converted to glucoronic acid and then to glucose. The removal of the organic complexing agent may result in less efficient absorption.

Medium-strength chelates protect the metal ion, facilitate its transport through the intestinal wall and release the metal ion in the bloodstream where it can then be bound to a carrier and transported to the cells. Some amino acids, peptides and proteins, when properly prepared, form excellent medium-strength chelates. Aspartate is one such amino acid.

Only certain minerals and trace elements can form coordinate covalent bonds with chelating agents. Non-metals, such as phosphorus and selenium, and singly-charged (monovalent) metals, such as sodium and potassium, cannot form chelates. Only multi-charged (multivalent) metals, such as calcium, magnesium, iron, zinc, copper, manganese and chromium form chelates.

The improved absorption of chelates can be seen in Table 2.2. Chelated copper is assimilated three to six times better than inorganic copper salts, chelated magnesium is assimilated two to three times better than inorganic magnesium salts, chelated iron is assimilated four to five times better than inorganic iron salts, and chelated zinc is assimilated two to three times better than inorganic zinc salts. Other organic salts such as gluconates and fumarates are absorbed better than the inorganic salts, but slightly less well absorbed than the most expensive peptide or amino acid chelates.

In the case of such elements as copper, zinc and manganese it may be more cost-effective to take organic complexes such as gluconates and fumarates. The same absorption may be obtained at much less expense by consuming a somewhat larger amount of the organic complex. In the case of magnesium, studies have shown that the aspartate is one of the best absorbed.

The fact that mineral chelates are both absorbed and utilized by the body has been proven by using radioactive minerals as tracers. (Iron is normally not radioactive, but it can be made to be so in the laboratory especially for the purpose of tracing its pathway through the body.)

Table 2.3 compares the incorporation of radioactively tagged iron from both inorganic iron sulfate and chelated iron.

Note that more of the chelated iron is retained, while more of the inorganic iron is excreted in the feces and urine.

Chelation therapy

Chelation therapy is a safe, nonsurgical technique that carries unwanted metal pollutants such as lead and cadmium out of the body and also removes free ionic calcium deposited in arterial plaques. This technique (also called chelation endarterectomy) is painless, safe, effective, and far less expensive than bypass surgery.

Chelation therapy is available from approximately one thousand physicians, many of whom belong to the American Academy of Medical Preventics (6151 West Century Blvd., Suite 1114, Los Angeles, CA 90045), and/or the American Holistic Medical Association (6932 Little River Turnpike, Annandale, VA 20003).

The procedure consists of administering a solution of the synthetic amino acid Na_2 EDTA (disodium ethylene-diamine-tetra-acetic acid) slowly into the bloodstream. As the compound flows through the arteries, the abnormal deposits of calcium are removed from the arteries as though a powerful magnet were pulling them out. As the EDTA flows through the body, it also binds up lead, mercury, cadmium and aluminum and carries them out. The health benefits of chelation therapy are considerable and have been described in *Supernutrition For Healthy Hearts* (Passwater, R. 1977. New York: Dial Press) and several other recent books.

TABLE 2.1 ASSIMILATION OF MINERALS IN RAT GUT (EXPRESSED AS PPM)

	Control	Organic fish meal chelate	Organic soybean meal chelate	Organic whey chelate	Inorganic carbonate	Inorganic sulfate	Inorganic oxide
Copper	trace	33	35	17	12	8	11
Magnesium	7	94	57	52	77	36	23
Iron	23	298	130	80	171	78	61
Zinc	14	191	191	126	87	84	66

Source: Ashmead, H. 1970. *J. Appl. Nutr.* 22(1&2):46.

TABLE 2.2 COMPARISON OF Fe_{59} RETENTION AND DISTRIBUTION FROM IRON SULFATE AND IRON AMINO ACID CHELATE IN THE RAT

Body part	cc/m/gm Iron sulfate	Iron amino acid chelate	% Inc.(Dec) amino acid chel./sulf.
Heart	63	151	140%
Liver	136	243	79%
Leg muscle	2	54	2,600%
Jaw muscle	14	138	886%
Brain	31	130	319%
Kidney	2	327	16,250%
Testes	20	109	445%
Blood serum	700	1,797	157%
Red blood cells	724	2,076	180%
Whole blood	1,355	4,215	211%
Feces	302,400	214,000	(29%)
Urine	490	370	(24%)

Data are shown as corrected counts per minute per gram of body portion being analyzed (cc/m/gm) Average of Rats.

Source: Ashmead, H., *et al.* 1974. *J. Appl. Nutr.* 26(2):5.

TABLE 2.3 CONVERSION TABLE TO DETERMINE THE AMOUNT OF "ELEMENTAL" MINERAL OR TRACE ELEMENT IN ITS AMINO ACID OR PROTEIN CHELATED FORM

Mineral	Chelated weight (commonly available)	Elemental weight contained in that chelated weight
Calcium	1000 mg	200 mg
Magnesium	500 mg	100 mg
Zinc	220 mg	22 mg
Iron	300 mg	30 mg
Manganese	500 mg	50 mg
Copper	125 mg	2.5 mg
Chromium	50 mg	1 mg

3

THE PROCESS OF HAIR ANALYSIS

Obviously, if there is more involved in nourishing your body than just food selection, you can never be sure how well you are nourished unless you monitor the body's mineral content. Are the proper nutrients still in the food you eat and do you efficiently absorb them? Only measurement of the trace element balance within your body will answer these vital questions.

How do you monitor your nutrient trace element balance and toxic metal pollution? Which specimen will tell the story—blood, urine, tissue biopsy or hair analysis?

Each method has strengths and limitations, and none should be relied upon as your sole mineral or trace element diagnostic tool. However, as an overall health indicator and as a measuring tool for biochemical mineral balance, hair analysis is the most convenient screening choice. Hair analysis can also be a most accurate method to monitor your exposure to certain toxic metal pollutants such as lead, cadmium or arsenic.[1]

Hair is like a strip of chart paper curling out of a scientific measuring instrument that is comparable to your body. It is permanently recording the past events of your trace element status. As your hair grows about one millimeter every three days or one-half inch per month, it takes protein from the blood and in the process, concentrates nutrient and toxic elements into the growing hair shaft. Elemental concentrations in the hair are often ten times or more greater than that in blood or urine.

Research has shown that for many elements hair more closely reflects body mineral stores than does blood or urine, particularly in cases of toxic metal accumulation. Often hair will show toxicity when blood and urine will not. The blood shows only what is present at the moment the blood is drawn while urine shows only what the body is eliminating, not what is stored. Hair grows slowly and analysis of hair levels will indicate the average levels in the body over a long period of time. The alternative to hair analysis is to obtain biopsy specimens from body organs. This requires surgery, is very expensive, is objectionable and would not be acceptable to most people. Hair analysis is not as accurate as surgical biopsy, but it provides an excellent screening measurement and is simple, safe and relatively inexpensive.

The advantages

Over 1500 citations in the world's scientific and medical literature attest to the usefulness of hair analysis as a screening diagnostic tool. Many of these references will be cited in our closing chapter as they pertain to the validity of hair analysis for each element discussed.

Hair analysis is proving to be invaluable to an ever-increasing number of nutrition-oriented health practitioners. Their clinical results further testify to the validity of hair analysis.

Hair analysis is an important screening tool that is cost-effective. If used properly, it will significantly extend the benefits of health care. If used improperly, it can cause overconcern, misdiagnosis, mistreatment or give false security. Hair analysis must be interpreted by a professional skilled in the interrelationships outlined in this book. To repeat, hair analysis by itself—just as blood analysis by itself—cannot be used to diagnose the presence or absence of disease. It is a helpful indicator, not a complete answer.

A novice could suggest that one trace element be inappropriately increased and this would have the effect of interfering with another trace element. For example, a zinc overdose could lead to a copper shortage.

Or the novice could conclude that a low iron level in the hair suggests the need for more dietary iron, which would prove to be a fatal mistake in the few people suffering from hemochromatosis. In fact, iron in hair has not been proven to correlate well with body stores of iron. Serum ferritin, a blood test, is far more accurate.

Or the novice could misinterpret high levels of hair zinc as indicating high zinc intake, when they really might indicate a low zinc intake and poor hair growth in a severely malnourished patient.

These complicating factors are explained in this book, but interpretation should be left to a health practitioner.

However, from the information contained in hair analysis, a health professional may tailor a specific nutritional program to restore the natural balance of the body.

Hair analysis has been found to be a valuable technique to identify subclinical signs of chronic diseases. When used with other tests, hair analysis provides accurate data that is not readily available by any alternative method, and, unlike blood or urine tests, hair analysis reflects systemic levels of mineral content and long-term retention of heavy metals.

Hair has several advantages as a specimen. It is:

■ biologically stable—stores easily, ships well, will not deteriorate
■ easy to obtain—non-traumatic, non-invasive
■ not buffered against changes as are blood and urine[8]
■ reflective of certain systemic mineral levels [9,10]
■ more easily and accurately measured than other specimens
■ in equilibrium with systemic activities and reflects metabolic balance over a period of time
■ a capsule of the body's general condition, not just a specific organ or tissue

Hair analysis for trace elements provides earlier detection of some diseases and some nutrient imbalances. Some clinicians are reporting that they can detect several diseases with great reliability, just by observing patterns of ratios of elements in the hair. These early findings may prove to be of great significance, but at this writing, our view is that this research needs further confirmation by several observers to prove its universality.

Table 3.2 contains recommendations following hair analysis for courses of action to be taken to correct abnormalities. Only those elements for which scientific evidence proves clinical significance are included.

If more precise, follow-up testing confirms a severe mineral or trace element deficiency we would recommend that doses of that mineral be taken at bedtime or on first awakening in the morning, well prior to breakfast, so that the excess quantities of that single element do not interfere with absorption of other essential nutrients contained with meals. In addition it is recommended that a balanced, multiple vitamin-mineral supplement be taken with each meal which contains the important essential nutrients in a physiologic ratio which approximates that found in nature and which does not contain a trace element in excess quantities which would block the uptake of other elements. Supplements containing approximately the following ingredients, as shown in Table 3.1, manufactured by a reputable company and formulated with a lengthy shelf life and in a readily absorbable form would be adequate:

TABLE 3.1 TOTAL DAILY INTAKE OF A BALANCED NUTRITIONAL SUPPLEMENT PROGRAM

Vitamin A (fish liver oil)	25,000 I.U.
Vitamin D (fish liver oil)	100 I.U.
Vitamin C (ascorbic acid)	1200 mg
Vitamin B1 (thiamine HCl)	100 mg
Vitamin B2 (riboflavin)	50 mg
Vitamin B6 (pyridoxine HCl)	100 mg
Vitamin B12	100 mcg
Niacin (vitamin B3, nicotinic acid)	50 mg
Niacinamide (vitamin B3)	150 mg
Pantothenic acid	500 mg
Folic acid	800 mcg
Biotin	100 mcg
Choline	50 mg
Inositol	100 mg
Para-amino benzoic acid (PABA)	50 mg
Vitamin E (d-alpha-tocopheryl acetate)	400 I.U.
Calcium	500 mg
Magnesium	500 mg
Potassium	99 mg
Iron	20 mg
Iodine	250 mcg
Copper	2 mg
Manganese	20 mg
Zinc	20 mg
Molybdenum	100 mcg
Chromium	200 mcg
Selenium	200 mcg
Bioflavonoids (rutin, hesperidine)	100 mg
Trace minerals (ocean grown sources)	100 mg

TABLE 3.2 HAIR ANALYSIS INTERPRETATION

Element	If this element is low your next step should be:	If this element is high your next step should be:
Calcium	1 Check for low dietary calcium intake. 2 Check for excess phosphorus intake from meats, food additives, soft drinks or other sources. 3 Eliminate sources of trans-fat (hydrogenated) in diet.	1 Rule out recent hair bleach or permanent wave as cause of erroneous elevation. 2 Determine if excessive, prolonged calcium supplementation has occurred. 3 Determine if excessive vitamin D is ingested regularly.

HAIR ANALYSIS INTERPRETATION (*cont.*)

Element	If this element is low your next step should be:	If this element is high your next step should be:
	4 Determine if vitamin D intake is adequate. 5 Assess whether gastric hydrochloric acid levels adequate. 6 Determine if any medications (antacids, laxatives, diuretics) are routinely taken which might impede absorption.	4 Evaluate dietary calcium/phosphorus ratio for possible relative calcium deficiency. 5 Reduce any excess phosphorus intake (meats, soft drinks, food additives). 6 Evaluate if protein intake is excessive. 7 Assess magnesium intake for adequacy.
Magnesium	1 Check for low dietary magnesium intake. 2 Check for excess dietary calcium or phosphorus intake. 3 Determine if any medications (antacids, laxatives, diuretics) or excess alcohol is taken which might impede magnesium utilization.	1 Rule out recent hair bleach or permanent wave as cause of erroneous elevation. 2 Evaluate adequacy of magnesium intake. 3 Determine if calcium/phosphorus ratio in diet is in proper balance. 4 Evaluate adequacy of vitamin B6 ingestion.
Zinc	1 Evaluate adequacy of dietary zinc. 2 Assess adequacy of vitamin B6 ingestion. 3 Assess adequacy of vitamin A ingestion. 4 Check for antagonism from excess lead, cadmium or copper exposure.	1 Rule out use of zinc-containing antidandruff shampoos as hair contaminant. 2 Check for extremely low dietary zinc intake. 3 Assess adequacy of vitamin B6 and vitamin A intakes. 4 Check for prolonged, excess zinc supplementation. 5 Possibly measure serum or urine zinc.
Copper	1 Assess adequacy of dietary copper. 2 Investigate possible excess zinc or manganese supplementation.	1 Rule out hair contamination from swimming pool use. 2 Rule out recent use of hair treatment or permanent wave as contaminant. 3 Investigate dietary copper exposure sources: drinking water, supplements, soft water from copper pipes. 4 Perform 24-hour urine copper determination, serum copper, ceruloplasmin (copper-binding protein). 5 May check other family members for heredity or environmental cause.

HAIR ANALYSIS INTERPRETATION (*cont.*)

Element	If this element is low your next step should be:	If this element is high your next step should be:
Chromium	**1** Assess adequacy of dietary chromium, and assess if foods high in refined carbohydrate are depleting chromium stores. **2** Reduce excess refined carbohydrate intake.	**1** Investigate occupational or other exposure source. **2** Evaluate 24-hour urine chromium.
Nickel	(Clinical significance of low nickel is unknown.)	**1** Rule out hair contaminant from recent bleach or permanent. **2** Investigate possible environmental sources. **3** Consider 24-hour urine or blood nickel measurement.
Lead	The lower the better. Lead is a toxic element.	**1** Identify and reduce sources of lead exposure. **2** If level is very high, rule out external contamination by checking pubic or axillary hair lead. Measure whole blood lead. **3** Can further assess exposure with provocative test using EDTA injection and measuring 24-hour urine excretion. **4** Ensure adequacy of protective essential nutrients; particularly vitamin C, calcium, zinc, selenium, chromium, manganese and fiber.
Mercury	The lower the better. Mercury is a toxic element.	**1** Identify and reduce sources of mercury exposure. **2** If level is very high, rule out external contamination by checking pubic or axillary hair mercury. **3** Can further assess exposure using dimercaprol (BAL) injection and measuring 24-hour urine mercury excretion. **4** Ensure adequacy of protective essential nutrients in diet, particularly selenium.

HAIR ANALYSIS INTERPRETATION (*cont.*)

Element	If this element is low your next step should be:	If this element is high your next step should be:
Cadmium	The lower the better. Cadmium is a toxic element.	1 Identify and reduce sources of cadmium exposure. 2 If level is very high, rule out contamination by checking pubic or axillary hair cadmium. 3 Further assess exposure with a provocative EDTA injection test, measuring 24-hour urine excretion. 4 Ensure adequacy of protective essential nutrients, particularly zinc, vitamin C, iron and fiber.
Arsenic	(The clinical significance of low arsenic is unknown.)	1 Identify and reduce sources of arsenic exposure. 2 Recheck level in pubic hair to rule out external contamination. 3 Consider 24-hour urine test or provocative chelation test with di-mercaprol (BAL), measuring 24 hour urinary arsenic output.
Sodium	1 Review dietary sodium intake for more appropriate assessment. Low hair sodium is not directly related to sodium intake.	1 Assess dietary sodium intake. Hair sodium does not correlate with sodium intake. 2 Determine if soft water high in sodium is consumed. 3 Consider possible hair contamination from heavy perspiration. 4 Determine if diuretic medication is taken. 5 Check for cystic fibrosis if clinically suspected.
Potassium	1 Evaluate dietary potassium intake and dietary sodium/potassium ratio for more appropriate information. Hair potassium does not correlate with dietary intake.	1 Assess dietary potassium level. 2 Determine if diuretic medication is taken.
Selenium	1 Ensure adequacy of dietary selenium intake.	1 Check for hair contamination from use of selenium-containing antidandruff shampoo. 2 Investigate for an occupational exposure.

Factors leading to misinterpretation

Modern analytical methods have been developed to accommodate the effects of many hair sprays, shampoos, hair colorings and other external contaminants. Residual effects of these absorbed pollutants can often be compensated for to assure findings which accurately reflect the body mineral content. There are exceptions to this. For instance, lead acetate is used in a number of gradual hair-darkening preparations and this results in a very highly elevated hair lead level despite any treatments by the laboratory. Shampoos which contain selenium, such as Selsun ®, always result in higher hair levels of selenium than would otherwise be obtained and in most cases the selenium is extremely high following use of these shampoos.

External copper contamination of hair from frequent use of swimming pools with a high content of copper in the water can result in elevated hair copper concentrations which do not truly reflect body content. Certain cold-wave or permanent treatments used on hair can affect copper and zinc levels.[5]

It is important that all preparations used on one's hair in the two months prior to analysis be listed on the submittal form which accompanies the hair specimen to the laboratory. Hair analysis laboratories keep detailed listings of those preparations which result in erroneous hair mineral concentration readings and this will usually be mentioned on the final report.

Hair analysis standardization

Trace-element analysis, like trace-element research, requires special techniques and ultra-clean laboratory facilities. It is not just a matter of purchasing sophisticated equipment; the entire facilities must be kept free of contamination. This is a difficult task requiring that the facility be designed from the start for trace analysis techniques.

Analysis for trace elements is difficult enough, but hair analysis for trace elements presents additional problems. Hairs that may be growing side-by-side often have different trace element contents because the hairs are in different stages of the growth cycle. Approximately a third of the head hairs are in a "resting" phase at any one time.

Differences in hair color and hair treatment compound the problems. It seems as if each laboratory has attempted to solve the various problems in different ways. Early in our use of hair analysis, we were frustrated by intra- and inter- laboratory variances on hair samples that we meticulously divided into multiple samples. We tried several methods of preparing standardized hair samples to determine the accuracy and precision of the various commercial laboratories.

There was no perfect solution, but the most meaningful standardization technique seemed to be that which was developed by the International Agency for Atomic Energy in Geneva. The major pitfall of this technique was that the hair samples had to be powdered to ensure homogeneity. (This is accomplished by freezing hair in liquid nitrogen and pulverization in Teflon® equipment.) Powdered samples should not be washed and require other sample handling variations.

The various techniques minimize the potential for interlaboratory comparisons. We felt that this handicapped the emerging technique. Each commercial laboratory wished to be the major laboratory, but defense of their own technique—and each was based on reasonable scientific studies—hindered the development of an industry-wide consistency which was slowing total growth and wider acceptance of this technique. Also, standards assure that a poorly qualified laboratory does not enter the scene and produce poor work.

We felt it was to the advantage of both physicians and laboratories to establish volunteer guidelines of standard practices. Thus a committee of experts, having no commercial laboratory ties, was formed. It was not our intention to force regulations upon anyone, but to help solidify this important clinical technique. The Hair Analysis Standardization Board was chaired by one of the authors and consisted of the following members:

CHAIRMAN: ELMER M. CRANTON, M.D.; Past President, American Holistic Medical Association; Editor, JOURNAL OF HOLISTIC MEDICINE: Charter Fellow: American Academy of Family Physicians; Diplomate, American Board of Family Practice. Many years of experience in active medical practice involving clinical applications of elemental hair analysis.

JEFFREY BLAND, Ph.D.; Associate Professor, Departments of Chemistry and Environmental Sciences, University of Puget Sound, Tacoma, Washington; Director, Belleview/Redmond Medical Laboratories; President, Northwest Diagnostics; President, Northwest Academy of Preventive Medicine; Chairman, Scientific and Technical Committee, National Academy of Clinical Biochemistry; Research Director, Western Academy of Biological Sciences; researcher, lecturer and author of many scientific studies concerning hair analysis.

A. CHATT, Ph.D. (formerly Chattopadhyay); Associate Professor, Trace Analysis Research Centre, Department of Chemistry, Dalhousie University, Halifax, Nova Scotia, Canada; researcher, author, lecturer and widely acknowledged expert in the field of hair analysis research.

ROB KRAKOVITZ, M.D.; Vice-President, Orthomolecular Medical Society; member, Board of Directors, International College of Applied Nutrition; many years experience in active clinical practice involving the use and interpretation of hair analysis.

JONATHAN V. WRIGHT, M.D.; author, lecturer and researcher in the field of nutritional biochemistry with many years of experience in the active clinical practice of medicine involving the use and interpretation of hair analysis.

Initial points of concern were sampling procedures, washing techniques, analytical procedures, normal ranges and clinical interpretation. (For a detailed description of hair analysis procedure, please see chapters 31 and 32.)

As this field is a state-of-the-art technique, any standards published here would probably be obsolete before publication. We suggest that in choosing a laboratory for performing hair analysis you should inquire if they conform to the standards established by the Hair Analysis Standardization Board, ASETL (American Society of Elemental Testing Laboratories) or other independent standardization boards. But in every case, you should require from the laboratory the exact procedures the laboratory follows for quality control, data interpretation and reporting procedures. It is recommended that specific references to published research be obtained to support any contradiction to the information contained in this book.

REFERENCES

1 Chattopadhyay, A., *et al*. 1977. *Arch. Environ. Health* 32(5):226–236.

2 Laker, M. July 31, 1982. *Lancet* II (8292):260–262.

3 Eilers, R.J. 1982. *West J. Med*. 126(5):423–424.

4 Gibson, R.S. 1980. *J. Hum. Nutr*. 34:405–416.

5 Chittleborough, G.A. 1980. *Sci. Total Environ*. 14(1):53-75.

6 Klevay, I.M. 1978. *Arch. Intern. Med*. 138(7):1127–1128.

7 Maugh, T.H. 1978. *Science* 202(4374):1271–1273.

8 Vitale, L. F., *et al*. 1975. *J. Occup. Med*. 17(3):155–156.

9 Jacob, R., *et al*. 1978. *Amer. J. Clin. Nutr*. 31(3):477–480.

10 Prasad, A., ed. 1976. *Trace Elements in Human Health and Disease*, vol. 1 & 2. New York: Academic Press.

11 McKenzie, J.M. 1978. *Amer. J. Clin. Nutr*. 31(3):470–476.

The macro-minerals

CALCIUM

PHOSPHORUS

MAGNESIUM

4

CALCIUM

The body contains more calcium than any other mineral, but quantity alone does not explain the importance of calcium to life and general wellbeing. Calcium is important to heart health, nerves, muscles, skin and, of course, strong bones and teeth. Calcium also helps relieve aches in muscles and bones, menstrual cramps, muscle spasms, nervousness, tension, tremors, insomnia and several other disorders in those individuals who have become calcium deficient over the years. Government surveys indicate that 60 percent of all Americans are getting *less* than the conservative RDA. There is strong evidence that many more could benefit from quantities greater than RDA.

Function

When calcium is mentioned, most people think of bones and teeth. While it is true that about 99 percent of all calcium in the body is in the bones and teeth, the remainder is extremely important to life. In fact, a hormone precisely regulates the amount of calcium in the blood of healthy people within 3 percent by borrowing calcium from bone or excreting it.[1]

The amount of calcium outside skeletal tissues may only be about 10 grams in the average person, but it regulates the heart beat, nerve transmission, muscle contraction and blood coagulation. Calcium helps control blood acid-alkaline balance, plays a role in cell division, muscle growth and iron utilization; activates certain enzymes, and helps transport nutrients through cell membranes. Calcium also forms a "cellular cement" called "ground substance" that helps hold cells and tissues together.

The heart beat is controlled by an electrical center called the "A-V" Node. Calcium is involved in the transmission of impulses in this center. Exercise improves the movement of calcium, the messenger to muscle cells, thus improving the contraction and relaxation of the heart and body muscles.[2] This may help explain why exercise reduces heart problems.

The calcium content of blood is about 10 milligrams (8.8–10.4 range) per 100 milliliters of blood. Calcium is present in several forms; free ions (5.5 mg/100 ml), bound to serum proteins (4 mg/100 ml) and complexed with phosphate and citrate (0.5 mg/100 ml). The blood level of calcium is maintained by several hormones (principally parathyroid hormone and calcitonin) and the active metabolite of vitamin D3.

The parathyroid glands, located on the thyroid, secrete the parathyroid hormone (parathormone). If the calcium level in the blood falls below normal, this hormone stimulates the release of calcium from bone and also stimulates the kidneys to absorb calcium that is being filtered through them on the way to excretion. At the same time, excretion of phosphorus is increased to maintain the proper calcium-phosphorus ratio. If the calcium level rises above normal, a thyroid hormone, calcitonin, goes to work stopping the release of calcium from bone. Circulating levels of these two hormones are adjusted automatically to maintain normal calcium levels in the blood. Many other hormones such as cortisol and insulin and those that affect growth can also influence calcium metabolism.

Much of the action of calcium is not due to the atoms or ions of free calcium, but due to the combination of calcium with certain enzymes. The key to the utilization of calcium is a protein called "calmodulin" which binds calcium and then interacts with the various enzyme system.[3,4] Now that calmodulin is being widely investigated, we are discovering that calcium may control even more life processes than ever imagined. "It may soon become more interesting to ask which cellular processes are not under calcium-calmodulin control than which are."[5]

Calcium has a calming effect on nerves due to its regulation of the permeability (degree of penetration) of the nerve cell membrane to sodium and potassium. Sodium, potassium and chlorine control the electrical charge distribution on the inside and outside membrane surfaces. This charge differential is called the "resting potential." When calcium ions are increased in the fluid around the nerve cell, it decreases the number of sodium ions, thus lowering the resting potential. A greater trigger (pain, stress, tension or other stimuli) would be required to "fire off" the nerve. Thus calcium has a calming effect on the nervous system.

Bones and teeth

The amount of calcium in a 155-pound person is approximately 1200 grams (2.6 pounds). The range is typically 1.5 to 2.0 percent of the total body weight.

Many people are surprised to learn that the calcium in bone and teeth is not permanent, but is constantly being deposited and then resorbed. In fact, the form of bone calcium may even change as we age.

Bone consists of calcium phosphate deposited within a soft, fibrous protein matrix. Calcium phosphate is the calcium "salt" of phosphoric acid which can be formed whenever dissolved calcium "ions" (atoms of calcium having an electrical charge of + 2) meet phosphate "ions" (atoms of phosphorus plus four atoms of oxygen, together having an electrical charge of − 1). This occurs frequently because the diet contains many sources of calcium and phosphate ions.

Calcium phosphate can be deposited in the skeletal tissue to be highly crystalline and complexed with calcium hydroxide to form a composition similar to the mineral hydroxyapatite, or the calcium could be noncrystalline. It appears that the calcium phosphate is mostly noncrystalline in early life and is superceded by the more brittle crystalline form in later life.[6]

Calcium is constantly being exchanged between bone and blood—more rapidly during early life and at a declining rate in later life. In an adult male, it has been estimated that about 700 mg calcium enter and leave the bones each day.[7]

The mineral content of bone is about 65 percent of the dry weight, with the protein matrix (mainly collagen) being approximately 35 percent. Fresh bone contains about 20 percent moisture. Besides calcium (24 percent) and phosphorus (10 percent), the other minerals with known biochemical function include sodium, magnesium, chlorine, molybdenum and zinc. Other minerals may accumulate, but at this writing they have no widely agreed-upon biochemical function. These include strontium, lead, fluorine, radium, barium, yttrium, uranium, plutonium, americium, cerium, zirconium, actinium, beryllium and gallium.[8]

Teeth have a higher proportion of mineral in relation to protein than bone. *Enamel* is approximately 99.5 percent mineral; *dentin* (beneath the enamel and surrounding the pulp) is about 77 percent mineral; and *cementum*, (the calcified covering of the root) is roughly 70 percent mineral. Enamel contains more minerals than any other tissue. It is 36 percent calcium and 17 percent phosphorus. It is not surprising that it is also the hardest tissue in the body. The protein of enamel is largely the very insoluble keratin, while the protein of dentin is collagen as in bone and skin.

Teeth can exchange minerals via interactions with saliva and the circulatory system, until mechanical damage or decay results. Unlike bone, damaged teeth do not seem to be able to repair themselves.

Aches and pains

Muscle spasms can be triggered by calcium deficiency. As mentioned earlier, a calcium deficiency increases the nerves' resting potential which can trigger muscle contraction. Muscle cramps, especially those which occur at night or at rest are temporary occurrences under hormonal control, but years of sub-optimal calcium intake often result in regularly occurring pains such as low back pain.

Leg and feet cramps so severe that they interrupt sleep can occur in the calcium-deficient person. Not all nocturnal leg cramps are due to calcium and/or magnesium deficiency. Some can be caused by poor circulation; often those cramps can be alleviated with vitamin E.[9,10,11] Sleep lowers the metabolic rate which in turn lowers the hormones that control blood calcium levels. The resulting drop in circulating calcium triggers the cramps. Sciatica, the pain felt at the back of the thigh and running down the outside of the leg, is due to an inflammation of the sciatic nerve. Sciatica also seems to have a relationship to calcium stress.

Even more serious pains are due to tetany. Tetany occurs when the serum calcium level drops below 7 mg/100 ml of blood. Tetany is characterized by intermittent muscle spasms and cramps, numbness and tingling of the extremities, nervousness, irritability and apprehension.

As we will discuss later, a partner of calcium, magnesium, is also very important in the nerve-muscle relationship, and a proper calcium-to-magnesium balance should be obtained.

Menstrual cramps may be related to calcium and/or magnesium deficiencies and many women have reported success in eliminating or lessening cramps by improving their calcium intake.

Arthritis and osteoporosis

Disturbances between bone and soft tissue calcium content result in pain, calcium deposits, osteoporosis (bone softening) and perhaps arthritis. Some of this bone calcium disturbance is due to dietary deficiency.

It is interesting to note that in a survey conducted by Mark Bricklin, editor of *Prevention* magazine, 1379 of 2959 respondents reported that calcium supplements either relieved or abolished musculo-skeletal "pains."[12] Vitamin D, which improves calcium metabolism, also has produced beneficial results.

The incidence of osteoporosis (literally "holey bones") is greater among persons having low dietary calcium intake.[13] In osteoporosis, bone decalcification occurs because calcium is "borrowed" from the bone to maintain the blood calcium level. Calcium is continuously being excreted from blood to urine. Blood calcium has higher priority over bone calcium because it is needed for the heart beat and nerve transmission.

Osteoporosis involves decreased bone mass, including both minerals and proteins. The chemical composition of the remaining bone is unchanged. (In osteomalacia, only the mineral content is lowered. Osteoporosis eventually causes a curvature of the spine because the spinal bones become fragile and collapse. This is often called a "dowager's hump." Studies have shown that postmenopausal women may lose from one to six inches in height.[14]

Postmenopausal women are especially subject to bone demineralization because of their decreased estrogen (female hormone) levels. Approximately 90 percent of postmenopausal women lose a significant amount of bone tissue, and 26 percent of women of sixty years of age have loss of height involving pain and deformity.[15] Four times as many women as men get osteoporosis.

According to a U.S. Public Health Service report, 30 percent of women over fifty years of age, seeking medical care were found to have osteoporosis. The survey found 20 percent of men over sixty-five had osteoporosis.

Osteoporosis accounts for some 8 million spontaneous bone fractures that occur in women every year. We all know how "elderly" women sometimes stumble and fall down, breaking their hips. Actually, the fracture occurs first in the majority of the elderly women with osteoporosis and then they fall.

Osteoporosis in men cannot be explained by estrogen level changes. It may be that men are protected by the type (not amount) of exercise and work they do and by the slower decline in testosterone (male hormone). The pressure that vigorous exercise or physical labor puts on bones maintains a better calcium balance regardless of sex.

In studies of the relationship of calcium intake to osteoporosis, mixed results have been obtained. There are several reports that calcium supplements have induced calcium retention and relieved osteoporosis symptoms.[16,78-82] This may reflect the fact that although the efficiency of absorption decreases with the amount of calcium in the diet, the total amount of calcium actually *retained* increases.[17]

Long-term dietary intakes of osteoporotic patients generally are lower than those of comparable healthy people. When these patients are given substantial increases of calcium in the diet (up to 1200 mg as a supplement), the calcium balance improves.[18,19] Dr. A. Albanese of the Burke Rehabilitation Center in White Plains, N.Y. has shown a positive correlation between low calcium intake and lower bone density and higher fracture rate in women over forty-five years of age. Two researchers have reported that demineralization of bone can be reversed with calcium supplements.[20,21]

In one study, sixty-one postmenopausal women were divided into three groups. One group (control group) received no treatment, another group received estrogen, while the third group received a daily supplement of 800 mg calcium. The untreated group continued to lose bone mass during the two-year clinical trial, while the estrogen group lost none. The calcium group did lose some bone mass, but not nearly as much as the untreated group.[22] Perhaps if they had taken more calcium, they would not have lost any bone mass. It should be noted that older people have poorer calcium absorption.[18,19]

A Veterans Administration Hospital study in Hines, Illinois led by Dr. Herta Spencer found that no demineralization occurred at a daily calcium intake of 1200 mg.[23] Dr. Spencer found that only some patients could achieve calcium balance on 800 mg, but all did on 1200 mg calcium per day.

A 1981 study on the effects of calcium supplementation on patients with osteoporosis was published in the *American Journal of Clinical Nutrition* (34:819–823) by Dr. C. J. Lee and colleagues at Kentucky State University. Twenty subjects over the age of sixty were selected. All had osteoporosis as measured by an X ray of the hand and all had a history of calcium intake of less than 500 mg per day. All remained on their regular diets, supplemented daily with three slices of processed cheese foods (360 mg calcium) and three capsules of dibasic calcium phosphate (350 mg calcium) with vitamin D. The regimen was continued for six months.

Eleven subjects had significantly increased bone density at the end of the study, and three showed no appreciable change. Six had decreased bone density and also had weight loss ranging from 4.5 to 11 pounds. This last finding suggests "a catabolic status of calcium produced by negative energy balance despite the increase in calcium intake." Based on this finding, the authors speculate that persons on reducing diets "may need to monitor calcium intake more closely than those who are not."

There were no significant changes in urinary calcium levels in this study, despite increased calcium intake. The authors conclude that this study demonstrates the benefit of calcium compounds and calcium-rich foods in more than half of the elderly women with osteoporosis in this study. The benefits were evident in a relatively short period of time. They note that more study is needed on the relationship between energy intake and calcium metabolism.

The best approach in preventing osteoporosis is to improve calcium balance before bone loss has progressed to high fracture-risk levels.[24] (See discussion of calcium to phosphorous balance, page 42 ff.)

Periodontal disease

Before the osteoporotic process removes mass from what we normally view as typical bones, the jaw bones which form sockets for the teeth (alveolar bone) are robbed first. This is because the alveolar bone is the most highly mineralized. If the dietary calcium deficiency continues, calcium is next removed from the ribs, vertebrae and the long bones.[25]

The decalcification of the tooth-socket bones leads to gum inflammation (gingivitis) and the loosening of teeth.[26] Dentists had long believed the process went the other way. Periodontal disease is the forerunner of osteoporosis. (This is not to imply that calcium deficiency is the only cause of periodontal disease.)

Dr. Lennart Krook of the State University of New York's College of Veterinary Medicine has thoroughly researched the relationship of dietary calcium deficiency to periodontal disease. After tracing the development of periodontal disease with animal studies, Dr. Krook tested calcium supplementation as a means of suppressing the disease. He found that 1000 mg calcium daily decreased the inflammation in every case; and in a number of cases, the inflammation disappeared completely, pocket depth was reduced and the teeth "tightened."

An encouragingly large number of dentists practice "preventive dentistry" relying heavily on proper nutrition, other dentists less so. Dr. Krook doesn't understand this. "Animals don't brush their teeth, but if they are properly fed they don't lose their teeth. So too with primitive peoples. Something more than proper oral hygiene must be at work. Also, diet, especially sucrose (sugar) intake, has been found to be a major factor in cavities, so the possible nutritional origins of dental problems is well established. Besides, even after dentists pull out a periodontal patient's teeth, thus removing all possibilities of plaque formation, the alveolar bone (teeth sockets) often continues to recede and dentists have to adjust the patient's dentures after a few years."[27]

Dr. Leo Lutwak, professor of medicine at the University of California at Los Angeles, showed that when the daily dietary calcium intake is *deficient* and when there is an excess in phosphorus intake, an imbalance occurs which demineralizes the tooth socket. (A chief source for excess phosphorus is the phosphate buffer in carbonated soft drinks and in phosphate food additives.)

Dr. Lutwak demonstrated that increased calcium intake can reverse the process, firmly reanchoring teeth in people with existing periodontal disease. In one study, ten patients were fed 1000 mg calcium a day for six months and showed a decrease in gum inflammation and reduction in tooth looseness.[28]

Heart disease

Calcium and magnesium deficiencies are strongly linked to heart disease. Calcium is used by the heart in the muscle contraction that produces the heartbeat, and magnesium repels the calcium to reverse the contraction to allow the heart to relax. A deficiency of both, or possibly either mineral causes abnormal heart rhythm and even spasms in the arteries. Some researchers estimate that as many as 50 percent of heart fatalities may be triggered by spasms in the arteries. Heart attacks are not caused only by clogged arteries.

The hazards of missing calcium often available in the water supply can be understood by the following discussion excerpted from *Supernutrition for Healthy Hearts*.[29]

Researchers around the world have observed that people living in hard-water areas where water is rich in calcium and magnesium have a much lower heart-disease death rate than those living in soft-water areas. Furthermore, one of the unfortunate properties of soft water is its usually higher content of sodium (table salt is sodium chloride) which can upset the potassium-sodium electrolyte balance. When this balance is disrupted, the heart cannot conduct the electrical stimulus that causes it to beat properly, and irregular heartbeat or heart failure results.

The first report of the link between soft water and heart disease was probably that of Japan's Dr. J. Kobayashi in 1957. Since 1957, many confirming reports have appeared, including those by Dr. Donald R. Peterson in Seattle, Dr. Gunnar Biorck of Stockholm, Dr. Margaret D. Crawford of England and Dr. Henry A. Schroeder of Dartmouth Medical School in Hanover, New Hampshire.

Dr. Schroeder's 1960 study of water supplies in 1315 U.S. cities showed that apparently the higher the calcium content of the water, the better. For example, the average hardness of water supplied to South Carolinians was 18 parts per million calcium, compared with 237 ppm for New Mexicans, and the heart-disease death rates among white males forty-five to sixty-four years of age was far higher in South Carolina (1107.5 per 100,000) than in New Mexico (563.4 per 100,000). There is, in fact, a much higher correlation between water hardness and low heart-disease mortality than between low dietary cholesterol and low heart-disease death rate.[30]

In 1966, Dr. Schroeder updated his study, finding similar correlation between water hardness and lower heart-disease death rates.[31] In 1968, Dr. Margaret Crawford and colleagues published similar results from a study of sixty-one English towns.[32]

Five years later, Dr. Crawford and her colleagues published a study of 289 men from twelve English cities, nearly alike except that six of the cities had hard-water supplies. Beyond a slight difference in lifestyle (the men in the soft water group participated in slightly more exercise), the men were fairly well matched. The important finding was that the heart-disease death rate was 50 percent higher in the towns with the softest water (720 to 862 heart-disease deaths per 100,000 in the soft-water towns compared to 499 to 597 in the hard-water towns). In addition, the men in the soft-water towns had higher pulse rates, higher blood cholesterol levels, and higher blood pressures.[33]

Current statistics from various authorities indicate that 70 percent of Americans drink soft water, and one estimate (unnamed in a brief filed against the EPA to act against soft water) is that 15 percent of the heart-disease deaths among those drinking soft water could be prevented by drinking hard water. This means, if the estimate is accurate, that about 10 percent of all heart disease in America could be prevented by switching to hard water.

I should point out that not all scientists are convinced that water "hardness" is a meaningful category, because different minerals can be present in two water supplies classified at the same level of hardness. Additionally, there are reversals in the link between soft water and heart disease. One example is the twin cities of Kansas City, Kansas (having hard water), and Kansas City, Missouri (having soft water). Here the heart-disease death rate is 36 percent lower in the soft water (50 percent softer) city. Another factor recently receiving attention is the "corrosiveness" of the water. Corrosive water picks up cadmium, lead and other toxic metals. Cadmium, according to a study by Dr. Henry Schroeder, raises blood pressure. And high blood pressure causes heart-disease complications.[34]

Tests with laboratory rats had indicated that rats having high blood pressure experienced a normalization of blood pressure when calcium was added to their diets.

Now Dr. David McCarron of the University of Oregon Health Sciences Center has noted that the patients he studied who had high blood pressure were getting 39 percent less calcium from dairy products and 22 percent less calcium overall than normal, non-hypertensive people.[35] Dr. Jose Villar of Johns Hopkins School of Medicine found calcium supplements reduced elevated blood pressure by 9 percent. It's not too surprising. It seems that a glass of milk helps keep you relaxed and your blood pressure down.

If soap lathers easily in your water, it is probably soft. Contact your local water department or the United States Geological Agency (or even the EPA) if you are interested in learning whether your local supply could be switched back to hard water. If such a switch is not possible, you should be especially sure your diet contains extra calcium and magnesium.

Calcium balance

A proper calcium balance is important in too many ways to list. It helps prevent kidney stones in patients with certain gastrointestinal, pancreatic and liver disorders. It lowers the absorption of harmful pollutants such as cadmium and lead. And on and on. The important point is that for you to be your healthiest, you should know how much calcium is in your diet. More important, you should determine your calcium balance in relation to other nutrients. The best way is by radiological examination of the density of the finger bones (phalanx 5-2), but hair analysis is more convenient. Beware, though, interpretation may not be straightforward. A high hair calcium can indicate low dietary calcium as will be explained later. Blood analysis is the last to show changes due to dietary calcium because blood calcium is under hormonal control. Blood calcium is more apt to reflect hormone output than true calcium balance.

There is more to calcium balance in the body than how much calcium you eat. Can you absorb calcium well? Are you excreting more calcium than is desirable because you are eating too much protein or phosphorus? Do you get enough vitamin D? Are other dietary factors making the calcium unavailable for your assimilation? Let's look at some of the factors that determine calcium balance: absorption, transport and excretion.

Calcium absorption takes place in the small intestine and is an energy requiring process, but not all of the calcium you eat is absorbed through the intestines. The efficiency of calcium absorption varies from person to person, and even varies with the ages of a person. It is generally true that while you are growing, your body is more efficient in extracting calcium from your food and transporting it to your bones than it will be when you are older.

Infants fed human milk absorb 50 to 70 percent of their dietary calcium, whereas adults absorb only 30 to 50 percent of the calcium obtained in a normal mixed-food diet.[36]

The amount of calcium absorbed also depends on other dietary factors such as vitamins C and D, protein, oxalic acid and phytic acid, as well as physical activity.

As dietary calcium intake increases, the body can receive its requirements without working so hard at calcium absorption. Thus the calcium absorption efficiency decreases although the total calcium absorbed increases.

On the other side of calcium balance is calcium excretion via urine, sweat and feces. Increased activity can lead to greater calcium loss through sweat.

Increased calcium intake leads to a greater percentage lost in the feces mostly because of a diminishing absorption efficiency. Calcium excretion via urine is influenced not by diet or calcium blood level, but by the efficiency of calcium reabsorption in the kidneys as controlled by parathyroid hormone and vitamin D.

To improve your calcium balance then, you should eat adequate calcium foods in balanced meals. The vitamins C and D and proper protein in the meal aid in the absorption of calcium. Too much calcium can interfere with zinc absorption and magnesium balance.

Improving absorption

Vitamin C significantly improves the absorption of dietary calcium.[37,38] Vitamin C is acidic: in older people, any acid, including hydrochloric acid, sometimes aids in absorption.

Vitamin D improves the absorption efficiency of calcium—during growth and possibly in later years as well—by assisting the production of the protein that transports calcium in the mucosal cells of the intestine. Vitamin D also helps mobilize calcium from bone and helps to reabsorb calcium in the kidney, preventing urinary loss.

Vitamin D3 (cholcalciferol) is converted in the liver to calcidiol which is the major circulating form of vitamin D3. Parathyroid hormone is transported to the kidney where it stimulates the production of the hormonal form of vitamin D3 called calcitriol from the calcidiol. Calcitriol is the active hormone that by itself stimulates the intestinal absorption of calcium. Calcitriol, in the presence of the parathyroid hormone, stimulates the mobilization of calcium from bone and the reabsorption of calcium in the kidney.

Protein deficiency lowers calcium absorption. If protein, especially the amino acid lysine, is present in adequate amounts along with the calcium, calcium absorption is greatly enchanced.[39,40] The reason for this is not clear, but it may be more closely related to the formation of the calcium protein carrier than to simply chelation or binding of calcium by protein constituents.

However, excessive dietary protein is debated as a possible negative influence on calcium balance. The debate is legitimate because of the difficulty in designing a "perfect" test in humans. The apparently conflicting results obtained thus far most likely are due to differences in calcium utilization between species of animals, the levels of calcium and the types of protein used in the experiments. There was evidence to suggest to some researchers that excessive nitrogen and/or sulfur from a high-protein diet increases the amount of acid formed in the body, which in a way "leaches" calcium out of bone.

Studies have documented that daily protein intake above 95 grams increases excretion of calcium in the urine.[41-46] Dr. Hellen Linkswiler of the University of Wisconsin has reported several experiments through the years. In 1974, Dr. Linkswiler demonstrated that in young men, calcium balance could be achieved with 500 mg daily provided the daily protein level was 47 g (grams). However, when the protein intake was increased to 142 g daily, 30 of the 33 young men could not achieve calcium balance even at 1400 mg calcium daily.[45] Dr. Linkswiler has estimated that consumption of 95 g protein daily along with 500 mg calcium would produce a bone loss of 21 g calcium yearly.

In 1979, Dr. Lindsay Allen and her colleagues demonstrated that dietary protein reduces the reabsorption of calcium in the kidney during a four-hour period after meals, thus increasing calcium excretion.[47]

Several researchers are currently thinking, in contrast to earlier theory, that normal amounts of sulfur-containing amino acids (cysteine and methionine) do not seem to increase calcium excretion any more than other amino acids. However, large amounts of purified sulfur-containing amino acids may significantly increase calcium excretion.[48,49]

Some researchers have noted that phosphorus intake also increases with protein intake, and that the calcium-to-phosphorus ratio is also a major factor in calcium balance.

Dr. Herta Spencer notes that in many of the experiments to measure the effect of dietary protein on calcium balance, the protein was increased but the calcium and phosphorus levels were rigidly held constant. In real life, when the protein level of the diet is raised, the phosphorus intake also increases. The increased calcium excretion effect of the protein may be offset by the increased calcium retention effect of phosphorus.[50] In normal human nutrition, phosphorus intake is generally correlated with protein intake, but calcium intake varies widely. Dr. Spencer found that a high protein intake derived from a high-meat diet had little effect on calcium balance.

Phosphorous ratio

As mentioned, increased phosphorous intakes have been thought to reduce urinary excretion of calcium and lower blood calcium levels.[51] Several researchers, however, have shown that at least in experimental animals, *excessive* intakes of phosphorus could lead to increased bone resorption and increased calcium loss in the feces.[52,53] It has been postulated that high phosphorous intakes in relation to calcium result in secondary hyperparathyroidism.[26,54]

The calcium-to-phosphorous ratio is widely recognized as an influence on calcium balance, but there is less agreement on the ideal range of numerical values. In laboratory animals, a calcium-to-phosphorous ratio of 2:1 appears to maximize calcium absorption and to minimize its loss from bone.[55,56]

The evidence for man is not as clear cut. The available evidence suggests that man can tolerate a much wider calcium-to-phosphorous ratio, between 2:1 and 1:2. Some have concluded that the preferred calcium-to-phosphorous ratio is above 1:1, whereas others have concluded that if the *diet* contains *sufficient* calcium, then calcium absorption is not affected by the calcium-to-phosphorous ratio.[57,58]

The question then becomes "How much calcium is *sufficient?*" The question is especially important because recent estimates indicate that the calcium-to-phosphorous ratio in the United States is about 1:1.5–2.8, with some individuals having a 1:4 ratio.[59-61]

Dr. Hellen Linkswiler commented on this concern.[61] "Larger amounts of phosphorus do not affect calcium absorption when dietary calcium intake is in the low to normal range. In some cases, phosphorus even *increases* calcium retention. Whether this increase reflects greater retention of calcium in the skeleton or soft tissue calcification is unknown."

Monkeys are related biochemically more closely than are mice, rats and dogs. Dr. Anderson fed monkeys a control diet with a calcium-to-phosphorous ratio of 1:0.4, while the experimental groups ingested diets with 1:2.1 and 1:1.4 calcium-to-phosphorous ratios. None developed bone disease during seven years of observation.[62]

However, seven years may not have been long enough to observe clinical symptoms of bone loss. The loss of bone mass is not detected by gross radiographic density changes until up to 30 or 40 percent of bone demineralization occurs.

Dr. Leo Lutwak of the University of California at Los Angeles Medical School suggests the ideal dietary calcium-to-phosphorous ratio is in the range 1:1 or 1:1.5 for adults.

Dr. Kim found that increasing phosphorous intake of healthy young men from 900 to 2400 milligrams per day did not affect calcium balance when calcium intake was 800 mg per day. Calcium absorption was depressed slightly when calcium intake was 2400 mg daily.[63]

Dr. Herta Spencer found absorption of calcium was unaffected by increasing phosphorus from 800 to 2000 mg daily at calcium levels ranging from 200 to 2700 mg daily. Thus phosphorus does not seem to affect calcium balance at normal intakes according to recent (1980) research. The same seems to be true for normal protein diets. However, the final word is not yet in. Phosphorus supplementation increased the calcium retention both in healthy and in demineralized persons. Four osteoporotic women given one gram phosphorous supplement showed improved calcium balance.[64] Healthy young men retained more calcium after their phosphorus intake was increased from 900 to 2400 milligrams per day while maintaining calcium intake at 800 milligrams.[47] Dr. Mark Hegsted showed that increased calcium retention occurs also with a high protein diet containing 500 mg calcium when the phosphorus was increased from 1010 mg to 2525 mg per day.[49]

However, it should be emphasized that increased retention is not always beneficial. It may well be—provided bone retention of calcium is involved. But it could be that soft tissue has been calcified. If the arteries, heart and kidneys are retaining the calcium, then it is detrimental to health. More research is needed before it can be recommended to increase phosphorus at this time.

Subjects on high phosphate diets have high levels of circulating parathormone suggesting that demineralization of the bones could be stimulated.[87] Dr. Hunter Heath of the Mayo Medical School in Rochester, Minnesota reported in *Medical World News* (Sept. 1981, p.71) that hyperparathyroidism is on the rise.

Keep in mind that most of the research indicates that adequate calcium must be present before extra phosphorus will increase calcium retention. It may be that at low calcium intakes, extra phosphorus increases calcium excretion. Dr. Leo Lutwak has shown that when the daily dietary calcium intake is deficient, excess phosphorus leads to demineralization of the jaw bone resulting in periodontal disease.

We emphasize a complete mineral balance. It is not just a simple matter of how much calcium, nor what calcium-to-phosphorous ratio, but a matter of total nutrition, and zinc, magnesium, chromium, manganese, molybdenum, etc., balance as well as calcium-to-phosphorous ratio. As a starting point, however, we are comfortable with a total daily calcium dietary intake of 1000 to 1200 mg, balanced by a total daily phosphorous intake of 800 to 1000 mg. The ideal magnesium, zinc and other minerals and trace elements will be discussed in their individual chapters.

While research continues on the calcium-to-phosphorous ratio, we feel it prudent to strive for a ratio between 1:1 or 1.5:1 in favor of calcium. If you exceed or undershoot the calcium quantities mentioned above, adjust the ratios of phosphorus and other minerals accordingly. Higher amounts of calcium can be used temporarily to reduce symptoms, but a balance should be restored to prevent future problems. We do not see any long-term problems with supplements providing 1000 to 1200 mg calcium, provided other minerals are kept in balance. We feel that most people will not need that much supplemental calcium if they maintain total mineral balance.

It is interesting to note that milk consumption has been declining and soft drink consumption has increased. In 1981, the per capita consumption of soft drinks was pegged at 39 gallons per year, up from 23 gallons in 1970. Soft drinks, especially colas, usually contain phosphoric acid to "buffer" the carbonation.

Salt

While humans do not seem to be seriously affected by increasing the phosphorous content of the diet provided they are receiving adequate calcium, we may have to keep an eye on our salt intake. Researchers at the University of Otago in New Zealand have found that excess salt increases calcium excretion via urine.[65]

Oxalic acid

Oxalic acid is present in beet greens, chard, rhubarb, spinach and cocoa. These foods are often cited as being rich in calcium, but unfortunately most of this calcium has been combined with the oxalic acid to form insoluble calcium oxalate. The calcium in these greens cannot be used by our bodies.[66-69]

Nutritionists have been concerned that some of the excess oxalic acid could combine with the calcium in other foods thus making that calcium unavailable as well. No lessening of calcium absorption has been noted due to oxalic acid in greens among children having an adequate calcium intake.[70] The same has been found for oxalic acid in cocoa and chocolate.[71,72] Phytic acid in bran cereals receives the same comments.[73]

Fluoride

Fluoride combines with calcium to form insoluble calcium fluoride. Several investigators are concerned about the increasing amount of fluorides in water and overall food supply, possibly decreasing calcium absorption in a population largely calcium deficient.[74,75]

Lactose

Lactose (milk sugar) aids calcium absorption. Milk contains both calcium and lactose which testifies to the wisdom of Nature in providing for the high calcium requirement of growing infants.

Exercise

People who are inactive tend to excrete more calcium than active people. Unless they are getting more calcium in their diet than is needed by active people, the net result is that inactive people lose bone mass. The rate of calcium loss is greatest in those confined to bed for exended time periods. According to Dr. Leo Lutwak, astronauts lose the same amount of calcium when they are under zero gravity. The conclusion is that bone health depends on compression of the long bones produced by standing, walking or running.

How much calcium?

Researchers have had difficulty pinpointing dietary calcium needs. People change their calcium absorption efficiency with changes in dietary calcium intake.

In general, if a person has been accustomed to a relatively high level of calcium intake, there is rejection by the intestine of a large portion of the calcium ingested. A decrease in dietary calcium leads immediately to a negative balance (calcium loss), but over a period of time the efficiency of intestinal absorption increases, fecal calcium loss is reduced in most individuals, and calcium balance may return. A reverse but similar type of adaptation occurs over long periods as an individual is shifted from an accustomed low level of calcium intake to a higher one. For these reasons, evaluation of calcium balance requires study over prolonged periods.[76,77] Unfortunately, some of the data used in determining recommended allowances have not been obtained from long-term studies.

The 1980 RDA recommends 800 mg calcium daily for adults. The FDA's USRDA is 1000 mg. The Food and Agriculture Organization and World Health Organization noted in 1962 that man has the ability to adapt to wide ranges of calcium intake and that intakes vary widely from country to country. They do not claim to define minimum or maximum calcium intakes but note that a range of 300 to 1000 mg seem to work in different cultures. They discussed a "practical allowance" of 400 to 500 mg per day.

However, there is strong evidence that the RDA may be too low for many American women past menopause. Higher calcium intake stopped bone loss in post-menopausal women in a study at Creighton University School of Medicine in Omaha, Nebraska. They were given a 1000 mg supplement of calcium daily, bringing the average daily calcium intake to 1500 mg.[24]

Postmenopausal women are generally in negative calcium balance at 800 mg daily due mainly to a high urinary excretion of calcium,[83,84] and the progressive decline in calcium absorption observed after the age of sixty years in both sexes, but more so in women.[19]

Dr. Albanese commented in the *Dairy Council Digest* that "the present RDA of 800 mg of calcium for adults from the Food and Nutrition Board is based on available data relative to mandatory endogenous losses and an absorption rate of 40 percent. While this amount may be sufficient for some individuals, it may provide little margin of safety for those individuals whose absorption coefficients are lower, *particularly the aging and the aged.*"[25] Dr. Roger Williams notes that people in an anxiety state may need five times the calcium required by the normal person, as their calcium can become tied up as calcium lactate.[85] Calcium consumption has been decreasing for twenty years. 1978 indicators are suggesting that this trend is being reversed.

Food sources

Among common foods, milk and cheese are the richest sources of calcium. Most other foods contribute much smaller amounts. In the United States, about 60 percent of calcium intake is derived from milk and dairy products.[86] Leafy green vegetables (excluding members of the goosefoot family such as spinach, chard and rhubarb that contain oxalic acid) rank next to milk and cheese products as good calcium sources. Broccoli is a decent calcium source, with citrus fruits and legumes ranked as fair sources. Meats, grains and nuts provide the least calcium. Table 4.1 ranks many foods in terms of calcium content.

TABLE 4:1 SOURCES OF CALCIUM

Milligrams (mg) per 100 grams edible portion (100 grams = 3½ oz.)

Kelp	1093	Globe artichoke	51
Swiss cheese	925	Dried prunes	51
Cheddar cheese	750	Pumpkin and squash	
Carob flour	352	seeds	51
Dulse	296	Cooked dry beans	50
Collard leaves	250	Common cabbage	49
Turnip greens	246	Soybean sprouts	48
Barbados molasses	245	Hard winter wheat	46
Almonds	234	Orange	41
Brewer's yeast	210	Celery	39
Parsley	203	Cashews	38
Corn tortillas		Rye grain	38
(lime added)	200	Carrot	37

SOURCES OF CALCIUM (*cont.*)

Milligrams (mg) per 100 grams edible portion (100 grams = 3½ oz.)

Dandelion greens	187	Barley	34
Brazil nuts	186	Sweet potato	32
Watercress	151	Brown rice	32
Goat Milk	129	Garlic	29
Tofu	128	Summer squash	28
Dried figs	126	Onion	27
Buttermilk	121	Lemon	26
Sunflower seeds	120	Fresh green peas	26
Yogurt	120	Cauliflower	25
Beet greens	119	Lentils, cooked	25
Wheat bran	119	Sweet cherry	22
Whole milk	118	Asparagus	22
Buckwheat, raw	114	Winter squash	22
Sesame seeds, hulled	110	Strawberry	21
Ripe olives	106	Millet	20
Broccoli	103	Mung bean sprouts	19
English walnut	99	Pineapple	17
Cottage cheese	94	Grapes	16
Spinach	93	Beets	16
Soybeans, cooked	73	Cantaloupe	14
Pecans	73	Jerusalem artichoke	14
Wheat germ	72	Tomato	13
Peanuts	69	Eggplant	12
Miso	68	Chicken	12
Romaine lettuce	68	Orange juice	11
Dried apricots	67	Avocado	10
Rutabaga	66	Beef	10
Raisins	62	Banana	8
Black currant	60	Apple	7
Dates	59	Sweet corn	3
Green snap beans	56		

Source: MineraLab, Inc.

TABLE 4.2 CALCIUM AND PHOSPHORUS CONTENT OF 100 GRAM POR-
TIONS OF SELECTED FOOD ITEMS* AND THEIR CALCIUM TO PHOSPHORUS
RATIO

Food Item	Calcium	Phosphorus	Ca:P Ratio
Liver, beef	8 mg	352 mg	1:44
Pork loin	12	234	1:20
Chicken breast	11	214	1:19
Frankfurter	32	603	1:19
Bologna	32	581	1:18
Fish, flounder, sole	12	195	1:16
Corn meal, degermed	6	99	1:16
Whole wheat flour	41	372	1:9.1
Potato	7	53	1:7.6
Peanuts	69	401	1:5.8
Beans, lima, mature	72	385	1:5.3
Lentils, mature seeds	79	377	1:4.8
Peas, green	26	116	1:4.5
Rice, white	24	94	1:3.9
Eggs, chicken	54	205	1:3.8
Bananas	8	26	1:3.3
Beans, white, mature	144	425	1:3.0
Almonds	234	504	1:2.2
Cottage cheese	94	152	1:1.6
Orange juice	11	17	1:1.5
Apples	7	10	1:1.4
Cheese, processed, American	697	771	1:1.1
Milk, cow's	118	93	1:0.8
Broccoli	103	78	1:0.8
Green beans	56	44	1:0.8
Brick cheese	730	455	1:0.6
Cheddar cheese	750	478	1:0.6
Swiss cheese	925	563	1:0.6
Spinach, fresh	93	51	1:0.5
Collard greens, fresh	203	63	1:0.3
Turnip greens	246	58	1:0.2

*These values are for unprocessed foods without prosphate additives.
*Calculated from *USDA Agricultural Handbook 8 ARS*

Source: MineraLab, Inc.

Calcium supplements

Government surveys show that far too many people still are not getting the optimum amount of dietary calcium. The most recent large scale survey, the Health and Nutrition Evaluation Survey (HANES), found that in the age group eighteen to forty-four years, approximately 60 percent of the diets provided *less* than the RDA for calcium.[89] The percentage of diets providing the full calcium RDA was 80 in 1955, 70 in 1965, *but only 39* in 1972.[90]

The biggest change in recent years has been in those receiving less than two-thirds of the calcium RDA. In 1955, 5 percent received less than two-thirds of the RDA; in 1965, 8 percent were below that mark; but in 1972 the percentage below two-thirds RDA jumped to 42.

The question then is how to optimize the diet by increasing its calcium content. The best answer is to add more calcium-rich foods; it is even better when high-calorie junk foods are replaced by wholesome nutritious foods. However, if you are already eating a wholesome diet and do not have junk foods to trade for good foods, you may find that adding extra calcium foods means more calories. The best advice here is to increase your physical activity to burn more calories so that more foods containing calcium can be added to your diet without creating a weight problem.

Another solution is to take calcium supplements which contain no calories. Time-honored favorites are bonemeal and dolomite. While these are popular and inexpensive, we feel that more efficient calcium supplements are available. Dolomite is poorly digested and only a few percent, if any, of the ingested amount actually is absorbed. You may take 100 mg, but the greatest bulk of that will pass through your system and be excreted. It's true, however, that some is better than none. But there are better alternatives. Chelated calcium and calcium compounds such as calcium lactate, calcium gluconate, calcium orotate and calcium carbonate are purer sources of calcium and are more easily dissolved and assimilated. Such compounds are assimilated in the tens of percents. Amino acid chelated calcium is 70–90 percent assimilated. These compounds are generally easier on your system.

Bonemeal contains phosphorus, and most people wishing to take calcium supplements desire to improve their calcium-to-phosphorus ratio. Thus bonemeal would be counter-productive.

We have also had good results with oyster shell and egg shell calcium supplements.

Hair analysis and calcium

Very little research has been done to determine the true significance of hair calcium in relation to calcium balance in other parts of the body. Many extravagant and scientifically unjustified claims have been made concerning the significance of hair calcium. Recommendations for dietary changes and supplements are often made solely on the basis of hair calcium, with no valid scientific basis for such recommendations.

This is not to say that significant information cannot be obtained from hair calcium levels. But the information must be interpreted in the context of many other variables which can have a major effect on hair calcium levels. Hair calcium concentrations diminish with age and are significantly lower in individuals with naturally gray hair. It is uncertain whether the low hair calcium is merely a normal characteristic of gray hair, in the presence of normal body calcium balance, or whether gray hair itself correlates with other abnormalities in the body which are related to calcium metabolism.

Various hair treatments such as cold-wave treatments (permanent waves) and bleaching can make interpretation of hair calcium much less reliable. Hair calcium concentrations usually increase following such treatments but can also decrease.

Recent research by Dr. Jeffrey Bland at the University of Puget Sound, Washington, documents the relationship of high hair calcium to subclinical hyperparathyroidism resulting in maldistribution of calcium out of bones where it should be increasingly concentrated in soft tissues, where calcium is normally in a much lower concentration.[88] This is the process which begins as periodontal disease, leads to osteoporosis and ends as diffuse soft tissue calcification—calcium in arteries, calcium in tendon sheaths and bursa (calcific bursitis) and calcium deposits building up throughout the body to the point where calcium deposits are visible on an X ray with a density comparable to that of bone. In simplified terms it can be stated that diffuse, ionized calcium builds up in the connective tissues of the body, much like cement, reducing the elasticity and increasing the rigidity long before it becomes visible on an X ray. As calcium builds up it also poisons enzymes and has an adverse effect on cellular metabolism. Recent research indicates that one of the earliest signs of this process may be elevated hair calcium.

A major difficulty in using hair calcium as a reliable means of detecting this metabolic abnormality is that the very people whose hair calcium would be expected to increase from early degenerative disease are those who develop gray hair and whose hair level of calcium, in the absence of soft tissue calcification, would be considerably lower. In such a person the otherwise elevated calcium may be reflected by a measurement in the normal range— that is, an increased calcium in the hair might merely raise the level from something below normal up into the normal range and be completely missed on interpretation. Much more research needs to be done in order to accurately assess and interpret hair calcium levels.

There is a clinical impression, not yet scientifically proven, that many individuals with low hair calcium have inadequate absorption of minerals in the digestive tract. This may be caused by insufficient hydrochloric acid in the stomach, by inadequate secretion of pancreatic digestive enzymes, by food allergies which can cause inflammation of the tissues in the digestive tract, and from a variety of other causes.

This means that hair calcium may raise suspicions of certain clinical abnormalities but that these abnormalities must be verified or excluded by other types of testing before a certain diagnosis can be made.

Much of what is stated concerning calcium also applies to magnesium. Calcium and magnesium generally tend to parallel each other as they increase and decrease in hair. This is not always the case and the exceptions are poorly understood. As is the case when testing for other hair elements, hair which has grown more than one and one-half inches from the scalp becomes much less reliable in determining calcium levels.

It has recently been reported that hair calcium concentrations correlate in direct proportion to the amount of sugar and sweets consumed.[91]

Elevated hair calcium levels lead to a clinical suspicion of metabolic calcium imbalance involving decreasing calcium in bone tissues and increasing abnormal deposits in soft tissues and connective tissues of the body. Hair magnesium is also usually elevated and these findings are frequently accompanied by decreased sodium and potassium concentrations in hair. This pattern has been related to the existence of allergies. In the presence of elevated hair calcium one should first assure that the hair has not been treated with any permanent waving techniques or bleaching which could cause an artificial elevation in the absence of other disease. The existence of a metabolic calcium disorder should then be further investigated with laboratory measurements such as ionized serum calcium; calcium excretion in a 24-hour urine collection; dental examination to exclude periodontal disease (dental X rays may provide an early warning sign in this regard); a careful dietary history with computerized analysis for calcium/phosphorus intake ratios, vitamin D intake and magnesium intake; a magnesium loading test with precise measurement of 24-hour urinary magnesium excretion after an injection of magnesium to assess the degree of magnesium deficiency; and a careful clinical history to determine presence or absence of symptoms of kidney stones, early periodontal disease, excessive tooth decay, bursitis, osteoporosis, adequate nutritional absorption, food allergies, coronary artery heart disease, hardening of the arteries of arteriosclerosis, and other clinical conditions possibly related to imbalances of calcium metabolism.

The remaining minerals in the hair analysis may well give further clues.

Elevated hair aluminum may be a sign of toxicity to the parathyroid gland, causing increased secretion of parathyroid hormone. Low levels in hair of several other elements would lead one to suspect malabsorption: zinc, copper, manganese, chromium, and selenium.

There are four metallic elements which are extremely important to the maintenance of an electrical potential across cell membranes. Calcium and sodium are minerals which exist primarily in the fluids surrounding the cells. Potassium and magnesium are in higher concentrations within the cells. Many types of cellular activity involve a reversal of electrical charge across the cell wall which is accomplished by movement of sodium and calcium from outside to inside the cell and of potassium and magnesium from inside to outside the cell wall. Equilibrium is then restored by energy requiring metabolic actions, much like a pump would pump water against gravity. The sodium and calcium are pumped from within the cell back into the fluids outside, and the potassium and magnesium are retrieved from the fluids surrounding the cell and are again concentrated within the cell membrane.

It might be stated in oversimplified terms that hair abnormalities of these four elements may indicate that a malfunction exists in the energy-consuming mechanisms which restore and maintain this delicate balance of concentrations against a diffusion radiant. More than that cannot be said at this time. Suspicions can be raised by imbalances of the hair concentrations of these four elements, but no exact diagnosis or conclusions can be made without more precise testing.

It must be kept in mind at all times that hair element analysis is a screening test and not a precise method of determining what is occurring in the body. Suspicions raised on hair analysis must always be confirmed by more precise and scientifically validated forms of testing before an exact diagnosis can be determined and before proper treatment can be initiated. A thorough medical history and physical examination will frequently provide an adequate basis for a diagnosis. The taking of a precise medical history and a thorough physical examination should certainly be foremost among those measures upon which a treatment plan is based.

Serum and blood levels of calcium and phosphorus are notoriously unreliable as methods of assessing calcium metabolism. Only in the most severe metabolic derangements do these tests show significant changes from the normal ranges.

Low hair calcium, especially when associated with low levels of magnesium and several other trace elemental nutrients, would lead one to investigate overall nutritional adequacy and to exclude disorders of absorption in the digestive tract.

In summary, hair calcium levels are quite variable and unreliable as a means of making a certain diagnosis. On the other hand, abnormalities in hair calcium can raise suspicions and lead to further diagnostic testing to confirm or exclude the presence of bodily imbalances. Normal hair calcium does not exclude such imbalances as a normal hair calcium can merely be an abnormal elevation in a person whose hair calcium would otherwise be low. For example, a person with gray hair or with calcium malabsorption or dietary inadequacy may also have increased soft tissue calcification.

Elevated hair calcium, especially when associated with elevated magnesium, would lead one to investigate for nutritional imbalances related to magnesium deficiency, phosphorus excess, vitamin D excess, or elevated body aluminum stores. Further testing would relate to a possible diagnosis of osteoporosis, periodontal disease, kidney stones, occlusive vascular disease, systemic sclerosis, bursitis and other disorders related to increasing soft tissue calcification and decreasing bone calcium. Low hair calcium, especially when associated with generally low levels of other elements, would lead to further investigations to exclude or confirm dietary deficiency or inadequate absorption and utilization within the body.

A carefully kept diet diary, listing all foods consumed over a seven-day period, and then analyzed by a computer which has been programmed with the content of forty or more known nutritional constituents in each food, can lead to a reliable assessment of dietary intake. Tests to determine adequacy of stomach secretion of hydrochloric acid and of pancreatic enzyme production can provide further clues to problems of malabsorption.

Individuals with known allergies or adverse reactions to specific foods frequently have impaired uptake by the digestive tract because of allergic inflammation of the tissues lining the intestines. One may be led to suspect any or a number of these other clinical conditions on the basis of abnormal hair calcium levels, but the diagnosis must await confirmation by more precise testing.

Case histories

F.M. is a seventy-year-old patient who suffered symptoms of severe burning in the feet causing great discomfort when walking and to a lesser extent at rest. He also had symptoms of coronary artery occlusion with anginal chest pains after walking only 100 feet on level terrain. He had multiple symptoms of food allergies and numerous known food intolerances. Hair analysis showed a very low calcium of 82 ppm (normal 200 to 600 ppm) with correspondingly low levels of magnesium, copper, manganese, zinc, chromium and selenium. The toxic metals were in the average range. Dietary analysis revealed adequate nutrition with no dietary deficiencies and a better than average balance among nutrients.

This patient was placed on an elimination diet and then was provoked with a variety of foods to determine which were causing adverse reactions. A number of symptoms related to the gastrointestinal system, and by eliminating certain foods, particularly milk products, wheat and yeast, bowel symptoms improved. It is assumed that absorption of nutrients was also improved.

He was supplemented with a balance of vitamins and minerals which included 1,000 mg calcium, 400 mg magnesium, 20 mg zinc, 20 mg manganese, 200 mcg selenium, 200 mcg chromium, other trace nutrients and relatively largé doses of the B-complex vitamins and vitamin C. B-complex has long been known to relieve symptoms of peripheral neuritis, the cause of painful feet in this patient.

On this regimen he immediately began to improve and within six months was no longer suffering with angina. He became able to wear shoes and walk normally without pain and without burning in his feet.

This case demonstrates an example of low hair calcium related to malabsorption which in turn was most likely caused by food allergy which was causing inflammation of digestive tract tissues. Treating the food allergies relieved that inflammation and improved absorption. The supplements provided larger-than-customary doses of most known nutrients in a balanced proportion, providing increased absorption even in the presence of absorptive impairment. B-complex vitamins by mouth in doses of 50 to 100 mg per day provided further relief of his neuritis. The fact that angina was relieved along with improvement of the burning feet would indicate that the chest pains were caused by spasm in the coronary arteries rather than irreversible blockage. Rebalancing of the essential nutrients, including calcium and magnesium, in addition to restoring optimal levels of all other nutrients, very effectively put an end to this arterial spasm and completely relieved those symptoms.

P.B.H. is a thirty-three-year-old married mother of several children. She had been told by her dentist that she had periodontal disease with gum infections and needed to have her teeth scraped and treated with extensive surgery by a periodontist. No mention was made of nutrition.

Her hair mineral analysis revealed calcium to be elevated at 1,100 ppm with a similar elevation in magnesium. Computerized dietary analysis revealed that the calcium/phosphorus ratio in her food intake was 0.7, indicating that significantly more phosphorus than calcium was contained in the diet. Even taking into consideration calcium supplements that were being taken, the calcium/phosphorus ratio remained the same because of equal amounts of calcium and phosphorus in the supplements. Her dietary intake of magnesium was 242 mg per day, which was less than the recommended daily allowance of 300 mg per day. She was not taking a magnesium supplement. She was taking a vitamin D supplement containing 1,000 units of activated ergosterol, vitamin D2, the synthetic form. Her hair aluminum was not elevated.

Dietary treatment of this condition consisted of correcting the dietary calcium/phosphorus ratio by giving a supplement containing 1,000 mg calcium per day and by counselling the patient to avoid carbonated beverages and processed food which might contain phosphate preservatives. Because her dietary protein was approximately double the recommended daily allowances, she was counselled to eat slightly less high protein foods and to stress the complex carbohydrate, high fiber foods such as whole grains and vegetables. The balanced supplement which was prescribed contained 400 mg magnesium and also contained adequate amounts of all of the other mineral nutrients and vitamin C to enhance connective tissue and ground substance integrity of her gums and of the periostial tissues surrounding the jaw bones. The synthetic vitamin D supplement was discontinued and she was supplemented with only 400 units per day of vitamin D3, the natural form, derived from fish liver oil. She was also counselled concerning foods and medicines which might contain aluminum, such as antacids and salt which "pours when it rains," because of the aluminum silicate drying additives.

On this regimen it is felt that her bone metabolism will slowly come back into balance and even if periodontal surgery is necessary to correct existing damage to the sockets of her teeth those corrections would be maintained through proper nutritional measures in the future. By starting at an early age, with the first signs of periodontal disease, it is hoped that osteoporosis, which would have inevitably occurred after menopause, can be prevented from occurring.

REFERENCES

1 Copp, D. H. 1970. *Ann. Rev. Physiol.* 32:61–86.

2 Anon. April 18, 1977. *Chem. & Eng. News* 17.

3 Means, R. and Dedman, A. May 8, 1980. *Nature.*

4 Miller, J. A. August 23, 1980. *Science News* 118:119–126.

5 Klee, C. B. *et al.* 1980. *Annual Review of Biochemistry.*

6 Posner, A. S. 1969. *Physiol. Rev.* 49:760–792.

7 Whedon, G. D. 1964. In: *Proceed. VI Internat. Congress on Nutr.,* Mills, C. and Passmore, R., eds. Edinburgh: Livingstone, pp. 425–438.

8 Mitchell, H. H. 1962. *Comparative Nutrition of Man and Domestic Animals,* vol. 1. New York: Academic Press, p. 461.

9 Ayres, S. and Mihan, R. 1969. *California Medicine* 111:87.

10 Cathcart, R. 1972. *J. Amer. Med. Assoc.* 219:216.

11 Ayres, S. and Mihan, R. 1972. *J. Amer. Med. Assoc.* 219:216.

12 Bricklin, M. February 1978. *Prevention* 3.

13 Wilson, E., Fisher, K. and Fuqua, M. 1965. *Principles of Nutrition.* New York: Wiley, p. 144.

14 Banner, E. June 1976. *Postgraduate Medicine.*

15 Anon. September 1977. *Geriatrics* 32(9):64.

16 Nordin, B. 1962. *Amer. J. Clin. Nutr.* 10:384–390.

17 Coulston, A. and Lutwak, L. 1972. *Fed. Proc.* 31:721.

18 Albanese, A. *et al.* 1975. *N.Y. State J. Med.* 326.

19 Bullamore, J. *et al.* 1970. *Lancet* 2:535–537.

20 Krook, L. *et al.* 1972. *Cornell Vet.* 62:32.

21 Lutwak, L. *et al.* 1971. *Isrl. J. Med. Sci.* 7:504.

22 Anon. September 24, 1977. *British Medical Journal.*

23 Spencer, H. 1974. *Amer. Family Physician* 10(2):141.

24 Spencer, H. December 1977. *Annals of Internal Med.*

25 Albanese, A. November-December 1976. *Dairy Council Digest* 47(6):34.

26 Krook, L. 1968. *Cornell Vet.* 58:59–73.

27 Anon. 1976. *Search* (State Univ. N.Y.) 1(3).

28 Anon. September 1975. *Food Product Development* 14.

29 Passwater, R. 1977. *Supernutrition for Healthy Hearts.* New York: Dial Press.

30 Schroeder, H. 1960. *J. Amer. Med. Assoc.*

31 Schroeder, H. 1966. *J. Amer. Med. Assoc.*

32 Crawford, M. *et al.* 1968. *Lancet.*

33 Crawford, M. *et al.* 1973. *Engineering Digest.*

34 Schroeder, H. J. 1978. *The Poisons Around Us.* New Canaan, Connecticut: Keats Publishing.

35 Anon. March 16, 1981. *Med. World News.*

36 Wilson, E., Fisher, K. and Fuqua, M. 1965. *Principles of Nutrition.* New York: Wiley.

37 Leichsenring, J. *et al.* 1957. *J. Nutr.* 63:425.

38 Lutwak, L. *et al.* 1964. *Science* 144(3622):1155–1157.

39 Hegsted, D. M. 1952. *J. Nutr.* 46:181.

40 Raven, A. M. *et al.* 1960. *J. Nutr.* 72:29.

41 Johnson, N. E. *et al.*1970. *J. Nutr.* 100:1425–1430.

42 Margen, S. *et al.* 1974. *Am. J. Clin. Nutr.* 27:584–589.

43 Anand, C. R. and Linkswiler, H. M. 1974. *J. Nutr.* 104:695–700.

44 Chu, J.-Y. *et al.* 1975. *Am. J. Clin. Nutr.* 28:1028–1035.

45 Linkswiler, H. M. *et al.* 1974. *Trans. N. Y. Acad. Sci.* 36:333–340.

46 Allen, L. H. *et al. 1979. Am. J. Clin. Nutr.* 32:741–749.

47 Allen, L. H. *et al.* 1979. *J. Nutr.* 109:1345–1350.

48 Block, G. D. *et al.* 1980. *Am. J. Clin. Nutr.* 33:2128–2136.

49 Hegsted, D. M. *et al.* 1979. *Fed. Proc.* 38:765.

50 Spencer, H. *et al.* 1978. *Am. J. Clin. Nutr.* 31:2167–2180.

51 Bell, R. *et al.* 1977. *J. Nutr.* 107:42–50.

52 Shah, B. G. *et al.* 1967. *J. Nutr.* 92:30–42.

53 Draper, H. H. *et al.* 1972. *J. Nutr.* 102:1133–1142.

54 Sie, T. L. *et al.* 1974. *J. Nutr.* 104:1195–1201.

55 Hegsted, D. M. 1973. *Modern Nutrition in Health and Disease*, Goodhart and Shils, eds. Philadelphia: Lea and Febiger, pp. 268–286.

56 Life Sciences Research Office. 1975. FASEB, SGOGS-32.

57 McBean, L. D. and Speckman, E. 1974. *Am. J. Clin. Nutr.* 27:603–609.

58 Wilkinson, R. 1976. *Calcium, Phosphate, and Magnesium Metabolism*, Nordin, ed. New York: Livingstone, pp. 36–112.

59 Food and Drug Administration. 1975. Compliance Program Evaluation, FY 74, 7320.08c.

60 Page, L. and Friend, B. 1978. *Bioscience* 28:192–197.

61 Linkswiler, H. M. and Zemel, M. B. May 1979. *Contemporary Nutrition* 4(5).

62 Anderson, M. P. *et al.* 1977. *J. Nutr.* 107:834–839.

63 Kim, Y. 1977. Ph.D. Thesis, Univ. Wis.

64 Goldsmith, R. S. *et al.* 1976. *J. Clin. Endocrinol. Metab.* 43:523–532.

65 Anon. 1980. *Mineral and Electrolyte Metabolism* 4(4).

66 Anon. 1962. *Nutr. Rev.* 20:46.

67 Fincke, M. L. 1941. *J. Nutr.* 22(5) 447–482.

68 Brine, C. L. *et al.* 1956. *J. Am. Diet. Assoc.* 31(9) 883–888.

69 Hammarsten, G. 1938. *Skand. Arch. Physiol.* 80:165–175.

70 Bonner, P. *et al.* 1938. *J. Pediat.* 12:188.

71 Bricker, M. L. *et al.* 1949. *J. Nutr.* 39:445.

72 Mitchell, H. H. 1964. *Comp. Nutr. Man and Domestic Animals*, vol. 2. New York: Academic Press, p. 681.

73 Wilson, E. *et al.* 1965. *Principles of Nutrition.* New York: Wiley, p. 142.

74 Reddy, G. S. *et al.* 1971. *Metab. Clin. Exp.* 20(7):642–656.

75 Courtney, A. M. *et al.* 1930. *Arch. Dis. Childhood* 5(25):17–22.

76 Malm, O. J. 1958. *Calcium Requirement and Adaptation in Adult Man.* Oslo: University Press.

77 National Research Council. 1968, 1974, 1980. *Recommended Dietary Allowances.* (editions 7–9). Washington, D. C.: National Academy of Sciences.

78 Gershon-Cohen, J. and Jowsey, J. 1964. *Metabolism* 13:221.

79 Harrison, M. *et al.* 1961. *Lancet* 1015.

80 Lutwak, L. and Whedon, G. D. April 1963. *Disease-a-month.*

81 Schwartz, E. *et al.* 1964. *Amer. J. Med.* 36:233.

82 Walker, A. R. P. 1965. *Amer. J. Clin. Nutr.* 16:327.

83 Nordin, B. E. C. 1964, 1976. *Calcium, Phosphate and Magnesium Metabolism* 1–35. Edinburgh: Livingstone Press.

84 Albanese, A. A. *et al.* 1973. *Nutr. Rep. Int.* 8:119.

85 Bricklin, M. March 1978. *Prevention* 38.

86 USDA. 1969. *Dietary Levels of Households in the U.S.*

87 Raines Bell, R. *et al.* 1977. *J. Nutr.* 107:42.

88 Bland, J. 1979. *J. John Basty College of Naturopathic Med.* 1(1):3–7.

89 *U. S. Health and Nutrition Examination Survey of 1971–1972.* Health Resources Administration, Public Health Service. 1972.

90 U. S. Department of Agriculture. *Household Food Consumption Survey.* Spring 1965. Agri. Res. Service USDA 12–17, 1968.

91 Maher, C. C. 1976. Dissertation, University of Michigan, 209.

5

PHOSPHORUS

Phosphorus, like calcium, has many functions in the body in addition to forming bones and teeth. Phosphorus is needed for the metabolic processes of all cells, to activate many other nutrients and to form energy-storage and releasing compounds. Our need for phosphorus is appreciable. We require an amount second only to calcium in terms of "mineral" requirements. Fortunately, phosphorus is widely distributed in the diet, and deficiency is rare. Not only is phosphorus plentiful, it is well absorbed (70 percent).

The phosphorous content of the body is approximately 1 percent of total body weight. Bones consist of about one-half as much phosphorus as the calcium content. The phosphorus in bone and teeth, like calcium, is in constant turnover. Phosphorus forms phosphate, the major anion (negatively charged electrical ion) in the body. Phosphate is an important part of cellular membranes and plays a role in transport through the membranes (permeability). Phosphorus combines with fat to form phospholipids, which are very important to the function of cellular membranes and to the nervous system.

Many of the B-complex vitamins are effective only when combined with phosphate in the body. A series of phosphorous compounds are formed in carbohydrate and fat metabolism. Phosphorous compounds are broken down and rebuilt during muscle contraction. Phosphorus is a component of several vital enzyme systems.

60

Two of the most important series of phosphorous-containing compounds are adenosine triphosphate (ATP) and nucleoproteins. Energy is stored and released in cells by the conversion from one member of the ATP group to another (adenosine monophosphate↔adenosine diphosphate↔adenosine triphosphate). Nucleoproteins are the major components in cell nucleii that control cell division, reproduction and heredity.

The parathyroid gland regulates blood phosphate level (2-4.5 mg/100 ml) and the rate of phosphate excretion from the kidneys.

The average daily intake of phosphorus of adults in the United States is about 1500–1600 mg.[1] The 1980 RDA is only 1000/mg. Thus deficiency is rare, but phosphorous depletion can occur as a result of prolonged and excessive intake of nonabsorbable antacids.[2] Aluminum, magnesium, strontium, and iron inhibit phosphorous absorption. This situation is characterized by weakness, weight loss, malaise and bone pain.

The more common problem involving phosphorus is matching the intake of calcium to that of phosphorus. Refer to the preceding chapter on calcium for a discussion on the calcium to phosphorous ratio and our comments on balancing phosphorous intake. Although there is active research "debating" the issue, it seems advisable to have a calcium-to-phosphorous ratio 1:1 or greater.

Recent research indicates that professional or world class athletes might have need for more phosphorus than suggested by the RDA. Strenuous exercise increases the excretion of phosphorus from the body for several hours afterwards.[3]

Food sources

Good food sources of phosphorus are fish, meats, poultry, eggs, legumes, milk and milk products, nuts and wholegrain cereals. Soft drinks often have phosphate buffers and some food additives contain phosphate. The per capita intake of soft drinks was 39 gallons in 1981. As a rule, our typical diets contain more phosphorus than ideal for our calcium-to-phosphorus ratio.

The phosphorous content of several foods is listed in Table 5.1.

Hair analysis and phosphorus

Hair phosphorus has little or no relationship to phosphorous metabolism in the body or to dietary phosphorous intake. Refer to the section on hair analysis ratios at the end of the next chapter (magnesium).

THE MACRO-MINERALS

TABLE 5.1 SOURCES OF PHOSPHORUS

Milligrams (mg) per 100 grams edible portion (100 grams = 3½ oz.)

Brewer's yeast	1753	Broccoli	78
Wheat bran	1276	Figs, dried	77
Pumpkin and squash seeds	1144	Yams	69
Wheat germ	1118	Soybean sprouts	67
Sunflower seeds	837	Mung bean sprouts	64
Brazil nuts	693	Dates	63
Sesame seeds, hulled	592	Parsley	63
Soybeans, dried	554	Asparagus	62
Almonds	504	Bamboo shoots	59
Cheddar cheese	478	Cauliflower	56
Pinto beans, dried	457	Potato with skin	53
Peanuts	409	Okra	51
Wheat	400	Spinach	51
English walnut	380	Green beans	44
Rye grain	376	Pumpkin	44
Cashews	373	Avocado	42
Beef liver	352	Beet greens	40
Scallops	338	Swiss chard	39
Millet	311	Winter squash	38
Barley, pearled	290	Carrot	36
Pecans	289	Onions	36
Dulse	267	Red cabbage	35
Kelp	240	Beets	33
Chicken	239	Radish	31
Brown rice	221	Summer squash	29
Eggs	205	Celery	28
Garlic	202	Cucumber	27
Crab	175	Tomato	27
Cottage cheese	152	Banana	26
Beef or lamb	150	Persimmon	26
Lentils, cooked	119	Eggplant	26
Mushrooms	116	Lettuce	26
Fresh peas	116	Nectarine	24
Sweet corn	111	Raspberry	22
Raisins	101	Grapes	20
Whole cow's milk	93	Orange	20
Globe artichoke	88	Olives	17
Yogurt	87	Cantaloupe	16
Brussels sprouts	80	Apple	10
Prunes, dried	79	Pineapple	8

Source: MineraLab, Inc.

REFERENCES

1 Page, L. and Friend, B. 1978. *BioScience* 28:192–197.
2 Lotz, M., Zisman, E. and Bartter, F. 1968. *New Engl. J. Med.* 278:409–415.
3 Steinhaus, A. (George Williams College) Unpublished Communication.

6

MAGNESIUM

Magnesium is closely related to calcium and phosphorus in body function. The average adult body contains approximately one ounce (20–28 grams) of magnesium. It is fifth in abundance within the body—behind calcium, phosphorus, potassium and sodium. Although about 70 percent of magnesium is contained in teeth and bones, its most important functions are carried out by the remainder which is present in the cells of the soft tissues and in the fluid surrounding those cells.

Next to potassium, magnesium is the predominant cation (positively charged ion) in cells. It is an essential part of many enzyme systems. The chief function of magnesium is to "activate" certain enzymes, especially those related to carbohydrate metabolism. Another major role of magnesium is to maintain the electrical potential across nerve and muscle membranes. Recent research indicates that magnesium controls many cellular functions.[1]

Magnesium is also involved in protein formation, DNA production and function, and in the storage and release of energy in ATP.

In nerve cells, calcium is the "stimulator" and magnesium is the "relaxor." Both, in correct balance, are essential to proper function. This is also true in heart health. As we have seen, calcium is responsible for heart contraction, and magnesium is responsible for heart relaxation which then allows for the next contraction or pumping action.

Little is understood about the complex magnesium compounds formed in bone and teeth, but it appears that most of this magnesium is not freely exchangeable and thus is not in dynamic equilibrium as are calcium and phosphorus.

The medical community has become more aware of the need for optimal magnesium intakes thanks to widely publicized reports of the relationship of magnesium deficiency to fatal heart disease and artery spasms. A review released in 1980 by the National Research Council of Canada related magnesium deficiency to heart disease, high blood pressure, urothiasis (urinary stones) and convulsions in infants. Both reports discuss declining intakes of magnesium caused by food processing, "softened" water and adverse effects of medications such as diuretics.

Heart disease

In discussion of calcium, we examined the correlation of "hard" water with a lowered heart disease death rate. Hard water supplies additional calcium and magnesium which are needed for proper heart function.

In addition to magnesium's role in allowing the heart to relax so that it may again contract for sustained pumping action, magnesium can lower high blood pressure, prevent arterial spasms and reduce the incidence of unwanted calcium deposits in arteries and heart valves.

It is not exactly clear just how magnesium prevents arterial spasms, but it is suggested that low magnesium levels in artery and heart cells allow unopposed calcium to cause contraction.

This concept supports the observations of five Welsh physicians who found that the hearts of heart disease victims contained about 30 percent less magnesium and more calcium than normal (unaffected) individuals.[2]

This observation confirmed earlier reports by others, including Dr. T. W. Anderson of the University of British Columbia.[3] A follow-up study by researchers at the State University of New York Downstate Medical Center in Brooklyn added even more information. Doctors Prasad Turlapaty and Burton Altura reported lower magnesium concentrations in the coronary arteries of heart disease victims.

When the researchers tested arteries from laboratory animals, they found that lower magnesium concentrations related to increased spasm in response to compounds that constrict arteries. The arteries become sensitized to constricting agents by magnesium depletion.

The researchers concluded that low levels of magnesium in arteries "could produce progressive vasoconstriction, resulting in coronary arterial spasm and, finally, sudden-death ischemic heart disease."[3]

The researchers suggest that risk from sudden death caused by heart attacks can be cut by 50 to 75 percent. They feel that too much emphasis has been placed on high cholesterol levels rather than low magnesium levels as a major cause of heart attacks.

The research that targeted arterial spasms as a cause of heart attacks, more so than cholesterol deposits, originated with a team of Italian physicians headed by Dr. Attilio Maseri of the University of Pisa. They found that in all seventy-six angina pectoris patients whom they examined spasms of the coronary arteries were frequently the cause of the angina pains. The blood clots related to heart attacks (coronary thrombosis) formed only *after* the arterial spasms, and they formed only where spasms had occurred.[4]

Irregular heartbeat such as ventricular fibrillation has also been linked to low magnesium levels by many researchers including Dr. Lloyd Iseri, Professor of Medicine at the University of California at Irvine.[5]

A review of the earlier research linking magnesium deficiency to heart disease has been presented by Drs. G. E. Burch and T. D. Giles of the Department of Medicine of Tulane University. They conclude, "It is apparent that magnesium plays an important role in cardiac homeostasis and that magnesium deficiency is capable of producing cardiac disease. . . . Magnesium deficiency will be found only when looked for, and thus the responsibility for prevention, detection and treatment resides with the physician."[6]

Cancer

Evidence is accumulating that magnesium has an anti-cancer effect. More precisely, magnesium deficiency increases one's susceptibility to cancer. Animal and epidemiological studies show an inverse relationship between dietary magnesium levels and the incidence of cancer.[7]

Several mechanisms have been proposed, including:
• magnesium enhances the fidelity of DNA replication
• magnesium at the cell membrane prevents changes that cause cancer
• magnesium on the cell membrane helps cells stick together in a normal fashion
• magnesium is required in more than thirty enzyme systems that deal with cell growth and division, which are disordered in cancer.

Dr. P. Bois of the University of Montreal has shown that magnesium deficiency in laboratory animals increases the incidence of spontaneous cancers.[8]

Dr. George Hass of the Rush-Presbyterian-St. Luke's Medical Center in Chicago has immunized laboratory rats against cancer but cannot do so if they are even marginally deficient in magnesium.[9]

These findings fit the general observation that people who are well nourished with vitamins and minerals have less cancer than those who are malnourished in the micronutrients.

Blood pressure

Georgetown University's Medical Researchers reported in *Angiology* (Oct. 1977) that persons with high blood pressure had an 11 percent decrease in blood pressure following magnesium therapy, whereas persons with normal blood pressure did not change. Both groups benefited from increased cardiac output and from greater efficiency of the heart muscle.

Energy

Magnesium sparks enzyme activity needed for energy production. Physicians are finding that many people with complaints of constant fatigue respond to supplements of magnesium together with potassium.

One study published in *Current Therapeutic Research* showed that eighty-seven of 100 persons complaining of constant fatigue experienced increased energy and strength within five to ten days after beginning magnesium and potassium supplementation.

In another study published in the *Journal of Abdominal Surgery*, 94 percent of the eighty subjects said their tiredness and weakness diminished within three days to two weeks after beginning magnesium and potassium supplementation.

Sleep, tension
and menstrual cramps

Persons taking magnesium and potassium supplements to improve their energy level also noted that they slept better and awakened without their usual morning exhaustion.

In another study involving more than 200 insomnia patients, Drs. W. Davis and F. Ziady of the University of Pretoria (South Africa) reported that 99 percent of all patients given magnesium supplements were helped.[10] They fell asleep more quickly, had uninterrupted sleep and awakened refreshed. They also found that anxiety and tension levels were diminished during the day.

Magnesium is a natural tranquilizer, that calms erratic nervous activity caused by magnesium deficiency. We have also noted that magnesium relieves severe menstrual cramps, and is an anticonvulsant in epileptic seizures.

Preventing kidney stones

Adequate magnesium intake keeps calcium from depositing in bone joints and in the soft tissues such as arteries. Magnesium also reduces kidney stone formation especially which contains calcium oxylate.

In a five-year study of 149 persons prone to recurrent kidney stones, Drs. Edwin Prien and Stanley Gershoff of Boston University found that magnesium supplements produced a dramatic reduction in kidney stone formation. The group averaged 1.3 stones before they took the magnesium supplements but averaged only one-tenth of a stone per person during the five years while taking magnesium supplements. Only seventeen individuals in the group of 149 developed stones.[11]

In a similar study Dr. Sverker Ljunghall, of the Uppsala Medical School in Sweden, found that kidney stones formed in only three of seventy high-risk persons taking magnesium supplements.[11]

Deficiency symptoms

Magnesium deficiency is seldom diagnosed because it is rarely looked for. However, it is far more extensive than previously thought.

Deficiency symptoms may include loss of appetite, irritability, weakness, insomnia, muscle tremor, tetany, twitching, numbness, tingling, confusion, disorientation, personality change, learning disability, apathy, memory impairment, skin lesions, elevated blood cholesterol, cardiovascular changes, tachycardia, elevated parathyroid hormone, pancreatitis and stress.

Not only is there a high incidence of less-than-optimal dietary intake, there are several medical conditions and medications that cause a "secondary" magnesium deficiency, which reduce the absorption of magnesium or increase the excretion.

Such conditions include alcoholism, malabsorption, diuretic therapy (water pills), burns, surgery, diabetic acidosis and coma, cirrhosis, hepatitis, hyperaldosteronism, hyperparathyroidism, Addison's disease, epilepsy, eclampsia, kidney disease and oral contraceptive use.

How much

How much magnesium is needed for optimal health and to balance the calcium, phosphorous and potassium intakes? The current RDA of the National Research Council is 350 mg for men and 300 mg for women. The FDA's USRDA is 400 mg.

Dr. Emanuel Cheraskin determined that the mean "ideal" magnesium consumption as determined by his analyses of individuals without clinical symptoms is 400 mg (range 300 to 530 mg).[12] Magnesium expert Dr. M. Seelig recommends a magnesium intake above 6 mg per kilogram of body weight per day. Thus Dr. Seeling is recommending 300 mg for a 110-pound person, 420 mg for a 154-pound person and 540 mg for a 200-pound person.[13]

A survey of college students in Montreal indicated an average 240 mg per day intake of magnesium (*Nutrition Reports International*, August 1978). Unfortunately, several other surveys indicate that large groups of people are not getting optimal amounts of magnesium in their food. Thus water content of magnesium (hardness) does become a critical factor to many individuals with marginal intake.

University of Wisconsin researchers found that a group of pregnant Wisconsin women had an average daily intake of 200 mg (range 100 to 333). Ninety-eight percent consumed less than the RDA and 79 percent consumed less than 55 percent of the RDA.[14] Unfortunately, pregnant women need more magnesium than others. The Food and Nutrition Board of the National Research Council states that the "average" American diet contains about 120 mg magnesium per 1000 calories of food intake. With today's sedentary lifestyle, our calorie needs have decreased. As an example, the Food and Nutrition Board recommends that the average female between fifty-one and seventy-five years of age consumes 1800 calories per day. Thus her daily magnesium intake would only be 216 mg. Similarly, the recommendation for the average male between fifty-one and seventy-five years of age is 2400 calories. The average man in this age group would be consuming only 288 mg magnesium daily. Certainly there is room for improvement.

Food processing refines out a large proportion of magnesium and it is not replaced by "fortification." When the wheat germ and bran are stripped away to make refined white flour, so is 85 percent of the magnesium. So called "enrichment" doesn't add back any magnesium.

The amount of magnesium absorbed from the diet varies with the amount consumed. The body absorbs about 80 percent of the magnesium in low-magnesium diets, 45 percent of typical diets, but only about 25 percent of high-magnesium diets.

Large amounts of calcium, vitamin D, protein or fats will decrease magnesium absorption. The absorption of magnesium resembles the mechanism for calcium absorption. There is evidence that they are the same. Thus both calcium and magnesium must compete for absorption and an excess or deficiency of one inversely affects the other.

About one-tenth to one-third of the ingested magnesium is excreted through the kidney which is the major regulator of body magnesium content. Unlike calcium, magnesium does not seem to be controlled by parathyroid hormone, although this is still debated. An inverse relationship has been noted between magnesium and aldosterone. Aldosterone probably affects intracellular magnesium more than blood magnesium levels do.

Magnesium is blood's most valuable mineral component. Replenishment from the body's limited magnesium stores is slow at best, and there doesn't seem to be any special activator. Therefore dietary magnesium is an essentially critical factor.

Food sources

The wide availability of magnesium in natural foods has misled many into believing that there is little problem with magnesium deficiency. However, food processing and declining calorie needs are making it more difficult to obtain optimal quantities of magnesium in modern diets.

Good sources of magnesium include green vegetables, whole grains, nuts and seeds. Table 6.1 lists the magnesium content of several foods.

TABLE 6.1 SOURCES OF MAGNESIUM

Milligrams (mg) per 100 grams edible portion (100 grams = 3½ oz.)

Kelp	760	Common beans, cooked	37
Wheat bran	490	Barley	37
Wheat germ	336	Dandelion greens	36
Almonds	270	Garlic	36
Cashews	267	Raisins	35
Blackstrap molasses	258	Fresh green peas	35
Brewer's yeast	231	Potato with skin	34
Buckwheat	229	Crab	34
Brazil nut	225	Banana	33
Dulse	220	Sweet potato	31
Filberts	184	Blackberry	30
Peanuts	175	Beets	25
Millet	162	Broccoli	24
Wheat grain	160	Cauliflower	24
Pecan	142	Carrot	23

SOURCES OF MAGNESIUM (*cont.*)

Milligrams (mg) per 100 grams edible portion (100 grams = 3½ oz.)

English walnut	131	Celery	22
Rye	115	Beef	21
Tofu	111	Asparagus	20
Beet greens	106	Chicken	19
Coconut meat, dry	90	Green pepper	18
Soybeans, cooked	88	Winter squash	17
Spinach	88	Cantaloupe	16
Brown rice	88	Eggplant	16
Dried figs	71	Tomato	14
Swiss chard	65	Cabbage	13
Apricots, dried	62	Grapes	13
Dates	58	Milk	13
Collard leaves	57	Pineapple	13
Shrimp	51	Mushroom	13
Sweet corn	48	Onion	12
Avocado	45	Orange	11
Cheddar cheese	45	Iceberg lettuce	11
Parsley	41	Plum	9
Prunes, dried	40	Apple	8
Sunflower seeds	38		

Source: MineraLab, Inc.

Magnesium supplements

If an analysis of your diet shows that you are deficient in magnesium, supplements are available to balance or enhance your dietary intake. The preferred supplement is chelated magnesium or magnesium aspartate followed by, in descending order of preference, magnesium gluconate, magnesium palmatate, magnesium chloride, magnesium sulfate and magnesium carbonate.

Hair analysis

The tissue content of magnesium is not represented accurately by hair analysis. Hair analysis for magnesium content possibly provides meaningful clinical information but only in relation to bone metabolism and hormone imbalances.

Hair magnesium tends to parallel hair calcium. Cellular magnesium concentrations, including red blood cells, white blood cells and skeletal muscle cells, are invalid as a measure of overall nutritional deficiency, according to Dr. Mildred Seelig.[13]

High magnesium level in the hair suggests bone wasting in the body (osteoporosis and/or periodontal disease) and the following confirmational steps should be taken. A thorough dental examination for early periodontal disease might be helpful. An "insurance" dose of magnesium in a balanced supplement could be taken as a preventive measure. A medical evaluation for adverse reactions to specific foods or a hormone imbalance may reveal unsuspected causes of fatigue or nervousness.

If the hair magnesium level is depressed, then there may be a total body deficiency of magnesium. This has not been proven as of 1982. The same can be true if the magnesium is normal or high in the hair. We do not believe that we can state from a hair analysis that magnesium is not deficient, regardless of what the hair levels are. We believe that if hair magnesium is depressed, a magnesium deficiency is a possibility and that if hair magnesium is elevated, in the absence of any recent cold wave, permanents or bleaching treatments, magnesium deficiency in the diet in relation to the phosphorus, calcium and aluminum imbalance should be suspected.

The following confirmational steps should be taken:

A more reliable method of evaluating a person's magnesium status is the determination of his/her 24-hour urinary output before and after a parenteral magnesium load, and evaluating the percentage retention in terms of renal function and blood (serum) magnesium levels.[14]

A recently developed technological advance will allow for much more accurate assessment of total body magnesium stores and will be available to practicing clinicians in 1983. This new procedure combines scanning electron microscopy with X-ray fluorescence to measure the levels of magnesium and other elements inside cells. Magnesium in cells gently rubbed from beneath the tongue has been found to correlate very accurately with magnesium in heart muscle cells. Intracellular magnesium-to-calcium ratios of cells from beneath the tongue accurately predict the risk of atherosclerosis, heart attack, stroke and perhaps even cancer.

Observations on ratios
(calcium, phosphorus, magnesium)

The following comments are based on scientific studies and clinical experience. We feel that they are well founded in clinical experience and research.

However, we also realize that new research will add to our knowledge and expand the usefulness of ratios between elements. Thus, our comments will serve as an initial foundation that can be extended in the future.

We suggest that you ask for verification of any extension of our comments. It is very easy to calculate ratios of hair minerals and suggest that these numbers are meaningful clinically. The proof is much harder to come by.

Usually when the calcium is elevated the magnesium is also elevated, and the degree that these elevations vary, one in respect to the other, has not been specifically worked out. We believe that when both calcium and magnesium are elevated in relation to other minerals that there is good scientific data to suggest the occurrence of widespread soft tissue calcification, usually ionic rather than in the form of precipitated deposits, or in the form of hydroxy apatite, which is the form seen on X rays as dense soft tissue calcium deposits. A suspicion of osteoporosis or periodontal problems, with subclinical hyperparathyroidism (ionized calcium slightly elevated even with normal to total serum calcium), can be formed if hair calcium and magnesium are elevated. The problem is that in an elderly population with gray hair reduced calcium and magnesium in hair (that is with both minerals below the reference range) can indicate the same problem.

Calcium and magnesium are both lower in patients with gray hair, so levels that would otherwise be elevated might be at a normal level in an elderly, gray-haired person. The point we are trying to make is that calcium and magnesium usually move together and it is the ratio of calcium and magnesium to their own reference range rather than the ratio of calcium to magnesium per se which is most significant clinically. Clinical experience has shown that patients (especially if younger than sixty-five) with occlusive arterial disease, arteriosclerotic heart disease, angina, congestive heart failure and other serious coronary artery disease symptoms seem to have a higher incidence of low magnesium with a normal to only slightly low calcium. This would certainly affect the calcium/magnesium ratio and would indicate cardiovascular pathology. The calcium/magnesium ratio is not as simply interpreted as some would indicate. The absolute levels of calcium and magnesium in relation to their own reference levels must be interpreted in conjunction with the ratio between these two minerals. Also important to consider is the fact that hair treatments such as cold-wave processing (permanents) and bleaching can both elevate calcium and magnesium and not necessarily in the same proportion, artificially altering this ratio. Women who have frequent hair treatments often have elevated calcium and magnesium in their hair on that basis alone. This is the same population which is most likely to have osteoporosis and metabolic causes for elevations of hair calcium and magnesium, which makes correct interpretation a difficult process without a very careful history of hair treatments in relation to the timing and method of specimen collection.

If the calcium/magnesium ratio is depressed, interpretation would depend on the absolute values—that is, whether calcium and magnesium are both elevated, whether calcium is normal and magnesium elevated, or if magnesium is normal and calcium depressed. As we have already seen, hyperparathyroidism (of a subclinical nature) can cause both calcium and magnesium to be either elevated, depressed or even in the normal range in an elderly gray-haired person who would have normally low calcium and magnesium and in whom an elevation would put these minerals back into a normal range.

Low hydrochloric acid production by the stomach may be responsible for a generalized malabsorption or diminished absorption of food nutrients, which would more likely cause both calcium and magnesium to be depressed rather than just a depressed calcium/magnesium ratio.

Recent work by Dr. Mildred Seelig in New York would certainly incriminate the excessive dietary consumption of phosphates in relation to calcium as a cause of progressive, subclinical, hyperparathyroidism throughout life, leading to increased bone absorption and diffuse soft tissue calcification in many, if not all, tissues of the body. We must consider that as the activity of the parathyroid gland increases, aluminum absorption from the bowel increases. Aluminum in turn contributes to increased parathyroid activity. What we have is a vicious circle. Dietary factors of inadequate magnesium (which enhances all of these metabolic defects), excessive phosphorus in relation to calcium intake, excessive vitamin D fortification of foods and perhaps absolute deficiency of calcium intake, all of which contribute to an increasingly active parathyroid gland, can lead to a very subtle increase in serum-ionized calcium and widespread "sludging" of the body metabolism because of diffuse calcium ions being deposited intercellularly and in connective tissue throughout the body. This leads to diminished tissue elasticity and increased cross-linkages causing tissue stiffness as well as metabolic poisoning—all contributing to degenerative diseases in a variety of syndromes. The increased parathyroid activity in turn causes an increased gut absorption of aluminum; the soft tissue deposits of aluminum can also cause neurological changes (recently incriminated in both Alzheimer's disease and Parkinson's disease) and are probably also a factor in increased connective tissue cross-linkages and decreased body flexibility.

If calcium is normal to somewhat low and magnesium is disproportionately low in relation to calcium, creating an elevated calcium/magnesium ratio, then suspect a high probability of cardiovascular pathology. If calcium and magnesium are both high, irrespective of the ratio between the two, then poor metabolic and cellular utilization of calcium, vitamin D excess, phosphate excess in relation to calcium and probable magnesium deficiency in conjunction with increased aluminum absorption are all to be considered. If calcium and magnesium are both high, irrespective of the ratio between the two, suspect osteoporosis and periodontal disease. If they are both low, also investigate for osteoporosis and periodontal disease.

Other than pointing to these preliminary and inconclusive interpretations, the calcium and magnesium levels in the hair are not good indicators of dietary intake. An exception might be in some cases wherein low hair magnesium is an indicator of low dietary magnesium. However as we stated before, magnesium deficiency in the diet potentiates all of the parathyroid, aluminum absorption disorders related to an inappropriate calcium phosphorous ratio and in that way magnesium deficiency in the diet can also cause elevated hair calcium and magnesium.

Hair phosphorus has little or no relation to phosphorous metabolism in the body or dietary phosphorous intake. Most people in our country have too much dietary phosphorus in relation to calcium which paradoxically causes an elevation in the calcium-phosphorous ratio in hair. Because hair phosphorus has not been shown to be an accurate indicator of phosphorous metabolism or body phosphorus, and because hair calcium elevates with too much phosphorus in the diet, we feel that the calcium-phosphorous ratio is not a reliable indicator. (A dietary magnesium deficiency can elevate hair calcium because of its effect on the parathyroid and increased soft tissue calcification, but this does not mean that a high calcium-phosphorous ratio in the diet or in the hair causes or is diagnostic of magnesium deficiency.)

Case histories

M. D. is a sixty-seven-year-old lady with chronic kidney disease; she is approaching end-stage kidney failure. She has known osteoporosis and thinning of her bones. Her hair analysis showed magnesium to be elevated at 230 ppm (normal 25 to 75) with calcium elevated at 1,200 ppm (normal 200 to 600). Little could be done to treat the bone condition because of her kidney disease, but she was cautiously given magnesium supplements within the tolerance of her capacity of her kidneys to handle any excess. Her spinal pain improved.

R. G. is a fifty-four-year-old male scientist who was having symptoms of angina or inadequate blood flow in the coronary arteries supplying the muscles of the heart. Extensive testing at a university hospital showed no arterial blockages. Hair analysis revealed a very low magnesium at 16 ppm (normal 25 to 75) with a slightly low calcium at 160 ppm (normal 200 to 600). The magnesium was disproportionately low in relation to calcium. He was treated with a broad spectrum multiple vitamin mineral supplement in physiologic ratios containing 400 mg magnesium aspartate per day. On this regimen he promptly improved and his exertional chest pains ceased. The clinical diagnosis was coronary artery spasm or atypical angina caused by mineral imbalances of the calcium/magnesium/phosphorous system. He became symptom-free and able to resume his normal activities on nutritional supplementation alone with no other medication.

REFERENCES

1 Rubin, H. September 1975. *Proceed. Nat. Acad. Sci.*

2 *Lancet.* October 4, 1980.

3 Turlapaty, P. and Altura, B. April 11, 1980. *Science* 208:198–200.

4 Maseri, A. *et al.* December 1978. *New Engl. J. Med.*

5 Iseri, L. September 8, 1976. *Med Tribune.*

6 Burch, G. E. and Giles, T. D. November 1977. *Amer. Heart J.* 94(5):649–657.

7 Blondell, J. M. August 1980. *Medical Hypotheses* 290(1041):863–871.

8 Bois, P. Report at Federation of American Societies for Experimental Biology, April 1981.

9 Clark, M. July 1965. *Prevention* 59–61.

10 Davis, W. H. and Ziady, F. 1976. Second Internat. Symp. Magnesium, Montreal.

11 Reports at the Annual Meeting of the American College of Nutrition, 1980.

12 Cheraskin, Emanuel. 1977. *IRCS Med. Sci.* 5, 588.

13 Seelig, M. 1980. *Magnesium Deficiency in the Pathogenesis of Disease.* New York: Plenum Medical Book Company.

14 Johnson, N. E. and Phillips, C. A. 1976. Second Internat. Symp. Magnesium, Montreal.

The electrolyte minerals

POTASSIUM

SODIUM

AND CHLORIDE

7

POTASSIUM

The vital tug-of-war between potassium and sodium in the body should be of interest to everyone. Although modern diets tip the balance in favor of sodium intake, our bodies contain more of the potassium. Typical diets supply 3–7 grams of sodium compared to only 1.5 to 5 grams of potassium. Primitive diets and unprocessed food diets consumed in non-industrialized nations normally supply the body with more potassium than sodium.

Our bodies normally contain more than twice as much potassium as sodium (typically 9 oz versus 4 oz). Sodium is relatively scarce in natural diets, which are rich in potassium. Thus the body has a better regulation mechanism to retain the "historically scarce" sodium, but poor regulation for retention of the "historically plentiful" potassium. And now modern man has decided to reverse the more natural dietary pattern.

About 98 percent of total body potassium is inside our cells. In fact, potassium is the principal cation (positive ion) of the fluid inside cells. This intracellular fluid has a potassium content more than thirty times the potassium concentration of the fluid surrounding the cells. The sodium-to-potassium ratio is 1:10 inside the cell and 28:1 in the extracellular fluid.

This concentration of potassium within the cells is not achieved by simple diffusion through the cell membrane. It is achieved by an energy-consuming process called the "sodium-potassium pump." As a result of this mechanism, the amount of potassium in the bloodstream or in hair may not accurately reflect the proper distribution or total supply of body potassium.

The kidney is the major regulatory mechanism controlling potassium balance. Although more than 90 percent of ingested potassium is absorbed from the gastrointestinal tract, the blood level remains relatively constant despite wide variations in intake.[1] Regulation of body potassium is dependent on elements in the system that maintain sodium balance. Magnesium helps hold potassium within the cells.

Potassium can be excreted via the gastrointestinal tract, but this loss is small except during diarrhea or kidney failure. Skin losses of potassium are trivial. Large volumes of sweat lead to only modest potassium losses.[2]

Function

Potassium is important in controlling the activity of the heart, muscles, nervous system and just about every living cell in the body.

Although sodium alone is believed by many to be the most important dietary determinant of blood pressure, variations in the dietary sodium-to-potassium ratio also affect blood pressure under certain circumstances. (This will be discussed in detail later.)

Potassium functions as an activator of enzymes and is involved in the use of amino acids. There is evidence that potassium is also involved in bone calcification.

The sodium-potassium pump through the cell membranes may also help other nutrients enter the cell. Potassium is needed to maintain cell integrity. If the potassium level dips in the cell, more sodium enters and interferes with cell metabolism, especially protein production.

Potassium is a co-factor in many reactions, especially those involving energy production and muscle building. Skeletal muscle contains six times more potassium than sodium.

Deficiency symptoms

Severe dietary deficiency is unlikely, but severe potassium depletion occurs with some diseases, with extensive burns and in general malnutrition. Moderate (subclinical) dietary deficiencies do occur, as well as major sodium-potassium imbalances.

Conditions bringing about potassium depletion include diuretic therapy (water pills), aspirin, prolonged laxative therapy, diarrhea, diabetic acidosis, cocorticosteroid therapy (cortisone or corticotrophic hormones), gastrointestinal disorders, cancer, and adrenal tumors which produce a hormone called aldosterone.

Deficiency symptoms can include weakness, irritability, edema, headaches, alkalosis, bone and joint pain and tachycardia or galloping heart.

Toxicity

Sudden increases in intake of potassium to levels about 18 grams (18,000 milligrams) per day may result in cardiac arrest. Kidney failure, dehydration and adrenal insufficiency can elevate blood potassium to toxic levels.

Heart rhythm

Potassium, like magnesium, affects heart rhythm. The over-refined "foods" necessitated by space travel were once low in potassium.

Apollo 15 lunar explorers David Scott and James Irwin both developed irregular heart rhythms due to potassium loss. NASA physician Dr. Charles Berry first noticed a few isolated premature heartbeats from Irwin when he was working hard on the moon. At lift-off from the moon, Irwin had a series of ten irregular beats. He suffered a series of abnormal heartbeats during three hours of transferring moon rocks to the Command Module. Scott's irregular beats occurred just before splashdown. He had taken aspirin to ease a shoulder pain, which increased his potassium loss.

Starting with Apollo 16, astronauts had potassium-enriched food and snacks added to their diets, and they were placed on a potassium-loaded pre-flight diet.

Blood pressure

Not all high blood pressure is due to the same cause. Some people may be genetically predisposed to blood pressure increases when they eat a diet with a high sodium–potassium ratio.

At the 1980 meeting of the American Physiological Society in Toronto, researchers told their peers of an important dietary link to high blood pressure. They suggested that people resist processed foods—not just because of their unnecessarily high salt content but also because of their low potassium content.

"We'd probably see some dramatic changes in the incidence of hypertension (high blood pressure) if Americans cut their salt intake to three grams (3000 milligrams) a day and started eating at least that much potassium," advised Dr. Harold Battarbee of Louisiana State University in Shreveport.[3] He noted, "Although potassium is plentiful in many fresh fruits and vegetables, it is almost entirely lost when they're canned or frozen." Potassium is one of the most soluble of all elements.

Dr. Battarbee and his colleague, Dr. John Dailey, knew that sodium gave their laboratory rats high blood pressure, but they found that increasing potassium intake prevented this blood pressure elevation. The salt (sodium) caused the levels of two neurotransmitters (nerve transmission compounds) to decrease, but the levels stayed normal with extra potassium.

This advice echoes that of Dr. George Miller of the Johns Hopkins School of Hygiene and Public Health: "It's not the amount of sodium you eat, but the amount of potassium."[4]

Dr. Miller and his research partner, Dr. Lewis Kuller of the University of Pittsburgh School of Public Health, studied 2000 people in three cities. They found that those with normal blood pressure tended to eat less salt and more potassium than those with high blood pressure. They deemed that the sodium-to-potassium ratio was a more accurate predictor of blood pressure than the amount of sodium alone.

Drs. Herbert Langford and Robert Watson found in the late 1960s that neither the amount of sodium nor the amount of potassium correlated with blood pressure. However, the sodium-potassium *ratio* clearly did correlate with blood pressure level.

The ratio of sodium to potassium determines water retention. A potassium deficiency allows more sodium to enter the cells. The additional sodium increases the water inside the cells, producing edema and damage.

A British study has confirmed that a high-potassium/low-sodium diet normalized blood pressure in patients having elevated blood pressure.[5] After going off the high-potassium/low-sodium diet, the patients again contracted high blood pressure.

Remember, not all people are sensitive to salt. It appears that there is a genetic predisposition to high blood pressure due to improper sodium-potassium balance. And it is always possible to find a small percentage of people responding in just the opposite fashion.

Energy

Blood sugar provides fuel for our immediate energy needs. When energy needs increase, the first energy reservoir is glycogen stored in muscles and liver. Glycogen is made from blood sugar and is the only fuel stored as carbohydrate. Because glycogen is carbohydrate, it can be quickly summoned from storage and converted back to blood sugar (glucose).

There is a limit to how much glycogen can be stored in muscle and liver. Once these reserves are filled, extra energy is stored as fat. Fat is more compact and can be stored in its own special containers—fat cells. However, the conversion from fat back to blood sugar involves many steps and is comparatively slow and inefficient.

Potassium is essential for the conversion of blood sugar into glycogen. A potassium shortage results in lower glycogen reserves and limited available energy. A potassium shortage also means that less blood sugar is utilized for conversion to glycogen; thus there is a tendency to high blood sugar and increased insulin need (even to overproduction of insulin, resulting in low blood sugar). High blood sugar is not energy-sustaining because it is quickly consumed when increased energy is needed or it is converted to fat by the increased blood levels of insulin. Energy sustenance requires a quick-acting, long-lasting reservoir.

It has been known since the early 1950s that low-potassium diets produce great fatigue and muscle weakness.[6] Magnesium is also involved in the energy process; thus a deficiency of either one will produce fatigue.

Fatigue forces you to reduce your activity, thereby conserving potassium. Remember that the hard work of the astronauts aggravated their potassium deficiency and led to abnormal heart rhythms. (Please refer to the preceding chapter on magnesium for a further discussion of this topic.)

Muscle strength

Potassium is a catalyst in enzymes involved in muscle contraction and coordination. The effect of potassium deficiency on the heart muscle is to cause irregular beats and even heart paralysis.

The weakness of the elderly correlates well with the severity of their potassium deficiency. Athletes should monitor their potassium intake. Heart patients taking digitalis medication are especially prone to adverse effects of potassium depletion.

Potassium needs

The 1980 RDA revisions recommend maintaining current average potassium intake levels (2000–6000 mg) while reducing the sodium intake in half. (The

THE ELECTROLYTE MINERALS

known need for sodium is 500 mg or less.) Kidney patients should consult their physician concerning their special needs.

FDA market basket surveys attempt to monitor typical food intakes. Average potassium levels for Adult Market Baskets in 1977 and 1978 were 4550 and 4735 mg per day, respectively. Milk provided the largest share of potassium, approximately 25 percent of the total.

TABLE 7.1 AVERAGE SODIUM AND POTASSIUM CONTENT IN MARKET BASKETS (mg/day)

	Infant	Toddler	Adult
SODIUM			
1977	885	1593	6697
1978	797	1685	6928
POTASSIUM			
1977	1551	1714	4549
1978	1590	1846	4735

Source: FDA

The optimal potassium intake is related to the sodium intake. Thus it is important to know not only the potassium level of your diet, but also the sodium level. Unfortunately, food tables are often misleading because improper food preparation removes potassium and food processing adds sodium. The skins of foods such as potatoes are potassium-rich, but they are often thrown away. Soaking and cooking in water leaches out potassium.

Dr. Battarbee believes that a potassium–sodium ratio of 1:1 would be beneficial, but others have suggested that 2:1 may be even better.

Table 7.4 compares unprocessed and processed foods in terms of the potassium and sodium content.

Food sources

Fresh fruits and vegetables are good potassium sources. One food that is high in potassium but often overlooked is buckwheat. Buckwheat contains 450 mg potassium per 100 g, and contains essentially no sodium.

Another high-potassium food is the parsley that most people push off their plate because they think it's just a decoration. Parsley has more than twice as much potassium as bananas (per unit weight) and only one-twelfth the calories.

Table 7.2 lists the potassium content of several foods.

Potassium supplements

Diets consisting largely of processed foods tend to have an undesirable potassium-sodium balance. The ideal solution of course is to replace much of the over-salted foods with potassium-rich natural foods. However, we realize that some will not make the change. Most people shun diets having less than four grams (4000 mg) of sodium. The second best advice is to balance the potassium-sodium ratio by cutting back on salt added at the table and taking potassium supplements. Both of the goals can be obtained simultaneously by replacing table salt (sodium chloride) with a salt substitute (potassium chloride). "Light salts" contain half potassium chloride and half sodium chloride.

Many persons on prescribed diuretics (water pills) may also be on prescribed potassium supplements. These prescribed supplements are much stronger than needed by the average healthy person to optimize the potassium-to-sodium ratio.

Using a potassium-based salt substitute in moderation should be sufficient for most people, but for those needing more moderate-level potassium liquids and tablets are available on prescription.

Potassium liquids are preferred because they are the gentlest on your gastrointestinal tract. Some prescribed tablets have enteric-coatings that remain intact in the stomach and do not dissolve until they are in the intestine. Earlier versions of such tablets were suspected of causing ulcerations in the intestines, but present forms are considered safe although expensive. Thus there is a tendency to prescribed liquid supplements despite the poor taste.

Non-prescription potassium tablets sold in health food stores and over the counter in drugstores are mild, but contain little potassium per tablet. Potassium is readily soluble; thus the form is not critical. Potassium does not chelate. Tablets marked "chelated Potassium" are a misnomer but still are good supplements.

Hair analysis

We believe that hair levels of potassium and sodium do not reflect dietary intake nor body stores of either. Certain drugs and diseases can elevate or depress hair sodium, but this is indistinguishable from the random fluctuations we have observed in healthy people.

This may be partially explained by the concentrating action of the sodium-potassium pump, and partially by the washing techniques used in sample preparation. Please refer to the discussion on sodium and potassium determination in hair at the end of the next chapter.

Much more research must be done before conclusions can be substantiated concerning hair concentrations of sodium and potassium.

TABLE 7.2 SOURCES OF POTASSIUM

Milligrams per 100 grams edible portion (100 grams = 3½ oz.)

Dulse (1 tsp. = approximately 242 milligrams)	8060	Mushrooms	414
		Salmon	410
Kelp (1 tsp. = approximately 160 milligrams)	5273	Potato with skin	407
		Collard leaves and stems	401
Blackstrap molasses (1 tsp. = approximately 146 milligrams)	2927	Dandelion greens	397
Brewers yeast, dry	1700	Fennel	397
Rice bran	1495	Brussel sprouts	390
Wheat bran	1121	Broccoli	382
Sunflower seeds, hulled	920	Liver, calves' or beef	380
Wheat germ	827	Kale	378
Almonds	773	Mustard greens	377
Raisins	763	Wheat, soft winter	376
Parsley	727	Banana	370
Sesame seeds, unhulled	725	Wheat, hard	370
Rice polish (note that rice bran contains potassium as rice polish)	714	Winter squash	369
		Ground round, raw	355
Prunes, dried	694	Carrots	341
Peanuts	674	Celery	341
Dates	648	Brains	340
Figs, dried	640	Pumpkin	340
Avocados	604	Beet root	335
Pecans	603	Chicken, light meat without skin, raw	320
Yams	600	
Beet greens	570	Beef kidney	310
Swiss chard	550	Persimmon, native	310
Parsnips	541	Cauliflower	295
Halibut	540	Nectarine	294
Chinese water chestnuts	500	Escarole	294
Spinach	470	Watercress	282
Rye grain	467	Apricot, fresh	281
Cashew nuts	464	Sweet corn	280
Buckwheat	450	Asparagus	278
English walnuts	450	Red cabbage	268
Collard leaves	450	Lettuce, all types except iceberg	264
Globe artichokes	430	Coconut meat, fresh	256
Millet	430	Cantaloupe, casaba, honeydew melons	251
Chicory greens	420	

SOURCES OF POTASSIUM (*cont.*)

Milligrams per 100 grams edible portion (100 grams = 3½ oz.)

Chicken, dark meat without skin, raw	250	Peas, podded	170
Okra	249	Blackberries	170
Tomato	244	Red raspberries	168
Sweet potato (compare with yams!)	243	Strawberries	164
Snap beans	243	Grapefruit juice, fresh	162
Papaya	234	Beef heart	160
Green cabbage	233	Cucumber	160
Onion, green	231	Grapes, slip skin	158
Wild rice	220	Pineapple	146
Eggplant	214	Lemon juice	141
Brown rice	214	Buttermilk	140
Sweet green peppers	213	Whole cow's milk	140
Peaches, fresh	202	Grapefruit pulp	135
Summer squash	202	Pear, fresh	130
Orange, peeled	200	Tangerine	126
Black raspberries	199	Apple	110
Figs, fresh	194	Chayote	102
Cherries	191	Apple juice	101
Mangoes	189	Eggs, whole	100
Orange juice, fresh	182	Watermelon	100
Goat's milk	180	Wine, unfortified	92
Lobster	180	Cranberries	82
Iceberg lettuce	175	Blueberries	81
Grapes, adherent skin	173	Cooked oatmeal	55
		Honey	10

Source: MineraLab, Inc.

TABLE 7.3 FOODS HIGH IN POTASSIUM (and low in sodium)

Food	Portion size	Potassium (milligrams)	Sodium (milligrams)
FRESH VEGETABLES			
Asparagus	½ cup	165	1
Avocado	½	680	5
Carrot, raw	1	225	38
Corn	½ cup	136	trace
Lima beans, cooked	½ cup	581	1
Potato	1 medium	782	6
Spinach, cooked	½ cup	292	45
Squash, winter	½ cup	473	1
Tomato, raw	1 medium	444	5
FRESH FRUITS			
Apple	1 medium	182	2
Apricots, dried	¼ cup	318	9
Banana	1 medium	440	1
Cantaloupe	¼ melon	341	17
Orange	1 medium	263	1
Peach	1 medium	308	2
Plums	5	150	1
Strawberries	½ cup	122	trace
UNPROCESSED MEATS			
Chicken, light meat	3 ounces	350	54
Lamb, leg	3 ounces	241	53
Roast beef	3 ounces	224	49
Pork	3 ounces	219	48
FISH			
Cod	3 ounces	345	93
Flounder	3 ounces	498	201
Haddock	3 ounces	297	150
Salmon	3 ounces	378	99
Tuna, drained solids	3 ounces	225	38

Sources: USDA Handbooks Nos. 456 and 8–1.

TABLE 7.4 SODIUM AND POTASSIUM (mg/100g) IN SOME UNPROCESSED AND PROCESSED FOODS

Unprocessed			Processed		
Food	Sodium	Potassium	Food	Sodium	Potassium
Flour, wholemeal	3	360	White bread	540	100
Rice, polished	6	110	Rice, boiled	2	38
Pork, uncooked	65	270	Bacon, uncooked	1400	250
Beef, uncooked	55	280	Beef, corned	950	140
Haddock, uncooked	120	300	Haddock, smoked	790	190
Cabbage, uncooked	7	390	Cabbage, boiled	4	160
Peas, uncooked	1	340	Peas, canned	230	130
Pears, uncooked	2	130	Pears, canned	1	90

Source: McCance and Widdowson's *The Composition of Foods*, H.M. Stationery Office, 1978.

TABLE 7.5 EFFECT OF PROCESSING AND COOKING ON FOODS

Sodium, milligrams per 100 grams

Food	Raw	Cooked
Bacon	680	1021
Bacon, Canadian	1891	2555
Barbecue sauce		815
Beef (all cuts)	65*	60*
Bread, white		507
Bread, wheat		529
Pickles		673-1428
Pudding mixes		99-447
Ham	1100	930
Potatoes		
French fried		236*
Hash brown		288
Mashed		301
Scalloped with cheese		447

*varies widely

Sodium, milligrams per 100 grams

Vegetables	Raw	Cooked	Canned
Asparagus	2	1	236 (a)
Beans, white	19	7	463
Baby foods (b)			170-290
Beans, lima	2	1	236 (a)

EFFECT OF PROCESSING AND COOKING ON FOODS (*cont.*

Sodium, milligrams per 100 grams			
Vegetables	Raw	Cooked	Canned
Beans, yellow or wax	7	3	236 (a)
Carrots	47	33	236 (a)
Corn, sweet	Trace	Trace	236 (a)
Peas, green	2	1	236 (a)
Soups			380-800
Spinach	71	50	236 (a)
Tomatoes	3	4	130

(a) Estimated average based on added salt in the amount of 0.6 percent of finished product.
(b) Most baby foods.

Source: *Composition of Foods, Raw, Processed Prepared.* Agriculture Handbook No. 8. Agricultural Research Service, United States Department of Agriculture, 1963.

TABLE 7.6 THE DIFFERENCE PROCESSING CAN MAKE

Menu I	Portion size	Potassium (milligrams)	Sodium (milligrams)
Roast beef	3 ounces	224	49
Potato, baked	1 medium	782	3
String beans, fresh	½ cup	95	2.5
Whole wheat bread, firm crumb	1 slice	68	132
Unsalted butter	1 tablespoon	4	1.4
Peaches, fresh sliced	½ cup	172	1
Milk, whole	1 cup	370	122
		1,715	310.9
MENU II			
Corned beef	3 ounces	51	802
Potatoes, hash brown, frozen	1 cup	439	463
String beans, canned	½ cup	64	159.5
White bread, soft crumb	1 slice	29	142
Butter	1 tablespoon	3	140
Peach pie	¼ pie	176	316
Milk, whole	1 cup	370	122
		1,132	2,144.5

Sources: USDA Handbooks, Nos. 456 and 8–1.

TABLE 7.7 POTASSIUM CONTENT BY FOOD COMPOSITE OF 3900-KCAL DAILY DIET COLLECTED IN FDA SELECTED MINERALS IN FOOD SURVEY

Food composite	1976[a] Potassium		1977[b] Potassium		1978[c] Potassium	
	mg	mg/1000 kcal	mg	mg/1000 kcal	mg	mg/1000 kcal
Dairy products	1311	336	1236	317	1254	332
Meat, fish, poultry	716	184	698	179	694	178
Grain and cereal products	519	132	535	137	565	145
Potatoes	910	233	836	214	874	224
Leafy vegetables	108	28	106	27	109	28
Legume vegetables	154	40	151	39	161	41
Root vegetables	59	15	57	15	60	15
Miscellaneous vegetables and vegetable products	127	33	150	39	165	42
Fruits	350	90	333	85	364	93
Oils, fats, and shortening	73	19	80	21	82	21
Sugar and adjuncts	64	16	63	16	59	15
Beverages including water	290	74	304	78	348	89
Total intake	4681	1200	4549	1167	4735	1213

[a]Mean value of 20–25 market basket collections.
[b]Mean value of 25 market basket collections.
[c]Mean value of 8 market basket collections.

REFERENCES

1 National Research Council. 1980. *Recommended Dietary Allowances*. (9th ed.) Washington, D.C.: National Academy of Sciences, p. 173.

2 Harvey, *et al*. 1976. *Principles and Practice of Medicine*. East Norwalk, CT.: Appleton Century Crofts, p. 96.

3 Anon. November 24, 1980. *Med. World News* 2

4 American Heart Association Conference (Spring 1978) Reported by Staines, L. 1978. *Prevention* 111.

5 *Lancet*. January 10, 1981 and January 17, 1981. (*Also see* October 22, 1982. *Science* 218:316–362).

6 Black, D. *et al*. 1952. *Lancet* 244.

7 McMahon, F.G. *et al*. July 5, 1982. *Med. World News* 21–23.

8

SODIUM AND CHLORIDE

Table salt is sodium chloride. Chloride (the chlorine ion) is essential as an electrolyte, but no known deficiencies have been reported with the exception of infants consuming only a commercial canned formula that was deficient in chloride. Chloride is readily obtained in nearly all foods, and is a component of table salt (sodium chloride).

There are many imbalances of chloride related to various medicines such as diuretics (water pills) and as a consequence of body fluid losses and replacement following injuries, burns or surgery. These iatrogenic conditions are beyond the scope of this book.

Chloride is not determined at this time by hair analysis, so no further discussion of this essential electrolyte is offered here.

The terms "sodium" and "salt" are often used interchangeably by nutritionists. They are not truly interchangeable in scientific terms, but the only practical problem caused by this practice is to cause confusion about the quantity. Only about 40 percent of the sodium chloride molecule is sodium. Therefore an ounce of salt contains 0.4 ounce of sodium. Most of our dietary sodium is from salt, but an appreciable amount is due to sodium nitrate, often used as a preservative in red meats, and monosodium glutonate (MSG), a flavor enhancer. Modern diets contain so much sodium that it is difficult to believe that dietary sodium was once scarce. Salt was once used as payment for goods or services. In fact, the word "salary" is thought to be derived from this practice.

The great esteem for salt may not have been principally for its value as a human nutrient. Its value was for its flavor enhancement, preservation of food and "licks" for cattle.

Still we should not lose sight of the fact that sodium is an essential mineral that our bodies regulate and conserve. The adult body averages a total content of over 100 grams of sodium, of which a surprising one-third is in bone. A small amount of sodium does get into cell interiors, but this represents only about 10 percent of the body content. The remaining 57 percent or so of the body sodium content is in the fluid immediately surrounding the cells, where it is the major cation (positive ion). The role of sodium in the extracellular fluid is maintaining osmotic equilibrium (the proper difference in ions dissolved in the fluids inside and outside the cell) and extracellular fluid volume. Sodium is also involved in nerve impulse transmission, muscle tone and nutrient transport. All of these functions are interrelated with potassium.

Virtually all sodium ingested in the diet is absorbed. Natural foods tend to be low in sodium and high in potassium, but processed foods are the opposite. Salt is normally added to enhance flavor by the food processing company, and potassium is often leached out by water during processing. Typical diets supply between 2300 and 6900 mg sodium daily.[1] Among some populations, adult humans are known to live normally for long periods with salt intakes exceeding 40 grams (40,000 mg).[1]

The body maintains the sodium concentration in the extracellular fluid by adjusting the water content. Excess sodium retention increases the fluid volume (edema) and low sodium leads to less fluid and relative dehydration.

When sodium intake is high, the level of adrenal cortex hormone, aldosterone, decreases in the blood, and the kidney is thus influenced to excrete more sodium in the urine. When the dietary intake of sodium is nil, the aldosterone level increases, and urinary excretion of sodium decreases to essentially zero. Kidney patients have trouble maintaining proper sodium levels. Blood levels of sodium reflect neither total body content nor clinical status.

Sweat removes sodium from the body. Working hard in hot weather can cause some adults to lose as much as 8000 mg sodium in a day. Whenever more than 2 or 3 quarts of sweat are lost, sodium should be replaced or nausea, vomiting, dizziness, cramps, exhaustion, apathy and circulatory failure could occur.

Please note, however, even then *we do not recommend salt tablets*. The most important factor is the replacement of the water. Salt tablets or high-salt solutions cause the water to remain in the stomach unduly long.

Weekend athletes should replace the salt during their next meal. Laborers and athletes can supplement their diet with a 0.1 percent solution for drinking water, if necessary.

Sodium and blood pressure

High blood pressure is a sign of several diseases. It is not one disease with one cause or one cure. Some people develop high blood pressure as a symptom that their potassium-sodium ratio is out of balance.

There is an inherited trait that makes the blood pressure in a portion of the population sensitive to dietary sodium. These persons often have increased blood pressure when sugar and salt are both high in their diets.

One study has found that a portion of patients having high blood pressure respond to salt in a unique manner. These individuals have higher sodium excretion, lower renin (a kidney enzyme that raises blood pressure by restriction of the blood vessels) activity and rated salt solutions significantly better tasting than persons having normal blood pressure.[2] The researchers suggest that the combination of high salt intake, lower renin activity and increased pleasantness of salt taste constitute a form of high blood pressure in which the biological mechanisms that regulate the sodium balance of the body are reset at a higher level.

Dr. Robert Kark, Chairman of the Department of Medicine at Rush Presbyterian-St. Luke Medical Center in Chicago, points out that the relationship between sodium and high blood pressure is not as clear cut as "common knowledge" tries to make it. Dr. Kark explains that although there is strong evidence between sodium intake and high blood pressure in *part* of the population, it is not a direct cause-effect relationship.

Keep in mind that another segment of the population experiences the opposite effect of sodium on blood pressure. A study by Dr. John Laragh, a cardiologist at Cornell University, of over one hundred patients with high blood pressure produced some interesting results.

Dr. Laragh found that severe salt restriction did work in about one-third of the patients. In about half of the cases, the low-salt diet had no effect at all on blood pressure. But in about 20 percent of the high blood pressure patients, the low-salt diet made their blood pressure go even higher.[3,4,5]

You can see the danger in prescribing a low-salt diet for everyone. High blood pressure patients should work closely with their doctor during any change in medication or diet to monitor the effect of that change on the *individual's* blood pressure.

Dr. Lawrence Krakoff, chief of the hypertension division of Mount Sinai Hospital in New York notes, "It is not common knowledge among doctors that restricting salt intake can actually make the blood pressure rise. If anything, the prevailing view among many physicians is that salt causes high blood pressure. That's not true at all."[3]

Dr. Aram Chobanian, director of the Cardiovascular Institute at the Boston University School of Medicine, explains the low salt high blood pressure effect as follows. "Cutting out salt can increase the amount of renin in the blood. And if your high blood pressure already is affected by the renin levels, then an increased renin level might make the blood pressure worse."[3]

Your renin level can be measured with a simple blood test. It is our view that the dietary potassium-sodium ratio is a factor in elevated blood pressure only in cases where renin is not. Our advice to high blood pressure patients is not to blindly follow a low-salt diet, but to find the cause of the problem. If it is dietary-related, then try a diet better balanced in the potassium–sodium ratio under the guidance of your physician for a month. If this helps, then full speed ahead. A high fat intake may also add to blood pressure elevations in some individuals.

We refer you to the section on high blood pressure in the chapter on potassium, for the evidence that the potassium-sodium ratio may be a key factor.[6]

Dietary sodium

We need not call attention to good food sources of sodium. Instead, we wish to point out unnecessary and hidden sodium in your diet.

Great excesses of sodium may leach calcium from your bones (see the chapter on calcium) and contribute to high blood pressure in genetically susceptible persons.

However, we do not recommend that the general public avoid nutritious foods solely on the basis of the amount of salt in those foods. Consider the overall nutritional contribution of the food.

One study reports that foods contributing most to the "possible average daily intake" of 7.1 g (7100 mg) salt *added to processed foods* were meat products (1.9 g), baked goods (1.8 g) and cheese (0.1 g), while snack foods contributed less than 0.05 g daily.[7]

FDA "market basket" surveys attempt to monitor typical food intakes. The average sodium content of Adult Market Baskets for 1977 and 1978 was 6700 and 6900 mg per day, respectively. Approximately 85 percent of the sodium comes from only four of the eleven commodity groups (excluding water): the grains and cereal products group and the sugar and adjuncts group each contributed nearly 30 percent. The other two major commodity group contributors are the dairy products group and the meat, fish and poultry group.

The market basket survey also found that the dietary sodium content based on a percentage of calories increased from infant to toddler to adult, while the potassium content declined.

Individual foods that are high in sodium include bread, crackers, celery, pasteurized cheeses, olives, bacon, peanut butter, pickles, pudding mixes, french fried potatoes and potato chips. It is encouraging that supermarkets as well as health food stores offer an increasing variety of these foods in salt-free or reduced-salt form.

Other unsuspected sources of sodium are softened water, red wines, some food additives and some medicines. What surprises many people, however, is the amount of sodium in processed foods compared to the amount in the same food before processing (see Table 8.3).

The Dietary Goal established by the U.S. Senate called for 5 g salt (2 g sodium) per day. Dr. Gaurth Hansen of Utah State University terms this inappropriate as it is almost impossible to plan an acceptable diet using that level as a guide.[8]

Toxicity

The average per capita intake of salt in the United States is clearly above the minimal nutritional need, but is within the range of physiologic accommodation by the *healthy* individual.

The SCOGS (Select Committee on GRAS Substance) report acknowledges that grossly excessive levels of salt can be acutely toxic and even fatal. There have been several instances reported in which fatal amounts of salt were inadvertently added to infant formulas when mistaken for sugar.[7]

Supplements

There is no need for supplementing the average diet. Heavy laborers and athletes may find a rare need to drink a 0.1 percent solution of salt water after extremely heavy work during unusually hot days. However, they normally need other minerals replaced before salt needs extraordinary replenishment.

Hair analysis

We do not believe the scientific or clinical evidence supports a meaningful interpretation of sodium content in hair at this time. Only limited published scientific studies have been performed on the clinical significance of hair sodium and potassium, and for that reason these elements are considered to be of only questionable clinical significance at this time. Hair levels of sodium and potassium are considered to be possibly significant in the presence of cystic fibrosis, celiac disease and hyperparathyroidism. Other than in those disease states, there is no scientific evidence of even possible clinical significance for sodium and potassium concentrations in hair.

This is an area where future research or procedural refinements might prove to be fruitful.

TABLE 8.1 SOURCES OF SODIUM

Milligrams (mg) per 100 grams edible portion (100 grams = 3½ oz.)

Kelp	3007	Turnip	49
Green olives	2400	Carrot	47
Dill pickles	1428	Yogurt	47
Ripe olives	828	Parsley	45
Sauerkraut	747	Artichoke	43
Cheddar cheese	700	Dried figs	34
Scallops	265	Lentils, dried	30
Cottage cheese	229	Sunflower seeds	30
Lobster	210	Raisins	27
Swiss chard	147	Red cabbage	26
Beet greens	130	Garlic	19
Buttermilk	130	White beans	19
Celery	126	Broccoli	15
Eggs	122	Mushrooms	15
Cod	110	Cauliflower	13
Spinach	71	Onion	10
Lamb	70	Sweet potato	10
Pork	65	Brown rice	9
Chicken	64	Lettuce	9
Beef	60	Cucumber	6
Beets	60	Peanuts	5
Sesame seeds	60	Avocado	4
Watercress	52	Tomato	3
Whole cow's milk	50	Eggplant	2
Salt, 1 tsp.	2132	Soy sauce, 1 tbl.	1319

The following foods contain large amounts of sodium chloride added during processing:

Canned or frozen vegetables	Luncheon meats
Cured, smoked, or canned meats	Salted nuts
Packaged spice mixes	Salted crackers
Bouillon cubes	Canned or packaged soups
Canned fish	Processed cheeses
Commercial peanut butter	Commercial salad dressings
Catsup, barbecue sauce	Meat tenderizers
Potato chips, corn chips, pretzels, etc.	

Source: MineraLab, Inc.
Selected values are given in the following tables (Table 8.2 and 8.3)

TABLE 8.2 SODIUM CONTENT OF SELECTED PROCESSED FOODS

Food	Amount	Sodium (mg)
Asparagus, canned	4 spears	141
Baby food, cereal	6 Tbs.	122-183
Beef with vegetables	3½ oz.	304
Mixed vegetables	3½ oz.	272
Bacon	2 slices	153
Beans, lima, canned	1 cup	401
Beans, green, canned	1 cup	562
Beef and vegetable stew, canned	1 cup	964
Beef, corned	3 oz.	1491
Bran flakes	1 cup	323
Bread	1 slice	130-180
Butter, salted	1 Tbs.	138
Cookies	1 average	30-40
Carrots, canned	1 cup	588
Cheese, creamed cottage	1 cup	560
Swiss	1 oz.	201
American	1 oz.	322
Chicken pot pie	1 pie (8 oz.)	932
Corn flakes	1 cup	251
Crackers, saltines	4	121
Cream substitute, dried	1 Tbs.	33
Frankfurter	1	499
Gelatin dessert	½ cup	61
Margarine, salted	1 Tbs.	138
Muffin	1 medium	176-200
Mushrooms, canned	1 cup	974
Peanut butter	1 Tbs.	97
Pie, apple	1 segment	473
Pizza	1 slice	525
Pork, cured	3 oz.	797
Potatoes, french fried, frozen	10 pieces	134
Potato chips	3 oz.	840
Salad dressing, Italian;	1 Tbs.	293
mayonnaise	1 Tbs.	84
Soup, chicken vegetable	1 cup	1030
Onion, from dry mix	1 cup	710
Tomato, canned	1 cup	313
Juice	1 cup	486
Ketchup	1 Tbs.	156
Tuna, canned	6½ oz.	1474

Source: U.S. Dept. Agriculture Handbook No. 456

TABLE 8.3 POSSIBLE AVERAGE DAILY INTAKE BASED ON LEVEL OF ADDITION OF SODIUM CHLORIDE TO FOOD BY FOOD CATEGORY

Food category	Level of addition (weighted mean) percent	Possible average daily intake 2-65 yr. g
Baked goods, baking mixes	1.31	1.8
Breakfast cereals	1.09	0.2
Grain products such as pastas or rice dishes	0.74	0.2
Fats and oils	1.43	0.2
Milk products	0.45	0.2
Cheese	1.00	0.1
Frozen dairy desserts, mixes	0.04	†
Processed fruits, juices and drinks	0.19	0.6
Meat products	2.49	1.9
Poultry products	0.33	0.1
Egg products	0.64	†
Fish products	0.96	0.1
Processed vegetables, juices	0.68	0.6
Condiments, relishes, salt substitutes	3.18	0.3
Soft candy	0.42	†
Sugar, confections	0.51	†
Sweet sauces, toppings, syrups	0.47	†
Gelatins, puddings, fillings	0.41	0.1
Soups, soup mixes	1.02	0.3
Snack foods	2.08	†
Beverages, nonalcoholic	0.04	†
Beverages, alcoholic	0.02	†
Nuts, nut products	1.12	0.1
Reconstituted vegetable proteins	7.27	†
Gravies, sauces	1.17	0.1
Dairy products analogs	0.64	†
Hard candy	0.41	†
Seasonings and flavors	50.53	†
		7.1

Calculated possible average daily intake of added sodium chloride for the age group, 2–65 + yr.
†Less than 0.05 g.
Source: *Sodium in Medicine and Health*, Edited by Campbell Moses, M.D. (Reese Press, Inc., Baltimore).

TABLE 8.4 FOODS HIGH IN SODIUM (and low in potassium)

Food	Portion size	Potassium (milligrams)	Sodium (milligrams)
Salt	1 teaspoon	trace	2,132
Soy sauce	1 teaspoon	22	1,123
Bouillon cube	1	4	960
HARD CHEESES			
Parmesan	2 ounces	53	1,056
American	2 ounces	93	812
Brie	2 ounces	87	356
Muenster	2 ounces	77	356
Cheddar	2 ounces	56	352
Colby	2 ounces	72	342
Swiss	2 ounces	64	148
Cottage cheese (2 percent fat)	½ cup	110	561
SNACK FOODS			
Pretzels, thin, twisted	10	10	1,008
Saltines	10	34	312
Potato chips	10	226	200
Peanuts, roasted, salted	¼ cup	243	151
PROCESSED MEATS			
Salami	3 ounces	170	1,043
Bologna	3 ounces	133	981
Frankfurter	3 ounces	136	1,003
CANNED SOUPS			
Chicken noodle	1 cup	53	1,049
Cream of mushroom (prepared with water)	1 cup	94	967
Tomato	1 cup	247	816
Vegetable beef	1 cup	162	896
CANNED VEGETABLES			
Beets	½ cup	142	200
Corn	½ cup	80	195
Lima beans	½ cup	188	200
Peas	½ cup	82	200

Sources: USDA Handbooks Nos. 456 and 8–1.

TABLE 8.5 SODIUM CONTENT BY FOOD COMPOSITE OF 3900-KCAL DAILY DIET COLLECTED IN FDA SELECTED MINERALS IN FOOD SURVEY

Food composite	1976[a] Sodium mg	mg/1000 kcal	1977[b] Sodium mg	mg/1000 kcal	1978[c] Sodium mg	mg/1000 kcal
NON-DISCRETIONARY						
Dairy products	717	184	704	180	792	203
Meat, fish, poultry	1000	256	952	244	921	236
Grain and cereal products	2036	522	2005	514	2002	513
Potatoes	65	17	75	19	82	21
Leafy vegetables	18	5	22	6	22	6
Legume vegetables	224	57	243	62	258	62
Root vegetables	16	4	18	5	17	4
Garden fruits	264	68	285	73	284	73
Fruits	74	19	66	17	75	19
Oils and fats	380	97	387	99	406	104
Beverages	9	2	17	4	24	7
Total non-discretionary	4803	1232	4774	1224	4886	1252
DISCRETIONARY						
Sugar, salt, and adjuncts[d]	1970	505	1923	493	2042	524
Total intake	6773	1737	6697	1717	6928	1776

[a]Mean value of 20–25 market basket collections.
[b]Mean value of 25 market basket collections.
[c]Mean value of 8 market basket collections.
[d]Includes the salt normally used in home food preparation and for seasoning at the table.

FIGURE 8.1 FACTORS INVOLVED IN HIGH BLOOD PRESSURE.

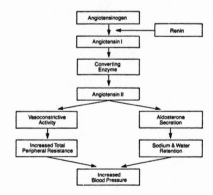

THE ELECTROLYTE MINERALS

REFERENCES

1 National Research Council. 1980. *Recommended Dietary Allowances.* (9th ed.) Washington, D.C.: National Academy of Sciences.

2 Bernard, R. A. *et al.* 1980. In: *Biological and Behavioral Aspects of Salt Intake*, Kare, M. *et al.*, eds. New York: Academic Press.

3 Kolate, G. April 1982. *Science.*

4 Laragh, J. August 1980. *Clin, Pharmacol. Therapeut.* (*Also see* April 12, 1982. *Science* 216 [4541]:38–9).

5 Anon. September 1, 1980. *Med. World News.*

6 Anon. 1980. *Mineral and Electrolyte Metabolism* 4(4).

7 Select Committee on GRAS Substances. 1979. *Evaluation of the Health Aspects of Sodium Chloride as Food Ingredients.* Bethesda, Maryland: Life Sciences Research Office, Fed. Amer. Soc. Exper. Biology.

8 *Food Product Development.* January 1979. 24.

Trace elements

IRON

ZINC

COPPER

MANGANESE

IODINE

9

IRON

Virtually all the atoms of oxygen used by the cells in the life process are brought to the cells by hemoglobin of red blood cells. Iron is a small, but most vital, component of the hemoglobin in 20,000 billion red blood cells, of which 115 million are formed every minute.

The essential functions of iron are oxygen transport and oxygen utilization. Hemoglobin helps accomplish the former and iron-containing enzymes help accomplish the latter function.

These vital functions depend on iron, yet the average adult body contains a mere 3.5 to 4.5 g (3500–4500 mg) of iron. That amount of iron is only one-tenth of a teaspoon.

The iron in the body is sometimes classified as one of two types—active component and stored component. The active component comprises about 75 percent of the iron, and includes hemoglobin (65–70 percent), myoglobin (3–5 percent), iron-containing enzymes, iron-containing cofactors and iron being transported by transferrin. Catalases, peroxidases and cytochromes are iron-containing enzymes. Myoglobin stores oxygen in muscles for use in contraction. The remaining 25 percent is stored in the form of ferritin and hemosiderin in the liver, spleen and bone marrow.

Once iron is absorbed into the body, it is carefully conserved by recycling. The major iron loss—though very small—is not not by excretion, but by cell loss from body surfaces or by bleeding. Of course during pregnancy some of the body storage of iron is transferred to the developing child.

If you stop to think about this for a moment, you can see the possibility that some atoms of iron may have been in your family for generations.

Deficiency/toxicity

Dietary deficiencies of iron are quite common, but it should be stressed that overdoses of iron supplements can be toxic. This is why chewable mineral supplements have "alleged" child-proof lids. When small children mistake vitamin-mineral pills for candy, a problem of iron toxicity can result.

As is often the case, deficiency symptoms and toxicity symptoms are similar. Deficiency signs can include fatigue, weakness, listlessness, lack of appetite, pallor, headache, long recovery period required after exertion, palpitation on exertion, infections, sore tongue, mouth inflammation, difficulty in swallowing, thin mis-formed fingernails (concave with length-wise ridges), cold extremities and craving for ice or dirt. Toxicity signs can include fatigue, loss of weight, headache, shortness of breath and dizziness.

Both iron deficiency and iron toxicity will be discussed in greater detail. But first, let's examine how iron is absorbed, transported and stored in the body, so that you can better understand why iron deficiency is so common, yet why some individuals have to worry about toxicity.

Absorption, transport, storage and excretion

Iron, in contrast with most other minerals, is regulated in the body primarily by absorption rather than by excretion. A number of studies have confirmed the critical importance of the gastrointestinal tract in controlling the total body iron.[1,2,3] Urine contains very small amount of iron, and the only iron found in feces is that iron unabsorbed from the diet.

Absorption is strongly influenced by the amounts of stored iron and the formation of red blood cells in the body. Factors such as the form of ingested iron, the nature of accompanying food, the composition of intestinal secretion, the products of digestion and the degree of alkalinity of the intestine can all affect the absorption of iron.

Normally 6 to 10 percent of the iron in food is absorbed, but iron-deficient individuals can absorb more than 15 percent. Persons with iron deficiency anemia may absorb 50 to 60 percent of the same amount of iron.

A blood donation of one pint means a loss of about 235 mg iron. A few days after a blood donation, the individual absorbs measurably more iron, but on an ordinary diet, it will take *many months* to fully replenish iron stores.[4]

The detailed mechanism of iron absorption is still somewhat controversial. It is generally agreed that iron is bound by receptors in the brush border of mucosal cells in the upper small intestine; transferred across the membrane by an unknown, but presumably energy-dependent process; transported to the basal surface of the epithelium by a carrier; and finally delivered to the iron-transporting protein, transferrin, in the plasma. The iron status of the individual, his red blood cell production rate, and other factors regulate the amount of iron transported across the intestinal mucosa. Transferrin transports iron to the bone marrow, liver or other tissues where it can be utilized for the synthesis of hemoglobin, cytochromes, ferritin, and other iron-containing compounds. Ferritin is an iron-storage molecule with a large iron-binding capacity. It exists as a ferric (iron) oxide complex and a protein shell (apoferritin). When saturated, each molecule can contain up to 4500 iron atoms, although it usually contains less than 3000. Ferritin provides a mobile reserve of iron to meet the varying needs of the body. Large amounts are found in the liver, spleen and blood-forming organs, and lesser amounts in other tissues which have no apparent iron-storage function. Blood ferritin has been used as an index of total body iron because it mirrors closely the quantity of iron stored in the tissues.

Another substance which functions as an iron-storage compound is hemosiderin. Its structure is ill-defined, being a relatively amorphous compound, containing up to 35 percent iron. Hemosiderin exists in the tissues as a brown, granular, readily stainable pigment; its iron is mainly ferric hydroxide. It has been suggested, on the basis of similar physical characteristics, that hemosiderin is formed from the denaturation and proteolytic cleavage of ferritin. Up to certain levels, both ferritin and hemosiderin are deposited in liver and spleen in roughly equal amounts.

Iron absorption is enhanced by ascorbic acid (vitamin C).[5] Ascorbic acid acts by "reducing" iron from a higher oxidation state (ferric form where iron has a valence of 3 positive electrical charges) to a lower oxidation state (ferrous form where iron has a valence of 2). (Valence concerns the number of electrons attached to an atom.) The lower form (ferrous) is much better absorbed. Ascorbic acid also acts to increase iron absorption by forming a "chelate" with iron. Twenty-five milligrams of ascorbic acid can increase iron absorption from a meal by 50 percent, while a gram (1000 mg) can increase iron absorption by 1000 percent when an individual is depleted.[6]

Iron is absorbed even better when both ascorbic acid and vitamin E are present.[7] Calcium aids iron absorption because calcium combines with phytic acid, oxalic acid and phosphate, thus keeping them from forming insoluble complexes with iron.[8] However, excessive calcium decreases iron absorption.

The type of iron in the diet can be classified as being either "heme" or "non-heme." The "heme" form is iron contained in a chelated structure that is a building block of hemoglobin. Thus, "heme" iron is readily absorbed.

A recent trend in estimating the availability of dietary iron for absorption is to consider the amounts of heme and non-heme iron separately. The amounts of heme and non-heme iron in any particular meal must be considered separately because of their different availability and susceptibility to influences from other dietary ingredients. Although the proportion of heme iron in animal foods varies, it amounts to an average of 40 percent of the total iron in all animal tissues, including meat, liver, poultry and fish. The remaining 60 percent of iron in animal tissues and all the iron of vegetable products are treated as non-heme iron. The absorption of this category is enhanced by two well-defined factors: ascorbic acid and the quantity of animal tissues present in each meal. On the basis of the concentration of these enhancing factors, meals can be classified as of low, medium or high availability of their non-heme iron. Non-heme iron from plant sources ranges in absorption rate from about 1 percent in spinach and rice, to up to 6 percent in lettuce, wheat and soybeans. If vegetables are eaten with some meat, the heme iron raises the absorption rate of the non-heme iron. Table 9.3 shows the iron absorption from various plant and animal foods.

Iron absorption is reduced by phosphates which can form insoluble complexes with iron.[9] Many soft drinks and some food additives contain phosphates which may tie up dietary iron. In fact, iron may complex with many compounds in food, thus reducing its absorptivity.[10] The absorption of iron is significantly less when given after a meal than when fasting. One study showed only 56 percent of that iron absorbed by a fasting individual was absorbed after a light meal.[11]

The oxalic acid in spinach reduces the availability of the iron. Copper deficiency,[12] tea[13] and antacids[14] reduce iron absorption.

"Iron-enriched" frozen bakery goods often are enriched with "elemental" iron (sometimes called reduced iron). This form of iron has been found to be insoluble and relatively unavailable after heating according to Dr. Kenneth Lee of the University of Wisconsin at Madison.[15]

Dr. James Cook of the University of Kansas has found that soy protein reduces iron absorption dramatically. Adding soy protein to meals has reduced the iron absorbed by as much as 92 percent.[16,17] At this writing, the FDA is seeking to replicate this research.

Researchers at Kansas Medical Center found a 51–74 percent decrease in iron absorption in the presence of 12 g bran added to a light meal. When 100 g of beef or 100 mg vitamin C was added to the same type meal, iron absorption was improved.[18]

Iron deficiency

Iron deficiency can cause severe symptoms before iron deficiency anemia results. Such iron deficiency is quite common, but the answer is not merely to take iron supplements. First, the cause of the iron deficiency should be determined. The cause could be a simple dietary deficiency, but it could also be the result of bleeding due to cancer, peptic ulcer, hemorrhoids, hiatal hernia, other gastrointestinal bleeding, heavy menstrual periods due to fibroids or other medical conditions that should be corrected.

Treat the cause—not the symptom. More iron could cure the iron deficiency, but it would only mask the more serious underlying problem.

Government surveys show that Americans are in a dietary decline in terms of meeting the RDA for iron. The U.S. Health and Nutrition Examination Survey (HANES) of 1968–70 indicates that approximately 95 percent of the children one to five years old and *females eighteen to forty-four years old* had iron intakes below the RDA.

In the 1955 and 1965 surveys, 90 percent of the population was obtaining the RDA for iron. By 1970, only 64 percent were able to obtain the recommended amount. Ten percent of the population was getting less than two-thirds of the RDA. Such low iron intakes deplete the body stores of iron and lead to impaired function of the iron-containing enzymes.

There are four situations in which iron intake is frequently inadequate in the United States: 1) in infancy because of the low iron content of milk and because the endowment of iron at birth is usually not sufficient to meet needs beyond six months; 2) during the periods of rapid growth in childhood and adolescence, because of the needs to fill expanding iron stores; 3) during the female reproductive years, because of menstrual iron losses; and 4) in pregnancy, because of the expanding blood volume of the mother, the demands of the fetus and placenta, and blood losses in childbirth. In order to provide for the necessary retention of 1 mg/day in adult males and postmenopausal females, and assuming an average availability of 10 percent of the food iron, an allowance of 10 mg/day is recommended. The allowance for women of childbearing age is set at 18 mg/day in order to meet the additional needs imposed by menstrual iron losses. The increased requirement during pregnancy cannot be met by the iron content of habitual diets in the United States, nor by the existing iron stores of many women; therefore, daily supplements of iron are recommended. These usually range from 30 to 60 mg/day; the amount should be determined by the physician administering prenatal care. Iron needs during lactation are not substantially different from those of nonpregnant women, yet continued supplementation of the mother for two to three months after childbirth is advisable in order to replenish stores depleted by pregnancy.

To provide a more precise definition of iron deficiency, investigators have attempted to relate it to the concentration of specific iron substances in the blood and tissue. Iron-deficiency anemia is a condition with small, pale red blood cells, depleted iron stores, plasma iron value below 40 micrograms per deciliter, elevated iron-binding capacity, and less than 15 percent saturation of transferrin, the iron-transporting protein. Infants and preschool children appear to be especially vulnerable to iron deficiency if transferrin saturation is used as the criterion. Almost half of one-year-old children from all income groups had a blood transferrin saturation less than 15 percent. About 10 percent of all children aged one to five years, and 14 percent of this age group in low income families, had "low" transferrin saturations.

The development of a sensitive assay for the iron-storage molecule, ferritin, has provided an additional promising technique to evaluate the iron stores in the body. The serum ferritin in patients with uncomplicated iron deficiency was less than 12 milligrams per liter, in contrast with 12 to 250 micrograms per liter in normal subjects, and as much as 10,000 micrograms per liter in patients with iron overload. In addition, red-cell protoporphyrin, the non-iron portion of heme, has been employed as a screening test for iron deficiency. Nevertheless, as pointed out in a recent review, no single test is without its pitfalls and even a battery of tests is not infallible in detecting iron deficiency.[19]

Keep in mind that there are several other kinds of anemias. Although iron deficiency anemia is the most common, there are folic acid-, vitamin B12-, and copper-deficiency anemias, plus lead poisoning anemia (a mild hypochromic microcytic anemia). Still other anemias can be caused by thyroid problems and a lack of some enzymes.

Iron toxicity

The toxicity of food iron is low, and harmful effects of daily intakes of 25 to 75 mg are unlikely in healthy persons.[20] However, there are a few individuals with genetic problems that make iron more toxic to them. There are also many cases of suspected iron overdosing each year due to children mistaking chewable vitamin and mineral tablets for candy or eating the iron supplements of their parents. Few cases result in actual symptoms of toxicity or require hospitalization, but unfortunately about twelve children die of iron poisoning each year.[21] Child-proof lids on supplements containing iron may help prevent such accidents.

The lethal dose of ferrous sulfate (a common iron supplement) for a two-year-old is near 3 g (3000 mg) (only about ten to twelve tablets). The lethal dose for adults ranges between 200 and 250 mg per each kilogram (2.2

pounds) of body weight. That's 12 to 15 g (12,000 to 15,000 mg) for a 132-pound person.

Other forms of iron are even less toxic as can be seen in Table 9.4

Subchronic and chronic toxicities of iron are characterized by disorders associated with excessive iron loading or storage in the body. The storage iron is predominantly in the form of insoluble hemosiderin, and an increase of iron storage is called hemosiderosis or simply siderosis. Under certain conditions, organs may contain grossly excessive amounts of storage iron and show evidence of damage. Such a condition is termed hemochromatosis. Semantic confusion results from the indiscriminate use of hemochromatosis and hemosiderosis as synonyms for iron loading.

The term *hemosiderosis* should be applied to conditions of increased iron stores confined mainly to the cells of the reticuloendothelial system and without obvious malfunction or disease which can be attributed to the presence of the iron. The term *hemochromatosis* should be applied when the organs containing excessive amounts of storage iron show evidence of damage, usually fibrosis. It is distinguished from hemosiderosis by well characterized clinical signs and symptoms, even though the total amount of iron in the body may be comparable in the two conditions.

Generalized hemosiderosis may result from chronic ingestion of large amounts of bioavailable iron, from repeated transfusions, and in certain microcytic hypochromic anemias, such as thalassemia.[22] Substantial iron overload resulting from dietary intake is rare.

Hemochromatosis is generally regarded as a disease entity characterized by extensive iron deposits in the liver, skin, heart, pancreas and spleen. Its etiology remains controversial. The typical patient with hemochromatosis will show portal cirrhosis, bronze pigmentation, diabetes mellitus, endocrinopathy, arthropathy and cardiac insufficiency. The normal control of iron absorption is faulty in these individuals, but the basic metabolic defect has not yet been identified. The dominant view regards hemochromatosis as a rare inborn error of metabolism, and considerable evidence supports this contention. One or more abnormalities in iron metabolism have been repeatedly recognized in 25 to 75 percent of first-degree relatives of patients with this condition. Siblings are often affected, and in a few cases overt disease has been detected in successive generations. Some have argued that hemochromatosis is always secondary to dietary, toxic, or other factors responsible for increased retention of iron.

The frequency of hemochromatosis has been estimated at 1 in 20,000 hospital admissions and at 1 in 7000 hospital deaths.

Ascorbic acid should be given only with extreme caution in patients with excess tissue iron.

Food sources

As previously discussed, iron absorption is dependent on many factors including the form of the iron in the food. Therefore, it is not merely how much iron is in a given food, but how much "heme" iron and "non-heme" iron, plus other absorption enhancing and inhibiting factors, are present. Such treatment of food values is beyond the scope of this book, but a good "average approximation" can be obtained by considering that an average of 10 percent of the total iron in the following table is absorbed.

TABLE 9.1 SOURCES OF IRON

Milligrams (mg) per 100 grams edible portion (100 grams = 3½ oz.)

Kelp	100.0	Artichoke	1.3
Brewer's yeast	17.3	Mung bean sprouts	1.3
Blackstrap molasses	16.1	Salmon	1.2
Wheat bran	14.9	Broccoli	1.1
Pumpkin and squash seeds	11.2	Currants	1.1
Wheat germ	9.4	Whole wheat bread	1.1
Beef liver	8.8	Cauliflower	1.1
Sunflower seeds	7.1	Cheddar cheese	1.0
Millet	6.8	Strawberry	1.0
Parsley	6.2	Asparagus	1.0
Clams	6.1	Blackberries	0.9
Almonds	4.7	Red cabbage	0.8
Dried prunes	3.9	Pumpkin	0.8
Cashews	3.8	Mushrooms	0.8
Lean beef	3.7	Banana	0.7
Raisins	3.5	Beets	0.7
Jerusalem artichoke	3.4	Carrots	0.7
Brazil nuts	3.4	Eggplant	0.7
Beet greens	3.3	Sweet potato	0.7
Swiss chard	3.2	Avocado	0.6
Dandelion greens	3.1	Figs	0.6
English walnut	3.1	Potato	0.6
Dates	3.0	Corn	0.6
Pork	2.9	Pineapple	0.5
Cooked dry beans	2.7	Nectarine	0.5
Sesame seeds, hulled	2.4	Watermelon	0.5
Pecans	2.4	Winter squash	0.5
Eggs	2.3	Brown rice, cooked	0.5
Lentils	2.1	Tomato	0.5

SOURCES OF IRON (*cont.*

Milligrams (mg) per 100 grams edible portion (100 grams = 3½ oz.)

Peanuts	2.1	Orange	0.4
Lamb	1.9	Cherries	0.4
Tofu	1.9	Summer squash	0.4
Green peas	1.8	Papaya	0.3
Brown rice	1.6	Celery	0.3
Ripe olives	1.6	Cottage cheese	0.3
Chicken	1.5	Apple	0.3

Source: SCOGS (Special commission on GRAS substances)-35, 1979. FDA 223-75-2004.

TABLE 9.2 CONTRIBUTION OF DIFFERENT FOODS IN THE U.S. DIET TO IRON INTAKE OF NORMAL ADULTS (20–34 yrs)

Food categories	Percentage of total iron intake	
	Males	Females
Meat, poultry, fish	46.3	43.1
Grain products	23.3	24.9
Eggs	6.7	5.2
Other vegetables, fruit	6.6	7.4
Legumes, nuts	4.5	4.1
Potatoes	3.7	3.4
Beverages other than milk and fruit juices	2.5	3.8
Sugars, sweets	2.1	2.2
Tomatoes, citrus fruit	1.5	2.1
Dark green, deep yellow vegetables	1.0	1.4
Milk, milk products	1.0	1.7
Fats, oils	0.7	0.6

Source: SCOGS—35, 1979

TABLE 9.3 IRON ABSORPTION FROM VARIOUS PLANT AND ANIMAL FOODS

	Food of Vegetable Origin							Food of Animal Origin						
	Rice	Spinach	Black Beans	Corn	Lettuce	Wheat	Soybean	Ferritin	Veal Liver	Fish Muscle	Hemo-Globin	Veal Muscle	Total	
Dose of Food Fe	2 mg	2 mg	3 to 4 mg	2 to 4 mg	1 to 17 mg	2 to 4 mg	3 to 4 mg	3 mg	3 mg	1 to 2 mg	3 to 4 mg	3 to 4 mg		Dose of Food Fe
No. Cases	11	9	137	73	13	42	36	17	11	34	39	96	520	No. Cases

Data were derived from a collaborative study of the Department of Botany and Medicine, University of Washington, Seattle, and Department of Pathophysiology, Instituto Venezuela de Investigaciones Cientificas at Caracas, Venezuela. Horizontal line represents the geometrical mean. Cross-hatched area shows limits of one standard error.

Source: Layrisse, M. and Martinez-Torres, c. 1971. *Prog. Hematol* 7, 137.

TABLE 9.4 ACUTE ORAL TOXICITY OF IRON COMPOUNDS

Compound	Species	LD_{50} (Lethal Dose) mg Fe/kg
"Reduced Iron"	Rat	98600
Ferrous carbonate	Guinea pig	2000
	Rabbit	2220
	Mouse	3800
Ferrous fumarate	Mouse	516-1100
	Rat	580-2500
Ferrous gluconate	Mouse	320-457
	Rat	865
	Guinea pig	350
	Rabbit	580
Ferrous sulfate	Mouse	150-305
	Rat	780
	Guinea pig	350
	Rabbit	600
Ferric ammonium citrate	Rabbit	560
	Guinea pig	350
	Mouse	1000

ACUTE ORAL TOXICITY OF IRON COMPOUNDS (*cont.*)

Compound	Species	LD$_{50}$ (Lethal Dose) mg Fe/kg
Ferric chloride	Mouse	440-500
	Guinea pig	200
	Rabbit	400
"Iron oxide"	Mouse	>15000
	Rat	>15000

Adapted from: SCOGS—35, 1979.

Food fortification

Iron is one of many nutrients stripped out during the processing of wheat to make refined "white" flour. A *few* of the nutrients (iron, vitamins, B1, B2, and B3) are *partially* replaced in so-called "enriched" flour.

The milling of wheat is said to have developed because of the need for a better process to remove impurities and foreign material from wheat. The milling process breaks open the wheat kernel and reduces the particles formed so as to separate the outer and inner portions of the kernel. Bran and germ are almost completely separated from the white interior portions of the kernel.

Soon it was discovered that the white interior, which is mostly starch, tastes better than the outside. People also developed a preference for the "purer" white flour for baked goods, so millers began to bleach it with chemicals.

The Council for Better Nutrition points out other motives for the refining of flour: "The wheat germ is removed primarily because it contains wheat germ oil which readily turns rancid. White flour has great resistance to spoilage. Neither insects nor microbes want it because its food value is gone."[23]

When they take the wheat germ and bran out of the flour, millers remove:

85% of the magnesium
60% of the calcium
76% of the iron
78% of the zinc
77% of the vitamin B1
80% of the vitamin B2
81% of the vitamin B3 (niacin)
50% of the pantothenic acid (a B-complex vitamin)
72% of the vitamin B6
86% of the vitamin E
27% of the protein.

In addition, milling robs you of goodly amounts of phosphorus, manganese, chromium, boron, sulfur, iodine, folic acid, choline, inositol and other vitamins and "minerals" and elements, known and unknown.

In all, about twenty-six vitamins and minerals *known* to be essential to human health are removed!

"Enrichment" consists in putting back about one-sixth of a cent's worth of synthetic vitamins B1, B2, and B3, plus a tiny bit of iron, often in the form of metallic iron filings, which are very poorly absorbed.

You might ask why the nutrients are removed in the first place. So called "enrichment" is like being mugged and having the thief leave you with change to make a telephone call for help.

In April 1970, the American Bakers Association and the Millers' National Federation proposed to the FDA that the amount of iron used for "enrichment" be increased. The FDA was also concerned with the deficiency of iron in the American diet noted by the White House Conference on Food, Nutrition and Health (1969) and the Ten-State Nutrition Survey (1968–70) conducted by the Department of Health, Education and Welfare. Both urged that corrective steps be taken. The Food and Nutrition Board of the National Academy of Sciences/National Research Council and the Council on Foods and Nutrition of the American Medical Association concurred in the view that iron deficiency is a problem in the general population.

The FDA agreed with the theory that changes in both dietary habits of consumers and methods of food processing (such as the use of other-than-iron cooking surfaces) has contributed to the diminishing amount of iron in the average diet. The Ten-State Nutrition survey noted a significant incidence of iron deficiency in certain population groups.

Grain products are selected as the most suitable vehicle to help increase the iron intake of American consumers, particularly women of childbearing age and children. Enriched flour constitutes two-thirds of all flour consumed in this country annually.

The FDA proposed the action for public comment on December 3, 1971 and there was opposition expressed to increasing the iron content of fortified foods. This opposition was based on the argument that the addition might increase the prevalence or severity of iron disorders, particularly the serious blood disorder, hemochromatosis.

At the FDA's request, the Federation of American Societies for Experimental Biology (FASEB) and the Council on Foods and Nutrition of the American Medical Association reviewed the safety question thoroughly. They concluded that the increased iron from enriched bread and flour would not jeopardize the health of normal individuals nor increase the incidence of hemochromatosis or other disorders.

After three years of study, on October 13, 1973, the FDA approved the increased level of iron fortification. The FDA Commissioner at that time, Dr.

Alexander Schmidt, said: "The amounts of iron to be added to flour and bread under this order are not great, and these amounts will not treat iron deficiency anemia. Neither will the added iron be harmful. We are concerned, however, that essential amounts of iron do appear somewhere in the diets that American citizens are now eating, and bread seems the most logical food to fortify."

The opposition to this FDA decision led to a hearing, held on April 1, 1974 before the ruling was to have gone into effect. More than a hundred physicians complained to the FDA that iron deficiency anemia was a minor and easily curable ailent in the hands of physicians, but the risk of the serious and incurable genetic disease, hemochromatosis, was unknown. One Cincinnati, Ohio physician argued, "The anemic woman should be going to the doctor, not the grocer."

A key point is that people should be eating foods from whole grains, not white flour.

The FDA action was overruled, and at this writing, the fortification levels are as listed in Table 9.5.

An interesting aside of this debate is that bread and cereals themselves impair the availability of iron.[24]

TABLE 9.5 AUTHORIZED IRON ENRICHMENT FOR FOOD PRODUCTS

Product	Iron enrichment levels mg/kg	Authorization
Bread, rolls, and buns	17.6–27.5*	21 CFR 136.115
Flour	28.6–36.3*	21 CFR 137.165
Self-rising flour	28.6–36.3*	21 CFR 137.185
Corn grits	28.6–57.2**	21 CFR 137.235
Corn meal	28.6–57.2**	21 CFR 137.260
Farina	not less than 28.6**	21 CFR 137.305
Rice	28.6–57.2**	21 CFR 137.350
Macaroni products	28.6–36.3**	21 CFR 139.115
Macaroni products with fortified protein	36.3**	21 CFR 139.117
Non-fat milk macaroni products	28.6–36.3**	21 CFR 139.122
Vegetable macaroni products	28.6–36.3**	21 CFR 139.135
Noodle products	28.6–36.3**	21 CFR 139.155
Vegetable noodle products	28.6–36.3**	21 CFR 139.165

* ". . . may be supplied by any safe and suitable substance."
** ". . . may be added only in forms which are harmless and assimilable."

Another consideration is the form of iron used in "enriching" flour and cereal. Dr. James Waddell, Executive Secretary Emeritus of the American Institute of Nutrition, commented:

Quite early, soluble iron compounds were recognized as having a deleterious effect on the storage stability of wheat flour and flour-containing mixes, especially under high environmental temperatures and high humidity. On the other hand, if the enrichment ingredients are added to the dough at the time of baking, ferrous sulfate presents no problems. When enrichment takes place at the flour mill, chemically inert reduced iron is frequently used. Manufacturers of pasta products object to the use of reduced iron because they believe it gives a greyish color to their white product; thus, they tend to rely on the insoluble phosphate salts both of which are light-colored. Similar considerations by manufacturers of other cereal products have led to use of one or another of the iron compounds. It is obvious that consideration of the relative bioavailability of the different iron sources has played little part in selecting the fortification agent.[25]

Iron supplements

The preferred forms of iron supplements are chelated iron, ferrous ascorbate, ferrous succinate, ferrous gluconate, ferrous fumarate or ferrous lactate. Ferrous sulfate is the form normally used and is effective, but we feel the others are "gentler" to your system, are unlikely to cause constipation, stool blackening and stomach upset.

Table 9.6 lists various iron salts in order of solubility. Iron salts should be the *ferrous* form, not *ferric*, which is much less soluble.

TABLE 9.6 ABSORPTION OF IRON SALTS

Salt	Absorption ratio[a]
Ferrous succinate	1.22
Ferrous lactate	1.06
Ferrous glycine sulfate	1.02
Ferrous fumarate	1.01
Ferrous sulfate	1.00
Ferrous glutamate	0.96
Ferrous gluconate	0.89
Ferrous citrate	0.74
Ferrous tartrate	0.64
Ferrous pyrophosphate	0.59

[a]Absorption of iron salt/absorption of ferrous sulfate.
Source: SCOGS—35, 1979.

There is quite a bit said about not taking iron supplements with vitamin E because iron destroys vitamin E. Yes, it can in the test tube. But have you noticed that whole wheat is a rich source of iron and vitamin E? Have you noticed that vitamin E and iron are both put in vitamin tablets that may sit on a shelf for a while, yet must maintain their labeled potency?

When vitamin E is protected from iron, there can be interaction, even when the two are together. Nature chelates iron in food or ties it up in a fashion that doesn't react with vitamin E. Manufacturers have learned to do the same.

If one takes chelated iron or one of the recommended organic ferrous salts, and also takes fair-sized amounts of vitamin E, there is little problem. It's convenient to take them both together. But if you are a purist, you may decide to take your iron on an empty stomach in the morning to get best absorption, and your vitamin E in the evening.

Hair analysis

Our opinion is that hair iron levels do not necessarily reflect the iron status of an individual, nor the dietary iron content. This conclusion is supported by the following two case histories and the medical literature.

A study by Dr. Paul Green and Joyce Duffield in Winnipeg, Manitoba concluded that the iron content of scalp hair gives no indication as to the state of the body iron stores in an individual patient: "While serial analyses of hair samples suggested that in some individuals the iron content of the hair fell when they became iron depleted and rose as iron stores were restored, this was not a consistent observation. Indeed, some individuals in whom the blood findings would strongly indicate iron depletion had [hair] iron values higher than average, whereas those with a surfeit of iron had values within normal range."

Case histories

G.D.H. was a forty-seven-year-old salesman who presented in May of 1978 extreme fatigue, weakness, diffuse aches and pains, poor concentration, chronic headaches and diminished sex drive. He had been to many clinics and seen many doctors without relief.

In March, 1978, a hair analysis showed hair iron to be 25 ppm (normal range 10 to 65 ppm for this laboratory). The laboratory interpretation indicated that the iron level was slightly below optimal concentration, in the lower half of the normal range. Because of this finding the patient had been taking iron, among his other supplements, to achieve an optimal body concentration.

In August, 1979, the iron content of his blood serum was found to be high at 203 mcg/dl. In the meantime, his sister died of pneumonia in another city.

Pneumonia is usually not a fatal disease in our culture because of readily available antibiotic therapy. An autopsy was performed which showed the sister to have the hereditary iron storage disease called hemochromatosis. An individual afflicted with hemochromatosis absorbs iron much more readily from the intestine than does a normal person. A normal diet containing only the recommended daily allowances of iron can lead to iron poisoning in a person who inherits hemochromatosis from his or her parents. Because of the familial nature of hemochromatosis, further testing was done on the surviving brother, G.D.H., who is described in this case history.

Serum ferritin, a protein in the bloodstream which closely correlates with body iron concentration, was measured at 853 ng (nanograms)/dl (normal range less than 313). He was then referred to a major university medical center where two subsequent tests confirmed the diagnosis of iron storage disease and organ poisoning with excessive iron burdens. He was given an iron chelating agent, deferoxamine, by injection, which caused iron to be excreted in the urine. His 24-hour urinary iron excretion was 3.5 mg (normal range less than 0.15 mg), a level twenty-three times higher than normal.

A liver biopsy was obtained using a needle to extract a tiny specimen of liver tissue. The pathologist who interpreted this specimen under a microscope after it had been treated with a special stain for iron pigment stated, "There are tremendous amounts of iron deposits in the liver."

A repeat hair analysis at this time by another laboratory showed iron concentration of 19 ppm (normal 20 to 50 ppm), and the laboratory's printed interpretation indicated marginal deficiency.

G.D.H. represents just one example of the lack of reliability of hair iron as an indicator of organ levels of iron in the rest of the body. Here is an individual who thought he was iron deficient, who felt badly from undiagnosed, early hemochromatosis, and who was poisoning himself by taking iron based on the results of a hair analysis.

Many hair analysis laboratories still recommend iron supplementation based on low hair iron. This is done in spite of contrary reports in the scientific literature as early as 1956.

How many other individuals with this hereditary type of iron poisoning have hastened the course of their illness by taking iron because of low iron on a hair mineral analysis? Fortunately, hemochromatosis is a rare disease.

N.A.S. is a fifty-eight-year-old lady who was first seen in August, 1980, for some routine medical problems. In the process of a medical evaluation she was found to be slightly anemic. The iron content of her blood serum was 40 mcg/dl (normal range 45 to 180) with an iron saturation of her blood protein of 12 percent (normal 15 to 55 percent). Serum ferritin, the protein which most closely correlates with body iron stores, was 26 ng/ml (normal 8 to 313), at the extreme low end of the normal range.

This patient had well-documented iron deficiency. A hair analysis done at this same time showed hair iron to be 29 ppm (normal range 20 to 55 ppm). This represents a case of iron deficiency anemia which would have been completely missed if the hair iron level had been relied upon as an accurate indicator of body iron stores.

REFERENCES

1 Bothwell, T. H. and Charlton, R. W. 1970. *Annu. Rev. Med.* 21:145–146.

2 Forth, W. and Rummel, W. 1973. *Physiol. Rev.* 53:724–792.

3 Linder, M. C. and Munro, H. N. 1977. *Fed. Proc. Fed. Amer. Soc. Exp. Biol.* 36:2017–2023.

4 Waddell, J. February 1974. *Food Prod. Dev.* 80–86.

5 Groen, J. *et al.* 1947. *Biochim. Biophys. Acta* 1:315. Also: Sayers, M. H. *et al.* 1973. *Br. J. Haematol.* 24:209–218. Layrisse, M. C. *et al.* 1974. *Amer. J. Clin. Nutr.* 27:152–162.

6 Greenberg, S. M. *et al.* 1957. *J. Nutr.* 63:19–31.

7 Cook, J. February 1978. *Food Nutr. News* 49(3)1.

8 Monsen, E. R. *et al.* 1978. *Amer. J. Clin. Nutr.* 31:134–141.

9 Bibeau, T. C. and Clydesdale, F. M. May 1976. *Food Prod. Dev.* 132.

10 Sharpe, L. M. *et al.* 1950. *J. Nutr.* 41:433–466.

11 Brise, H. 1962. *Acta Med. Scand.* 171:39–45.

12 Wintrobe, M. *et al.* 1953. *J. Nutr.* 50:395–419.

13 Freeman, S. *et al.* 1942. *Amer. J. Physiol.* 137(4):706–709.

14 Lee, K. April 1981. *Amer. Chem. Soc. Meet.*, Atlanta.

15 Anon. March 1981. *Food Prod. Dev.* 18.

16 Anon. February 2, 1951. *Food Chem. News* 32–34.

17 Anon. 1977. *Nutr. Rev.* 35:271–274.

18 Simpson, K. M. *et al.* 1981. *Amer. J. Clin. Nutr.* 34:1469–1478.

19 Finch, C. A. and Nonsen, E. R. 1972. *J. Amer. Med. Assoc.* 219:1462–1465.

20 Nat. Res. Council, Nat. Acad. Sci. Subcom. on Iron, Wash., D.C., 1977.

21 Aldrich, R. A. 1958. In: *Iron in Clinical Medicine*, Wallerstein and Mettier, eds. Berkeley, CA: Univ. Cal. Press.

22 Bulletin Council Better Nutr. (Ohio) 6. April 1, 1979.

23 Lee, K. and Clydesdale, F. M. 1979. *CRC Crit. Rev. Food Sci. Nutr.* 11:116–153.

24 Mervyn, Len. *Minerals and Your Health.* 1981. New Canaan, CT: Keats Publishing, pp. 91–94.

25 Waddell, J. February 1974. *Food Prod. Dev.*, p. 82.

Also see Finch, C.A. 1982. *New Eng. J. Med.* 307(27):1702–1703.

10

ZINC

We have only recently begun to understand the roles of zinc in health. Perhaps there are two reasons for this delay. The biggest reason is that accurate and sensitive analytical procedures for zinc were difficult until the widespread availability of a relatively new scientific instrument called an atomic absorption spectrophotometer in the late 1960s. Accurate and sensitive measurements are essential when dealing with trace minerals consumed in milligram quantities.

The second reason that zinc was not researched with zeal is that many nutritionists *assumed* that since zinc was widely distributed in soil, there would be no deficiency (it is the twenty-fifth most abundant element, making up 0.004 to 0.01 percent of the earth's crust).

Zinc was known to be essential to rats and assumed to be essential to humans as long ago as 1934.[1] However, it was not until 1963 that human zinc deficiency was reported in the medical literature.[2] In 1974 zinc was included in the National Academy of Sciences Recommended Dietary Allowances.

We do know that the major functions of zinc are enzymatic. There are now over seventy metallo-enzymes known to require zinc for their functions.[3] The main biochemicals in which zinc has been implicated as necessary include: 1) enzymes and enzymatic function, 2) protein synthesis, and 3) carbohydrate metabolism. It has been suggested that the vital role zinc plays in DNA synthesis explains the rapid onset of biochemical changes following the induction of zinc deficiency.

Protein composes the building blocks of each cell in the body. Within each cell is a small biochemical "factory" which manufactures protein from the constituent amino acids. The sequence in which these amino acids are connected together is determined by coding contained on the genes and chromosomes in the form of DNA (deoxyribonucleic acids). The DNA coding on genes and chromosomes forms the template or pattern from which very complex and large protein molecules, such as those which make up enzymes and connective tissues within the body, are manufactured. This pattern is taken from the DNA coding and transposed onto a sequence of RNA molecules which are hooked together in long chains (polymerized). The enzyme which translates the protein manufacturing code from the DNA chromosome to the RNA pattern upon which the protein molecules are manufactured is called "DNA dependent RNA polymerase."

This enzyme depends upon zinc for its function and is the enzyme which limits the rate at which protein can be made within the body. In zinc deficiency states, the reduced function of this enzyme is one of the first to be noticed. Reduced protein manufacture by cells slows the rate of healing, slows the production of replacement enzymes and other essential protein molecules within the body and in general prevents optimal health and healing. Antibodies, the essential molecules of the body's immune system, are also composed of protein and are compromised by zinc deficiency by this same mechanism—as well as through other mechanisms.

Three enzymes appear to be extremely sensitive to zinc deficiency—alkaline phosphatase in the bone, carboxypeptidase in the pancreas, and deoxythymidine kinase in the subcutaneous connective tissue.[3]

Zinc is a constituent of insulin and male reproductive fluid. Zinc is necessary for the proper metabolism of alcohol, to get rid of the lactic acid that builds up in working muscles, and to transport carbon dioxide in the blood and to transfer it to the lungs.

The concentration of zinc in the bone is higher than most other tissues. Normal tissues typically rank in terms of zinc concentration as follows: prostate, eye retina, liver, kidney, muscle, bone, testes, pancreas, heart, spleen, lung, brain, adrenal.

The "average" adult body contains approximately 2 to 2½ g zinc, but the body pool of biologically available zinc appears to be small and to have a rapid turnover, as evidenced by the prompt appearance of deficiency signs.[4]

The most prominent signs of zinc deficiency are loss of appetite, failure to grow, skin changes, impaired healing of wounds and decreased taste acuity.[4] Zinc deficiency in pregnant animals, even when transitory, can result in birth defects and behavioral disturbances in the offspring.[5] The human fetus may also be vulnerable to birth defects due to maternal zinc deficiency.

Body balance

Approximately 20 to 30 percent of ingested zinc is absorbed, but absorption is complicated by several factors.[3] A zinc-deficient person might absorb 50 percent of a meager zinc intake. Animal sources are more easily absorbed than plant sources, especially plant seeds.[6,7] Absorption studies of zinc are difficult to perform because most of zinc excretion is via the gut and it is difficult to distinguish between non-absorbed and excreted zinc. However, it is known that certain food substances interfere with zinc absorption. Among these are dietary fiber, phytic acid, other chelating agents, calcium and phosphorus. In animal studies, a high calcium intake in the presence of a high phytic acid (breads, cereals, soybeans) intake appears to have a synergistic effect in decreasing zinc absorption.[8]

Dr. Herta Spencer, of the Hines VA Medical Center in Illinois, points out: "In studies in *man*, using radioactive zinc as the tracer, no significant difference in zinc absorption could be demonstrated when the calcium intake was increased tenfold from 200 to 2000 mg per day. The high calcium intake in this study had a very low phytic acid content and was given in three to four divided doses. The use of divided doses, as would be expected to be the case when a high calcium diet is consumed, is pointed out because the effect of a single large dose of calcium may differ from the effect of multiple smaller doses on the intestinal absorption of zinc."[8] A large single dose of calcium is reported to decrease the intestinal absorption of zinc in man in the absence of phytate.[15]

A low-protein diet containing limited meat with food items rich in phytic acid would have little of the dietary zinc available for absorption and would be grossly inadequate in terms of zinc status.[8] High dietary fiber content may also interfere with the availability of zinc for absorption.[6,9,10] Pronounced zinc deficiency is known to occur in populations whose zinc intake is far in excess of the RDA but is derived exclusively from vegetable sources.[4] Vitamin B6 increases zinc absorption significantly.

The effect of vitamin D is not clearly understood as studies have indicated that vitamin D: decreases zinc absorption;[11] makes no significant change;[12] leads to increased bone uptake;[13] and has an unknown effect not related to any of the above.[14] It appears that low-zinc diets may be adversely affected by vitamin D, but not zinc-adequate diets.

A brief note regarding the role of zinc on absorption of other minerals and toxins is that excessive zinc can decrease copper, iron, calcium, lead and cadmium absorption because they all compete for similar binding sites.[3] It is possible that zinc decreases to some extent the amount of selenium absorbed.

Absorbed zinc is excreted mainly via the feces due to the loss of the pancreatic juice into the gut.[15] Negligible amounts are excreted by the liver into bile.[16,17] Some zinc is also lost in urine and sweat. The average daily zinc loss, on an otherwise well balanced diet containing 12 to 15 mg (the RDA) zinc, is 1 to 2 mg zinc excreted in the feces, 0.5 mg excreted in urine, and 0.5 mg lost in sweat.[3] Excessive sweating can eliminate 2 to 3 mg zinc in a day.

Alcohol increases the urinary excretion of zinc.[18] This is due to the increased need for the zinc-containing enzyme, alcohol dehydrogenase. Since the fetus and newborn are dependent on the mother for zinc supply, alcoholism in the mother leads to severe zinc deficiency in the child. This is called fetal alcohol syndrome and is characterized by prenatal and postnatal growth deficiency, small jaw, joint deformities, cleft palate, heart and kidney abnormalities and other defects.[3]

Surgery, burns, injury or weight loss substantially increases the urinary excretion of zinc. Increased salt intake or the use of diuretics decreases urinary concentration but the total quantity involved or the mechanism governing the urinary excretion of zinc is not clear.[19]

Sugar (sucrose) increases zinc excretion because the zinc-containing hormone insulin is required to maintain the resulting blood sugar (glucose).

As mentioned earlier, clinical research involving zinc has lagged, but already we are aware of the role of zinc against many conditions detracting from health. The subject deserves a book by itself; we can only cover the highlights here.

Pregnancy and child health

The first cases of human zinc deficiency were discovered by examining dwarfs in Egypt and Iran.[20,21] Both groups of dwarfs were eating substances that decreased the absorption of zinc. The Egyptian dwarfs were subsisting chiefly on cereals and unleavened bread high in phytic acid, while the Iranian dwarfs consumed a clay that tied up zinc. Both groups of dwarfs grew in stature and matured sexually when fed zinc supplements.

Normal growth is only part of the concern for adequate zinc for expecting mothers and youngsters. Zinc-deficient diets during pregnancy result in a high rate of miscarriages, and joined toes or fingers and hydrocephalus (fluid excess in the brain) in the baby. The children have a greater incidence of birth defects including reduced learning capacity, underdeveloped genitalia, reduced immune status, allergies, scoliosis, (sideways curvature of the spine) and kyphosis.[22,23] Zinc deficiency is also linked to mongolism.[24] We have discussed the role of alcoholism causing birth defects due to increased maternal zinc excretion in the preceding section on zinc excretion.

A potentially fatal genetic defect causing an absorption disorder, AE (acrodermatitis enteropathica) can be reversed in a few days by supplementing the lactating mother with zinc or supplementing the "formula."[25] By the way, zinc deficiency leads to stretch marks.

Returning to infant growth, a study at the University of Colorado Medical Center shows the importance of zinc to normal growth. In a six-month clinical trial, researchers provided the parents of thirty-four infants with a supply of a widely used milk formula, which contained a trace of zinc. Another group of parents of thirty-four babies was given the same commercial milk formula supplemented with zinc so as to contain three times as much as otherwise. These babies averaged approximately a 10-percent improvement in length and weight.

Zinc is needed not only for sound bones in the developing children but also for sound teeth. Experiments conducted at the Mississippi Agricultural and Forestry Experimental Station in 1980 suggest that zinc strengthens tooth enamel and reduces cavities.

Intelligence and behavior

In animal experiments in 1975, Dr. Harold Sandstead and his colleagues at the U.S. Department of Agriculture's Human Research Laboratory in Beltsville, Maryland, showed that zinc deficiency in the last trimester of pregnancy produces off-spring with smaller than normal brains.

When the learning ability of the males was tested, those from zinc-deficient mothers were rated at 35 percent of peak performance, compared to 80 percent among males from mothers adequately nourished with zinc.

A surprising finding was that the females born to the zinc-deficient mothers were violent and aggressive. Both the learning disability and violent behavior have been described by other researchers.[26,27]

Dr. H. Ronaghy tested the effect of zinc supplements on illiterate nineteen- and twenty-year-old Iranians. As mentioned earlier, zinc deficiency is aggravated in Iran due to the prevalence of phytic acid from unleavened bread and even a zinc-binding clay in the diet of many Iranians. Dr. Ronaghy noted a marked differential in scholastic performance after one year of zinc supplementation compared to a matched group not receiving the zinc supplements.[27]

The IQ of young children suffering from AE showed dramatic spurts while being cured. One child had his IQ jump from 89 to 98 in a week, and to 109 in a year, according to the article published in the *Journal of Pediatrics* (Sept. 1978) by the University of Colorado Medical Center researchers. They also report that a twelve-year-old girl became sociable and talkative within hours of taking zinc. She had shunned friends and school and had been tutored at home. In a few months she rose to the top of her class.[28]

Dr. Adon Gordus of the University of Michigan found a strong positive correlation between the zinc nutrition of college students and their scholastic rankings.[29]

Healing

A series of clinical trials led by Drs. Walter Pories and John Henzel, beginning in 1966 at the U.S. Air Force Hospital at the Wright-Patterson Air Force Base in Ohio and continuing through the 1970s at the Department of Surgery at the University of Missouri in Columbia, show that zinc speeds healing. Looking back on the discovery, it is easy to suggest that it should have been more apparent. The ancient Egyptians had used zinc preparations (calamine, zinc oxide) on the skin to promote healing. (Some zinc is absorbed through the skin—especially injured skin.) The researchers were aware of the use of zinc in farm animals to speed healing, especially of leg ulcers. They also knew that a 1953 study by Dr. Pories showed zinc promoted healing of burns.[30]

Drs. Pories and Henzel reasoned that zinc could speed healing because of its role in the synthesis of protein and nucleic acid. They also realized that a significant portion of the population might have low zinc stores based on a U.S. Department of Agriculture study revealing that thirty-two of fifty states had zinc-deficient soil.

In a twenty-man study, they found that zinc supplements increased the rate of healing threefold.[31] The days required for the healing of a surgical procedure decreased from eighty in the non-supplemented group to forty-six days in the zinc supplemented group. Larger wounds healed 43 percent sooner with orally administered zinc. They also found that zinc supplements promote healing only moderately during the first fifteen days, but vigorously thereafter.

The zinc supplement available at the time was zinc sulfate which was used principally as an emetic (to cause vomiting). The supplement was given in a dose of 220 mg zinc sulfate three times a day. No toxic side effects were observed during periods ranging from forty-three to sixty-one days.

During the study they noted that surgical patients have a fall in zinc stores during the early postoperative period. Radioactive tracer studies showed that zinc from the supplement migrates into the wound on a temporary basis, moving elsewhere before the time of complete scarring (100 days).[32,33,34]

They also found that zinc-deficient patients have impaired wound healing, and that urinary excretion of zinc increases after weight loss, burns or surgery.[35,36]

Further studies elucidated that healing wound fluid and blood zinc levels continued to bring zinc to the wound site. They also noted that heavy exercise increased blood zinc levels.[37]

Dr. Thomas Sedlacek, of the University of Pennsylvania, found that zinc supplements cut the number of days by two-thirds that women were hospitalized after gynecological surgery. He concluded, "At current rates, a decrease in hospital stays of this magnitude represents a savings of about $4000 for each patient."[38] Seventy-five percent of the women not receiving zinc supplementation had their surgical wound break open, whereas only 20 percent of those receiving the zinc supplements had this complication.

Dr. Fredric Pullen of the University of Miami School of Medicine found that zinc supplements accelerated healing after tonsillectomy.[39] Twenty-one of twenty-four patients receiving nearly 500 mg zinc a day were completely healed within two weeks, compared to only thirteen of twenty-two patients not receiving the zinc supplements.

There is strong evidence that zinc plays a role in bone metabolism and that supplemental zinc could be beneficial to bone healing.[40]

Immunity and cancer

Zinc deficiency impairs immunity to disease. Dr. Robert Pekarek of the U.S. Department of Agriculture's Human Nutrition Laboratory in Grand Forks, North Dakota, found that zinc deficiency impairs one limb of the immune system, the cell-mediated system that helps fight viral, parasitic and mycotic infections, neoplastic (abnormal tissue formation) diseases, and diseases in which the body produces antibodies to its own proteins.[41,42]

The thymus is responsible for immune T-cell production, and zinc deficiency can cause thymus gland damage.[43,44] The ways in which zinc deficiency affects immune response is beyond the scope of this book, but has been elaborated on in the scientific literature.[45]

In 1975, an article in the *Journal of the National Cancer Institute* reported that zinc supplementation reduced the incidence of cancer in mice injected with sarcoma cancer cells. In rats fed nitrosamine, a cancer-inducing chemical, 80 percent of those deficient in zinc developed cancer compared to only 30 percent of those on an adequate zinc diet.[46]

Patients with esophageal cancer were found to be zinc-deficient. This fits the observation that tissues in pigs having a known zinc-deficiency-related disease resemble tissues from human esophageal cancer. Also, alcoholics have a relatively high incidence of esophageal cancer, and alcohol increases zinc excretion.

Heart disease and the zinc-copper ratio

Conflicting opinion has been expressed by researchers regarding the role of zinc and zinc-to-copper ratio in heart disease. One group relates low dietary zinc intake with heart disease, another group believes that a combination of zinc and copper deficiency is related to heart disease, while a third group believes that the ratio of zinc to copper is the important factor. We believe a close look at the facts will end the confusion.

Zinc and copper have separate actions, competing interactions, and complementary interactions. Zinc and copper compete for absorption, and they both are incorporated into molecules such as superoxide dismutase.

Let's begin with the research of Dr. J. Henzel and his colleagues at the Department of Surgery of the University of Missouri Medical Center in Columbia. This is the same research team that has been studying the role of zinc in the healing process.

While studying various patients in terms of healing, Dr. Henzel noticed that some heart patients taking zinc seem to improve faster than normal. The research group decided to test this observation by giving zinc supplements to twenty-four patients with inoperable atherosclerosis and having severe symptoms.

The patients were re-evaluated with treadmill walking, exercise electrocardiograms, arteriograms, plethysmography and ultrasonic flowmeter (Doppler), and blood tests at subsequent examinations. There was distinct improvement in eighteen of the twenty-four patients receiving 150 mg of zinc daily, after three to ten months.[47]

Of the eighteen having distinct improvement, eight were rated "excellent," eight "good," and two "moderate." The criteria for the "excellent" rating included being able to work full time, no symptoms from any activity and doubling of treadmill exercise performance. The criteria for the "good" rating include being able to perform all "necessary" activity and a doubling of treadmill exercise performance.

The researchers noted that 52 percent of the patients had sub-normal blood zinc levels and 18 percent had low-normal blood zinc levels. No consistent relationship was observed between patient response and elevated blood zinc levels following supplementation. The improvement appeared to be more related to duration of therapy, rather than to the degree of increased zinc level in the blood.

The researchers also commented that the single most impressive result of long-term zinc supplementation was the diminution in or elimination of claudication (severe limping) pain.

The researchers were surprised to note such improvement although the arteriograms did not reveal evidence of increased collateral circulation. They also noted that a number of the patients who exhibited improvement did so in spite of diminished perfusion pressure (arterial pressure) in the leg. The researchers concluded, "This particular observation, together with the repeated subjective-objective documentation of increased foot warmth, new distal extremity hair growth, and distal 'pinkness,' all suggest improvement in tissue metabolism and respiration."

It remains to be defined whether or not blood flow is actually enhanced at the micro-vessel level by zinc or if the response is due to zinc-augmented tissue metabolism. Most likely several zinc enzymes (such as carbonic anhydrase, lactic acid dehydrogenase and alkaline phosphatase) increase cellular activity, thus promoting nutritive tissue metabolism.

A research group at the Kettering Laboratory of the University of Cincinnati Medical Center has found that experimental animals deficient in zinc and copper form fatty deposits in their arteries more readily.[48]

The zinc-copper ratio theory has been advanced by Dr. Leslie Klevay of the U.S. Department of Agriculture's Human Nutrition Laboratory in Grand Forks, North Dakota.

The interactions between dietary zinc and copper are not fully understood, but the following has been determined. Dietary zinc and copper compete for absorption. Excessive zinc intake can lead to a copper deficiency.[49,50] Dietary zinc has no effect on the amount of copper excreted by the body or retained in the body, but increasing dietary zinc increases blood zinc levels which in turn tends to decrease blood copper levels.[51]

In 1973, Dr. Klevay found that an increase in the zinc-copper ratio raised the blood cholesterol level in rats.[52] An increased zinc-copper ratio can be achieved by either increasing the dietary zinc level or decreasing the dietary copper level or both.

In 1975, Dr. Klevay compared coronary heart disease death rates from forty-seven American cities with data on the average amounts of zinc and copper in the milk in each of those cities. The ratio of zinc to copper in milk differs from area to area due to the feed concentration of each mineral varying with the availability of each in the area's soil. Dr. Klevay found a definite correlation between high zinc-copper ratios and higher death rates from heart disease.[53] Incidentally, the zinc-copper ratio in human milk is lower than in cow milk.

Dr. Klevay has also determined that the copper content of many foods is lower today than in the 1940s and that many people are eating less than the RDA of 2 mg.[54]

We can speculate that increased zinc levels in the blood can increase the amount of the retinol-binding protein that carries vitamin A, and that vitamin A in turn could raise blood cholesterol levels.[55] But such a cholesterol elevation in itself would not necessarily be a factor in heart disease or detrimental in any way.

Although Dr. Klevay has built an early impressive array of data to support his hypothesis that the zinc-copper ratio is related to heart disease, later evidence has tended to put the blame on copper deficiency and absolve zinc.

There has been one small scale study, involving only twelve male patients, that indicated increased zinc intake had no effect on total cholesterol or low-density lipoprotein cholesterol, but lowered the protective high-density lipoprotein cholesterol.[56] Later studies by this same group [57] did not confirm this small study, and in the light of the observation that a more frequent pattern of cholesterol change is that when the total cholesterol is unchanged and either the low-density or high-density lipoprotein shifts, there is an opposite shift in the remaining lipoprotein.

The second study by the researchers at the School of Medicine of the University of New Mexico and the Albuquerque VA Hospital involved feeding laboratory rats a standard feed containing a fixed amount of copper to which they added zinc to give zinc-copper ratios of 0.7, 1.3, 7 and 33.[57] They found no differences in blood cholesterol or high-density lipoprotein cholesterol. They concluded that dietary zinc and zinc-copper ratios such as used in their experiments have little effect on lipid (fat) metabolism in rats.

The effects of different amounts of dietary zinc and copper on cholesterol metabolism in laboratory rats were investigated by researchers at the Bureau of Nutritional Science in Ottawa.[58] The levels of zinc and copper used by the research team headed by Dr. Peter Fischer were comparable to normal mixed North American diets. The dietary changes did affect the blood levels of zinc and copper, but did not affect the liver cholesterol, total blood cholesterol or high-density lipoprotein. The researchers concluded that dietary zinc and copper at levels likely to occur in normal mixed diets are not significant factors in cholesterol metabolism.

The test involved normal diets, but what about zinc-supplemented diets?

Dr. Jeanne Freeland-Graves of the University of Texas studied the effect of altering the dietary zinc-copper ratio on blood cholesterol and high-density lipoprotein cholesterol in thirty-two women.[59] Zinc supplements were given for sixty days to achieve zinc-copper ratios of either 3, 13, 21, or 64. The blood plasma zinc levels increased in proportion to the amount of the supplement, but no uniform nor sustained response of blood cholesterol and high-density lipoprotein cholesterol was observed as the zinc-copper ratios were manipulated. However, they did find that blood copper levels were significantly related to blood cholesterol levels. They concluded that blood cholesterol levels in women are more influenced by copper than by zinc. The lower the copper level, the higher the cholesterol.

A similar conclusion was reached by a team of researchers at Colorado State University.[60] They concluded that no correlation was observed between dietary zinc and cholesterol level, but they too noted that copper level affected cholesterol level, i.e., low dietary copper produced a high cholesterol level. They also noted that this effect was abolished by copper supplementation.

Thus it appears that most of the recent research supports the thesis that zinc does not affect total cholesterol or any of the lipoprotein-bound cholesterol. However, this research, and most of Dr. Klevay's observations, supports the observation that low copper levels elevate blood cholesterol and that low dietary copper may be a risk factor in heart disease. Even though zinc, per se, does not cause a problem, the fact that excessive zinc can interfere with copper absorption must be kept in mind. If adequate copper is in the diet, the normally encountered ratios of zinc to copper are unimportant. If inadequate copper is present, then zinc concentration may become a factor by diminishing the absorption of copper and aggravating the copper deficiency.

Blood cholesterol levels are not necessarily related to cholesterol deposits in arteries. We have little to go on because laboratory mice and rats do not readily develop atherosclerotic plaques (cholesterol deposits) with simple dietary manipulation and laboratory animals, more often than not, fail to approximate the fibrous-type plaque observed in humans having clinical signs of heart disease.

However, a rabbit study at the Sinai Hospital in Detroit not only absolves zinc as a problem, but indicates that zinc is protective against atherosclerotic plaque formation. The researchers fed diets that are known to produce plaques to two groups of rabbits. One group also received extra zinc. At the end of three months, the aortas of the rabbits were examined and it was learned that the oral administration of zinc was found to significantly inhibit the formation of plaques.[61]

In cases where atherosclerotic plaques have reduced the blood circulation, zinc supplements restored normal metabolism, although not necessarily improving blood flow. One such example was given as an introduction to this section.

Zinc levels in the blood decrease for two to three days after heart attack.[62] This may be because zinc is being used in healing the heart. Studies have shown that raising the blood level of zinc protects against heart damage after a heart attack.[63]

Zinc decreases absorption of the pollutant cadmium. Cadmium is linked to increased blood pressure, atherosclerosis and stroke. Zinc concentrations within cells protect against the toxic effects of cadmium which has already been absorbed. That is, that zinc-cadmium ratio within kidney tissues has a definite bearing on high blood pressure. Higher levels of cadmium can be tolerated in the presence of adequate zinc. Small levels of cadmium can be more toxic in zinc deficiency states.

Thus we see that zinc heals the heart and reduces plaque formation, that copper deficiency increases blood cholesterol and may be a heart disease risk factor, and that zinc and copper both are required to build the critical enzyme superoxide dismutase. Yet we know that zinc can interfere with copper absorption and vice versa. Is it any surprise that our knowledge of the possible roles of these nutrients in heart disease has been slow in coming?

Sex, fertility and the prostate

Earlier we mentioned that zinc deficiency in childhood impaired the development of the sex organs and secondary sexual characteristics. In adulthood zinc is vital to the glands that govern libido—the ovaries in women and the testes in men. Even a marginal zinc deficiency can lower one's libido.

Research at a Michigan Veteran's Administration Hospital showed that zinc-deficient diets lower the levels of the male hormone testosterone. In the study, the testosterone levels returned to normal in most of the men when zinc supplements were given. However, not all the men responded, but this may be that they needed more time on the supplements and/or a greater zinc intake. These findings were confirmed by a research group at Rutgers University.[64]

The Michigan researchers also noted that diets even moderately deficient in zinc reduced sperm counts, and in some cases the reduction was sufficient enough to classify the men as being sterile in two to fourteen months. In two to twenty months after taking zinc supplements, the sperm counts returned to normal.

The prostate gland contains more zinc (550 mcg/g) than any other organ in the male. There must be a reason for a concentration of zinc in this organ that weighs about an ounce and is sized somewhere between that of a large olive and a small walnut. The gland consists of three lobes that surround the urethra near the base of the penis. Its only known function is to make the seminal fluid for ejaculation and to add it to the semen in the prostatic urethra.

There are three diseases common to the prostate, and two of them may be related to zinc deficiency. Prostatitis is an inflammation of the prostate gland that affects younger men more than older men. Benign prostatic hypertrophy is an enlarged prostate gland that affects older men more than young men. The third common disease of the prostate gland is cancer.

All three diseases can lead to serious consequences, and a physician should be consulted whenever the symptoms appear. We do not encourage "waiting to see if it goes away" or trying zinc supplements for a few months to see if that cures it. If you guess wrong, any infection might spread or cancer could go from treatable to non-treatable. Prostate trouble signs include pain or difficulty in urination or sexual function.

Studies by Dr. Irving Cook and others at various Chicago hospitals have shown that many men having prostatitis have abnormally low levels of zinc in their prostates and semen. In a study of 200 men having prostatitis not caused by bacterial infection, zinc supplements relieved the symptoms in 70 percent of the men.

Enlarged prostate-glands affect 10 percent of forty-year-old and 80 percent of eighty-year-old men.[65] There is no reason for the prostate to enlarge with age. Actually, it is the urethral glands inside the prostate that enlarge and cause the prostate (especially the middle lobe) to constrict the urethra.

A small clinical trial determined that zinc supplements brought the relief of symptoms to all nineteen patients having benign prostatic hypertrophy, but more importantly returned the prostate to normal size in fourteen of the nineteen.[66]

The Chicago studies led by Dr. Bush found that although men with enlarged prostates had normal blood zinc levels (which is not a really good measure of zinc status), they responded well to zinc therapy. More than 70 percent had shrinkage of the prostate to normal or near-normal size.[67] The amount of zinc used in the above studies was 50 to 150 mg per day.

Skin, acne and vitamin A

Zinc is important to skin health in many ways. There is an appreciable amount of zinc in skin but the most important factor may be the role zinc plays in transporting vitamin A to the skin: vitamin A is vital to skin health.

Zinc deficiency interferes with the production of a protein complex that carries vitamin A from the liver into the bloodstream.[68,69] This protein complex is called retinol-binding protein. Zinc deficiency leads to low blood levels of vitamin A due to the impaired ability to mobilize vitamin A from the liver in the form of the vitamin A-retinol-binding protein complex.

Increasing the amount of vitamin A in the diet does not necessarily increase the amount of vitamin A circulating in the bloodstream. The added vitamin A may be stored in the liver if there is no more available retinol-binding protein to carry it in the blood. The critical factor is how much vitamin A reaches the skin via the bloodstream.

Some researchers have reported good results in treating acne with zinc. However, acne is not a simple disease having one cause. We believe it is ill-advised to try to self-treat serious acne. The condition may not be caused by poor nutrition and may become worse and require more dramatic treatment, or lead to scarring. Nutritional changes can be made simultaneously with whatever recommendations are made by a dermatologist.

At one time dermatologists favored using oral doses of the antibiotic tetracycline for acne. Unfortunately, zinc interferes with the absorption of tetracycline. Now most dermatologists favor topical application of a lotion of the antibiotics erythromycin or clindamycin. Thus the problem of zinc interference is avoided and both may be administered concurrently. In fact, under normal conditions it would be wise to improve your vitamin A and zinc status as a nutritional adjunct.

An alert Swedish physician treating a patient for another ailment in the

Uppsala University Hospital noticed that the patient's acne improved after treatment with zinc supplements. Dr. Gerd Michaelsson led a research group that then tested the theory. They conducted a clinical trial in which sixty-four patients were given oral zinc (135 mg) and vitamin A in doses many times the RDA.[70]

The researchers kept track of the number of pimples on each patient. After only four weeks, there was significant improvement among those receiving the zinc supplements. After twelve weeks of zinc supplementation, the results were astounding. The patients taking zinc showed an 87 percent improvement. In this Swedish study, nine patients who did not respond to tetracycline treatment had excellent results with the zinc supplements.

·The improvements obtained with zinc supplements applies to both adolescent and adult acne. Women on oral contraceptives should note that the Pill reduces the amount of zinc in the blood.[71]

Other skin problems such as boils and body odor have responded dramatically to improved zinc status.[72,73] A particularly difficult disorder is the skin ulcer. Poor circulation often produces thin skin that is easily irritated and then ulcerated. Both patients and physicians tend to accept the presence of an ulcerated leg with a grim stoicism born of years of unsuccessful treatment.[74] It used to be that most leg ulcers took around eleven weeks to heal, irrespective of treatment. However, Dr. Latafat Husain, of the University Department of Dermatology, Western Infirmary in Glasgow, Scotland, found that zinc better than halved the healing time. In a double-blind, placebo controlled clinical study of 104 patients, Dr. Husain noted the time required for complete healing took only an average of thirty-two days for the patients receiving zinc supplements, compared to seventy-seven days for those not receiving the zinc supplements.[75] The amount of zinc was 150 mg given in three daily doses.

Both venous and arterial (chronic ischemic) leg ulcers respond to zinc supplements even though blood circulation is poor and the zinc level of the blood may be in the normal range.

Dr. Knut Haeger, of the University Hospital in Malmo, Sweden, produced total healing in forty days with 136 mg zinc daily.[76] In a double-blind study 97 percent of the zinc-supplemented patients with venous leg ulcers were completely healed as compared to only 58 percent of the patients not receiving the zinc supplements.

Later Dr. Haeger found that this level of zinc supplementation also sped the healing rate in ischemic leg ulcer patients by more than 100 percent.[77]

If zinc helps wound healing and leg ulcers, will it help gastric ulcers?

Ulcers

Zinc not only helps leg ulcers as we have just discussed, but also helps gastric ulcers heal. Dr. Donald Frommer of the Department of Gastroenterology at the Prince of Wales Hospital in Sydney, Australia found that zinc sped the healing of gastric ulcers.[78] Again, this is true even in patients who show no signs of zinc deficiency.

In a double-blind, placebo-controlled clinical trial complete healing of gastric ulcers was obtained in three weeks by 40 percent of the zinc-supplemented (150 mg) group compared to 13 percent in the non-supplemented control group. It should be noted that all patients in the zinc supplemented group had some degree of healing compared to only 75 percent of the control group.

It seems that any type of wound or skin problem or lesions inside the digestive tract may respond to zinc supplementation.

Rheumatoid arthritis

Studies have shown that rheumatoid arthritis patients have lower than normal levels of zinc in their blood. This observation suggested to Dr. Peter S. Simkin of the University of Washington at Seattle that perhaps restoring zinc levels of the blood to normal would be beneficial.

Dr. Simkin gave supplements containing 50 mg zinc to patients with active rheumatoid arthritis that did not respond to conventional drug therapies. These patients were matched against similar patients not receiving the zinc supplements. However, both groups continued to receive their drug therapies throughout the clinical trial.

After twelve weeks the patients taking zinc supplements fared better in all clinical measurements than those not receiving the zinc supplements. Joint swelling decreased by 26 percent in the zinc group compared to no change in the control group. Morning stiffness decreased significantly in the zinc group, but not in the controls. The zinc-supplemented patients significantly reduced their time required to walk a 50-foot course, whereas the others did not. More important, the zinc-supplemented group reported improvements with each visit to the clinic.[79]

Taste

As we grow older we seem to lose our sense of taste and develop a preference for spicier foods to obtain more flavor. One of the reasons for decreased taste and smell acuity is the loss of zinc stores as years of marginal zinc deficiency add up.

Drs. Robert Henkin and R. Aamodt of the Taste and Smell Clinic at the National Institutes of Health have found that zinc supplements restore taste in many people.[80] Copper and nickel may also be involved in maintaining normal taste and smell acuity.

Drs. Henkin and Aamodt studied approximately 4000 people ranging in age from twenty-five to eighty-one with taste and smell problems. Their one common denominator was low blood levels of zinc. They all responded well to zinc supplements.

Sickle-cell anemia

Dr. George E. Brewer of the University of Michigan has found that zinc supplements ease the pain of sickle-cell anemia and decrease the number of abnormal blood cells.

Senile dementia

A link between dietary zinc and senile dementia is proposed by F.M. Burnet, in the journal *Lancet*.[81] He hypothesizes that additional dietary zinc might prevent or delay the onset of dementia in some people.

Mr. Burnet bases his hypothesis on the involvement of zinc metalloenzymes in DNA replication, repair and transcription. Apparently, when zinc is removed, these enzymes lose activity. Mr. Burnet suggests that senile dementia may be linked with the body's loss of ability to make zinc available for insertion into newly synthesized enzymes. He hopes that his admittedly speculative idea will spur further investigative research.

You can see that zinc is important to our health in many ways. Yet we are seeing evidence of zinc deficiencies more often. What is causing this trend?

Food sources

Zinc can be found in many foods provided zinc is in the soil in adequate amounts to be taken up by the plants that we eat or feed to farm animals. Normally, meat, liver, eggs and seafood are good sources of available zinc, whereas wholegrain products contain zinc in a less available form. Table 10.1 lists typical zinc levels of foods. However, food tables are not reliable indicators of dietary zinc, because zinc content varies from region to region in line with the soil content.[8] Plants need only fifteen or so elements for growth and health, whereas people need approximately twenty-three elements. We depend on plants carrying along elements that we need, but they don't. Some would have you believe that the plants wouldn't grow without zinc or other elements essential to man, but nonessential to plants. There are wide areas within the United States in which the soil is deficient in available zinc and where the appearance of spontaneous zinc deficiency in farm animals has necessitated zinc enrichment of feeds.[82]

Dr. Frank Viets of the U.S. Department of Agriculture has noted soil deficits of zinc in at least thirty states and has found the deficit growing during the last two decades.[83] He predicts that unless zinc is replaced in the soil on a large scale, more and more people will develop symptoms of zinc deficiency.

Another concern is that fertilizers overloaded with phosphorus, potash and nitrogen decrease the absorption of trace elements by plants.

Zinc content of food being so variable is only one part of the problem. The biological availability of zinc in different foods also varies widely. Pronounced zinc deficiency is known to occur in populations whose zinc intake is far in excess of the RDA but is derived exclusively from vegetable sources.[4] We have already mentioned that phytic acid (phytate) and dietary fiber are of the greatest practical importance because they prevent zinc from being absorbed. After a period of debate on the issue, researchers have now concluded there is no reasonable doubt that phytic acid binds zinc, and when in sufficiently high concentration in the diet, decreases the availability of zinc.[9,84–86]

TABLE 10.1 SOURCES OF ZINC

Milligrams (mg) per 100 grams edible portion (100 grams = 3½ oz.)			
Fresh oysters	148.7	Haddock	1.7
Ginger root	6.8	Green peas	1.6
Ground round steak	5.6	Shrimp	1.5
Lamb chops	5.3	Turnips	1.2
Pecans	4.5	Parsley	0.9
Split peas, dry	4.2	Potatoes	0.9

SOURCES OF ZINC (*cont.*)

Milligrams (mg) per 100 grams edible portion (100 grams = 3½ oz.)

Brazil nuts	4.2	Garlic	0.6
Beef liver	3.9	Carrots	0.5
Nonfat dry milk	3.5	Wholewheat bread	0.5
Egg yolk	3.5	Black beans	0.4
Whole wheat	3.2	Raw milk	0.4
Rye	3.2	Pork chop	0.4
Oats	3.2	Corn	0.4
Peanuts	3.2	Grape juice	0.3
Lima beans	3.1	Olive oil	0.3
Soy lecithin	3.1	Cauliflower	0.3
Almonds	3.1	Spinach	0.2
Walnuts	3.0	Cabbage	0.2
Sardines	2.9	Lentils	0.2
Chicken	2.6	Butter	0.2
Buckwheat	2.5	Lettuce	0.2
Hazel nuts	2.4	Cucumber	0.1
Clams	1.9	Yams	0.1
Anchovies	1.7	Tangerine	0.1
Tuna	1.7	String beans	0.1

Black pepper, paprika, mustard, chili powder, thyme, and cinnamon are also high in zinc.

Source: MineraLab, Inc.

Thus, we have zinc-depleted soil and phytic acid tying up zinc so that we can not rely on the food tables as evidence we are absorbing adequate zinc.

However, let's assume for a moment that the food tables (Table 10.1) do reliably indicate zinc nourishment. With today's trend towards a less active lifestyle, we must reduce caloric intake in order to maintain desired weight. Try to design a practical weekly diet plan that contains more than 85 percent of the zinc RDA (15 mg) and yet provides only the calories needed to maintain your desired weight. This is a tough problem even for experienced dieticians.

Now we have three complications: zinc-depleted soils, phytic acid and low-calorie diets. But there are more problems: food processing and preparation.

The refining of foods usually results in a decrease in the zinc content.[87] During the milling process of wheat to make flour, up to 80 percent of the zinc may be lost.[88–90] Bread made from white flour has less zinc than whole-wheat bread, corn starch contains much less zinc than corn kernels, canned beans lose 60 percent of the zinc contained in fresh beans, canned tomatoes 45 percent, canned spinach 40 percent, and so forth.[90–92]

During food preparation, the corrosive action of acid foods in contact with galvanized metal increases zinc content in foods, but with the increased use of stainless steel, aluminum, plastic, and plastic-coated cooking utensils, this source of zinc has decreased.[19]

With all these factors affecting zinc nutriture, it is no wonder that recent evidence suggests that marginal states of zinc nutrition do exist in segments of the United States population.[4] A 1973 study suggested that the average zinc content of diets consumed by American adults was between 10 and 15 mg.[93] However, a 1979 survey found the average intake was only 8.6 mg per day, with the range being 6 to 12 mg per day.[94] Some hospital diets contain only 30 percent of the RDA for zinc.[8]

There are other causes of zinc deficiency than sub-optimal dietary intake. Table 10.2 lists various causes Diuretic usage, alcohol and a high calcium intake are examples of zinc lowering factors.

Zinc deficiency is difficult to detect by blood tests. Unless dietary zinc is low or poorly absorbed for a long period of time, plasma zinc tends to stay within the "normal" range.[95,96] Acute zinc deficiency can often be detected by white opaque spots on fingernails.[97]

TABLE 10.2 CAUSES OF ZINC DEFICIENCY IN HUMAN SUBJECTS.

Dietary	Excessive intake of phytate, fiber, polyphosphates, clay and laundry starch, and alcohol
Malabsorption	Pancreatic insufficiency, steatorrhea, gastrectomy, intestinal mucosal disease
Cirrhosis of the liver	
Renal disease	Nephrotic syndrome, renal tubular disease
Renal dialysis	
Chronically debilitating diseases	Neoplastic diseases, chronic infections
Psoriasis (skin loss)	
Burns	
Parasitic infections (chronic blood loss)	
Iatrogenic	Penicillamine therapy, total parenteral nutrition, surgical trauma
Genetic	Sickle cell disease, acrodermatitis enteropathica
Pregnancy	
Diuretic use	
Alcoholism	

Toxicity

The toxicity of zinc is fairly low and occurs with the ingestion of 2 grams or more. However, this dosage usually causes vomiting. Zinc can decrease copper absorption, so care must be taken not to use large amounts of zinc supplements if a copper deficiency is possible. In other words, ensure adequate copper if taking zinc supplements above 45 mg daily.

When zinc is taken in doses larger than the RDA of 15 to 20 mg per day, to replete zinc deficiency states as documented by testing, take the extra zinc at bedtime or on first arising in the morning, at least two hours before breakfast or several hours after the evening meal, to allow the zinc to be absorbed without competing with other minerals for uptake sites in the intestine. In this way zinc deficiency can be repleted without competing with copper and other essential trace nutrients and without the possibility of creating a deficiency state which did not exist prior to supplementation with zinc.

Hair analysis

Many studies have been published in the peer-reviewed scientific literature to document the clinical significance of low hair zinc concentrations as a reliable, simple and easily obtainable method of assessing body zinc stores. Hair has been found to be more reliable than blood testing as a method of detecting zinc deficiency. There are a few conflicting reports in the medical literature, but most of those reports were studies in which circulating blood levels of zinc were used in comparison with hair zinc, assuming that the blood zinc was an accurate indicator of zinc deficiency. That has since been disproved (Strain, 1966; Reinhold, 1966; Hambidge, 1972; Hambidge, 1973; Amador, June 21, 1975 *Lancet*; Hambidge, 1976; Prasad, 1976; Lin, 1977; Greger, 1978; Adkin-Thor, 1948–1951, 1978; Dogru, 1979; Bradfield, 1980).

There also exists conflicting data in the literature which did not find a correlation between hair zinc and body zinc stores. This apparent contradiction has since been explained by additional studies in which it has been shown that in very severely zinc-depleted patients, zinc-dependent enzymes slow protein production to such an extent that hair grows extremely slowly. In such a case zinc concentration in the hair becomes high because of slow hair growth and greater time for uptake of zinc by the hair because of its longer stay in the hair follicle, even in the presence of low zinc in surrounding tissues. In a study published in the *American Journal of Clinical Nutrition* by Drs. Pekarek, Sanstead and other investigators in 1979, a case was described of a seventeen-year-old male patient with severe brain injury who had been fed intravenously and with artificial tube feedings for a prolonged period during a coma. This individual became severely zinc-deficient and hair analysis showed hair zinc to be elevated. When zinc was added to his feedings, hair began to grow much more rapidly, causing an initial rise in hair zinc and then a rapid fall to subnormal levels followed by a slow return to normal hair zinc levels as body stores of zinc were gradually replaced. Similar observations were made by Dr. Erten in Turkey in 1978.

It has also been found that patients with diabetes have a lower hair level of zinc, on the average. Zinc is an essential component of insulin. These studies describe the juvenile onset type of diabetes which is caused by an absolute deficiency of insulin.[98]

To summarize the interpretation of hair zinc: low hair zinc levels most likely indicate a deficiency of total body zinc stores. An exception might be in patients who have had hair bleaching or cold-wave treatments or in elderly patients with gray hair in whom normal zinc levels might be slightly lower than in younger patients with darker hair pigmentation. On the other hand, normal or high hair zinc does not eliminate the possibility of zinc deficiency. If an individual is so severely zinc-deficient that protein manufacture is slowed, the slower growth of hair can lead to an elevated hair zinc concentration, even with total body zinc deficiency. Also individuals with zinc deficiency may suffer from dandruff or eczema and may be using a zinc-containing shampoo which may give an artificially normal or high zinc level in hair. Hair analysis is a screening test and, although a suspicion of deficiency or toxic states may be raised by hair concentrations, more specific testing must be done to confirm a clinical diagnosis and before beginning any treatment which might incur additional risk.

Case histories

D.C. is a five-year-old girl who was growing very slowly. Her height and weight were in the fifth percentile for her age, despite the fact that her parents were of average to slightly greater than average size. A careful medical history revealed the presence of food allergies which could easily have been causing an intestinal malabsorption of not only zinc but other essential nutrients required for proper metabolism. Hair zinc was low at 12 ppm (normal 160–240 ppm for this laboratory).

Dietary changes were recommended to eliminate allergic foods such as milk, and supplementation was begun with a broad spectrum vitamin-mineral preparation containing zinc in a proper physiologic ratio with other minerals. Within two months the patient's appetite improved and her growth accelerated. Within a year she was within the twenty-fifth percentile for her age in both height and weight and was rapidly catching up with other children in her age group. In this case, zinc therapy in safe, low doses was felt to be diagnostic as well as therapeutic. Because of the unreliability of blood levels of zinc in the diagnosis of zinc deficiency it was felt that to give safe doses of zinc therapeutically in a preparation with other minerals was a safe approach to treatment. It must be remembered that when additional zinc is given there must be a proper amount of copper, manganese, selenium and other micronutrients to avoid inhibition by zinc of the uptake of these other substances. If zinc is given in still larger concentrations, it is safest to give the extra zinc at bedtime, long after the last meal of the day and quite separate from the balanced multiple vitamin and mineral preparation, so that there is no competition for uptake sites on the intestine and no decrease in absorption of other minerals which might be adequate before treatment but which could be blocked in their absorption by simultaneously giving high doses of zinc.

B.G., a sixty-eight-year-old male patient suffered with symptoms of enlargement of the prostate gland with decreased ability to empty his bladder. He also had diminished taste sensation and white spots on his fingernails. Hair analysis showed decreased zinc at far below the lower limits of the normal reference range. He, too, was treated with a balanced multiple vitamin-mineral preparation with zinc in a proper ratio with other micronutrients taken following each meal. He was given 40 mg of zinc separately at bedtime on an empty stomach, in addition to the 20 mg of zinc in the vitamin-mineral following each meal, for a total of 60 mg of elemental zinc supplementation per day.

On this regimen his sense of taste improved and his urinary symptoms were gradually relieved. His fingernails became stronger and the white spots disappeared. In this case the administration of zinc, in combination with a balanced multiple vitamin-mineral preparation, was diagnostic as well as therapeutic.

REFERENCES

1 Todd, W. R. 1934. *Amer. J. Physiol.* 107:146–156.

2 Prasad, A. S. *et al.* 1963. *J. Lab. Clin. Med.* 61:537–549.

3 Prasad, A. S. March/April 1981. *Nutrition Today* 10.

4 National Research Council. 1980. *Recommended Dietary Allowances.* (9th ed.) Washington, D.C.: National Academy of Sciences.

5 Food and Nutrition Board (NRC). 1970. *Zinc in Human Nutrition.* Washington, D. C.: National Academy of Sciences.

6 O'Dell, B. L. 1969. *Amer. J. Clin. Nutr.* 22:1315–1322.

7 O'Dell, B. L. and Savage, J. E. 1960. *Proc. Soc. Exp. Biol. Med.* 103:304–306.

8 Spencer, H. and Kramer, L. November/December 1980. *Food and Nutr. News* 52(2) 2.

9 Oberleas, D. and Prasad, A. S. 1976. In: *Trace Elements in Human Health and Disease*. New York: Academic Press, pp. 155–162.

10 Reinhold, J. G. *et al. Trace Elements*, Oberleas and Prasad, pp. 163–180.

11 Whiting, F. and Bezeau, L. M. 1958. *Can. J. Anim. Sci.* 38:109–117.

12 Wasserman, R. H. 1962. *J. Nutr.* 77:69–80.

13 Becker, W. M. and Hoekstra, W. G. 1966. *J. Nutr.* 90:301–309.

14 Chang, I. H. *et al.* 1969. *Metabolism* 18:625–629.

15 Pecoud, A. *et al.* 1975. *Clin. Pharm. & Therap.* 17:469.

16 McCance, R.A. and Widdowson, E. M. 1942. *Biochem. J*, 36:692–696.

17 Sheline, G. E. *et al.* 1943. *J. Biol. Chem.* 147:409–414.

18 Sullivan, J. F. and Lankford, H. G. 1962. *Amer. J. Clin. Nutr.* 10:153–157.

19 Halstead, J. A., Smith, J. C. and Irwin, M. I. 1974. *J. Nutr.* 140(3) 345–378.

20 Prasad, A. S. *et al.* 1963. *Arch. Intern. Med.* 111:407.

21 Halstead, J. A. 1970. *Trans. Amer. Clin. Climat. Assoc.* 82:170–176.

22 Hambidge, K. M. *et al.* 1972. *Pediat. Res.* 6:868–874.

23 Hurley, L. S. and Swenerton, H. 1966. *Proc. Soc. Exp. Biol. Med.* 123:692–696.

24 Halstead, J. A. and Smith, J. C. 1970. *Lancet* 1:322.

25 Portnoy, B. and Molokhia, M. 1974. *J. Derm.* 91:701.

26 Oberleas *et al.* July 1971. *Psychopharmacology Bulletin*.

27 Ronaghy, H. A. July 10, 1972. *Chem. Eng. News*.

28 Also reported by Gottlieb, W. January 1979. *Prevention* 94.

29 Gordus, A. 1974. ACS national meeting, reported in *Prevention* 186 (January 1975).

30 Strain, W. H. *et al.* 1953. *Univ. Rochester Reports*.

31 Pories, W. J. *et al.* January 21, 1967. *Lancet* 121–124.

32 Pories, W. J. *et al.* 1967. *Clin. Med.* 74:21–26.

33 Pories, W. J. *et al.* 1967. *Annals of Surgery* 165(3) 432–436.

34 Henzel, J. H. *et al.* 1967. *Archives of Surgery* 95:991–999.

35 Henzel, J. H. *et al..* 1970. *Archives of Surgery* 100:349–357.

36 Lichti, E. L. *et al.* 1971. *Amer. J. Surg.* 121:665–668.

37 Lichti, E. L. *et al.* 1971. In: *Trace Subs. Envirn. Health* IV Hemphill, D., ed., U. Missouri.

38 Sedlacek, T. U. *et al.* 1976. *Gynecologic Oncology* v. 4.

39 Pullen, F. W. 1974. In: *Clin. App. Zinc Met.*, W. J. Pories, ed. Springfield, IL: Thomas.

40 Calhoun, N. R. *et al.* September 1974. *Clin. Orthopedics* 103:213–234.

41 Pekarek, R. S. April 1976. Fed. Amer. Soc. Exp. Biology Annual Meeting, Atlantic City, New Jersey.

42 Pekarek, R. S. *et al.* 1979. *Amer. J. Clin. Nutr.* 32:1466–1471.

43 Fraker, P. J. *et al.* 1977. *J. Nutr.* 107:1889.

44 Luecke, R. W. *et al.* 1978. *J. Nutr.* 108:881.

45 Good, R. A. *et al.* 1979. *Clin. Bull.* 9(1) 3.

46 Newberne, P. M. and Fong, Y. Y. February 11, 1978. *Sci. News* 113(6):88.

47 Henzel, J. H. *et al.* In: *Clin. App. Zinc Metabolism*, W. J. Pories, ed. Springfield, IL: Thomas, pp. 336–341.

48 Reported in *Let's Live* 17–18, May 1975.

49 Prasad, A. S. *et al.* 1978. *JAMA* 240:2166–2168.

50 Sandstead, H. H. 1978. *JAMA* 240:2188–2189.

51 Taper, L. J. *et al.* 1980. *Amer. J. Clin. Nutr.* 33(5) 1077–1082.

52 Klevay, L. M. and Hyg, S. D. 1973. *Amer. J. Clin. Nutr.* 26:1060.

53 Klevay, L. M. April 1975. American Chemical Society Meeting, Philadelphia, PA.

54 Klevay, L. M. April 1976. FASEB Meeting, Anaheim, CA.

55 Erdman, J. W. and Lachance, P. A. 1974. *Nutr. Reports Int.* 9(5):319–329.

56 Hooper, P. L. *et al.* 1980. *J. Amer. Med. Assoc.* 244(17):1960–1961.

57 Woo, W., *et al.* 1981. *Amer. J. Clin. Nutr.* 34(1):120–121.

58 Fischer, P. W. F. *et al.* 1980. *Amer. J. Clin. Nutr.* 33(5):1019–1025.

59 Freeland-Graves, J. H. *et al.* 1980. *Nutr. Rep. Int.* 22(2):285–293.

60 Harvey, P. W. *et al.* 1981. *J. Nutr.* 111(4):639–647.

61 *Bulletin on Sinai Hospital of Detroit.* 1975. 23:81.

62 Lekakis, J. and Kalofoutis, A. 1980. *Clin. Chem.* 26(12):1660–1661.

63 Singal, P. K. *et al.* 1981. *Lab. Invest.* 44(5):426–433.

64 Marmar, J. L. *et al.* 1975. *Fertility and Sterility* 26:1057.

65 Lattimer, J. K. July 1976. *Executive Health* 12(10):1–6.

66 Lawson and Fischer. 1951. *Canadian Medical J.*

67 Bush, I. M. *et al.* Amer. Urological Assoc. Meeting (1972) and AMA Meeting (1974).

68 Smith, J. E., Brown, E. D. and Smith, J. L. 1974. *J. Lab. Clin. Med.* 84(5):692–697.

69 Smith, J. C. May 31, 1975. *Lancet.*

70 Michaelsson, G. *et al. Arch. Derm.*

71 May 1977. U. of Cal. study reported in *Prevention* 63.

72 *Lancet.* December 24 and 31, 1977.

73 *Arch. Derm.* September 1977.

74 Rivin, S. 1958. *Lancet* 1363.

75 Husain, S. L. May 31, 1969. *Lancet* 1069–1071.

76 Haeger, K. *et al.* 1972. *J. Vascular Dis.* 1.

77 Haeger, K. *et al.* 1974. *J. Vascular Dis.* 3.

78 Frommer, D. J. November 22, 1975. *Med. J. Australia.*

79 Simkin, P. S. September 11, 1976. *Lancet.*

80 Henkin, R. I. and Aamodt, R. L. July 26, 1971. *J. Amer. Med. Assoc.*

81 July 1981. As reported in *Food Development* 10.

82 Food and Nutrition Board. 1970. *Zinc in Human Nutrition.* Washington, D. C.: National Academy of Sciences.

83 *Medical World News.* August 4, 1972.

84 Reinhold, J. G. *et al.* 1976. In: *Trace Elements in Human Health and Disease,* vol. 1, Prasad, A. S., ed. New York: Academic Press, p. 163.

85 Oberleas, D. *et al.* 1962. *J. Animal Sci.* 21:57.

86 O'Dell, B. L. and Savage, J. E. 1960. *Proc. Soc. Exp. Biol. Med.* 103:304.

87 Mertz, W. 1970. *Fed. Proc.* 29:1482–1488.

88 Czerniejewski, C. P. *et al.* 1964. *Cereal Chem.* 41:65–72.

89 Schroeder, H. A. 1971. *Amer. J. Clin. Nutr.* 24:562–573.

90 Schroeder, H. A. *et al.* 1967. *J. Chronic Dis.* 20:179–210.

91 Osis, D. *et al.* 1972. *Amer. J. Clin. Nutr.* 25:582–588.

92 Miller,W. J. and Miller, J. K. 1963. *J. Dairy Sci.* 46:581–583.

93 Sandstead, H. H. 1973. *Amer. J. Clin. Nutr.* 26:1251–1260.

94 Holden, J. M. *et al.* 1979. *J. Amer. Diet. Assoc.* 75:23–28.

95 Hambidge, K. M. 1972. *Pediatr. Res.* 6:868–874.

96 Sandstead, H. H. *et al.* 1980. *Clin. Res.* Also see Greeley, S. and Sandstead, H. H. 1980. *Contem. Nutr.* 5(4):1–2.

97 Pfeiffer, C. C. 1975. *Mental and Elemental Nutrients.* New Canaan, CT.: Keats Publishing, pp. 231–235.

98 Amador. December 6, 1975. *Lancet* 1146.

11

COPPER

Copper has been an enigma, but recent research has shed some light on its mysteries. Copper is essential to life and is found in all body tissues. Copper deficiency leads to a variety of abnormalities, including anemia, skeletal defects, degeneration of the nervous system, reproductive failure, pronounced cardiovascular lesions, elevated blood cholesterol, impaired immunity and defects in the pigmentation and structure of hair.[1,21] However, since copper is involved in many body processes throughout the body, it is difficult to discover all of the copper-involved functions or to uncover the more subtle effects of marginal copper deficiency.

The range of optimum copper intake may be narrow, as preliminary evidence suggests that excessive copper may produce subtle detrimental effects before gross toxicity is observed.

An average 155-pound adult has 75 mg copper (range 50 to 120 mg) with about one-third of that fairly evenly divided between the liver and brain, one-third in the musculature, and the remaining third dispersed in other tissues.[2,3] More than a dozen enzymes have been found to contain copper.[4] The best studied of the more than one dozen copper-containing enzymes are superoxide dismutase, cyctochrome C oxidase, catalase, dopamine hydroxylase, urincase, tryptophan dioxygenase, lecithinase and other monoamine and diamine oxidases. Copper, itself, is catalytic in the oxidation of vitamin C, and there are indications that an enzyme yet to be isolated, ascorbate oxidase, contains copper.[5]

Much of the earlier research on copper dealt with how copper promotes iron absorption and utilization. Several attractive mechanisms that explain copper's essential role in iron absorption, transport and incorporation into red blood cells have been proposed, but the question of how it is accomplished is unresolved.[6] Copper deficiency causes bone demineralization.[5]

However, the function of copper in maintaining the integrity of the cardiovascular system may be more important than its role in forming red blood cells. Copper-deficient animals and people having a genetic defect impairing copper utilization (Menkes' disease) have twisted blood vessels and massive internal hemorrhages. This probably results from a collagen protein defect in the blood vessels. Copper-deficient aortas contain less "mature" elastin and a higher proportion of soluble collagen than normal.[7]

Absorption, storage and excretion

Absorption of copper occurs primarily in the stomach and upper small intestine. Absorption is probably mostly due to simple diffusion, although an undetermined amount of copper may be transported through the intestinal walls by metallothionein which also may transport zinc and cadmium.[8] This would explain their antagonistic relationship. Mercury, lead, vitamin C, sulfides, raw meat, silver and possibly calcium and molybdenum also decrease the absorption of copper.[6,8] Amino acids and fresh vegetables may increase copper absorption.

The interactions of zinc, copper and iron have been reviewed by Dr. George Davis.[9] Typically, about 30 percent of ingested copper is absorbed. In diets containing 2 to 5 mg copper, typically 0.6 to 1.6 mg would be absorbed.

Absorbed copper is transported in combination with albumin to the liver where the copper is then incorporated into a blue protein called ceruloplasmin. The normal level of copper in the blood is 100 mcg, of which approximately 90 percent is in ceruloplasmin.[6] There is an indication that when the quantity of ceruloplasmin is adequate, it inhibits the intestinal absorption of copper.[10]

The liver controls copper storage and excretion. Excess copper is excreted via the bile,[11] although as the copper intake increases, the amount retained also increases.[12]

The amount of copper stored in the liver is approximately 30 percent of the total body copper content. About 80 percent of copper excretion is via the bile, about 15 percent diffuses into the intestine, and the remainder is excreted in the urine.

Heart disease

The complex interrelationship between zinc and copper with heart disease was discussed in the last chapter. In essence, a copper deficiency leads to an enlarged heart, weak blood vessels and elevated blood cholesterol. A zinc excess aggravates the problem of copper deficiency. Please refer to the preceding chapter for details.

Arthritis

Do you remember the fad of wearing copper bracelets to reduce the pain of arthritis? This fad of the mid- and late-1970s was based on folklore. Anyone who claimed that the copper bracelets reduced arthritic pain was quickly reminded of how arthritis is unpredictable and often "comes and goes," or the placebo effect—that merely believing something will work often makes pain disappear.

Surely objective, scientifically controlled experiments would show that copper bracelets for the purpose of reducing the pain of arthritis is a fraudulent concept. We could find no controlled studies in the U.S. literature— probably because *everyone knows* that they couldn't work. And we could only find non-professional newspaper accounts of controlled studies in Australia.[13]

Dr. Ray Walker of the University of Newcastle in New South Wales found that thirty-one of forty arthritis patients felt better wearing the copper bracelets. Seventeen patients said there was less pain while they wore the bracelets and fourteen others reported that they were unwilling to carry on for two months without the bracelets.

Dr. Walker was a skeptic and wanted to disprove the suggested link. He had authentic-looking "imitation copper" bracelets made out of aluminum. One group wore copper bracelets and the other group wore look-alike bracelets. Although patients in both groups improved, many more in the copper bracelet group improved.

Dr. Walker discovered that the copper bracelets lost an average of 13 mg per month. The copper dissolves in sweat and is absorbed through the skin. Another skeptic, a columnist in a scientific journal, investigated the issue after a scientist reader reported beneficial effects of a copper bracelet on his wife.

She had been wearing it, but gave it up because it tarnished and stained her skin green. The scientist thought that perhaps fatty acids in the skin might be dissolving the oxide on the surface of the bracelet, producing fat-soluble copper soaps that could be absorbed through the skin.

The columnist tried the bracelet himself and his arthritis pains were alleviated. The skin under the bracelet became green. He licked the place and got the metallic taste of copper salts. Water would not remove the stain. He had to use soap to get it off. He decided that indeed the copper was migrating into the body through the skin.

Still believe there is nothing to it? Well, keep in mind that superoxide dismutase is being considered as an anti-inflammatory drug for use in arthritis. Superoxide dismutase is an enzyme containing copper and zinc.

Dr. Knud Lund-Olesen of Ringe City Hospital in Denmark has given superoxide dismutase to 200 arthritis sufferers. He remarked in a recent newspaper interview, "It's a real breakthrough . . . [superoxide dismutase] has proved safe and effective in all the patients we gave injections."

According to Dr. Kerstin B. Menander-Huber, medical director of Diagnostic Data Inc., [superoxide dismutase] proved to be "significantly more effective than placebo, as effective as gold, and without side effects."

Dr. James L. Goddard, former Assistant Surgeon General of the U.S., labeled superoxide dismutase "a remarkable substance" for treating arthritis which affects more than 22 million Americans.

It appears that injectable superoxide dismutase will relieve the morning stiffness, pain and swollen joints in about 85 percent of arthritis patients. Oral superoxide dismutase should also be of benefit, but it is destroyed by stomach acid and must be specifically formulated to pass through the acid stomach into the alkaline small intestine without losing potency.

Do we think copper bracelets are helpful? We don't know, but we feel that superoxide dismutase production in the body is. Copper deficiency would limit superoxide dismutase production. If a copper-deficient person absorbs copper through the skin, then normal amounts of superoxide dismutase may be produced and inflammation and pain reduced.

Other copper-complex compounds have been found to be anti-inflammatory.[14-17] Aspirin, phenylbutazone, indomethicin, dexamethasone and others combine with the copper in the tissue of the stomach lining. The sequestered copper is then transported to the site of the inflammation.[18] Theoretically, one 5-grain aspirin tablet can tie up three times as much copper as our entire body contains.[19]

The localized depletion of copper from the stomach lining by copper-sequestering drugs may allow inflammation in the stomach and small intestine that can lead to ulceration.

Ulcers

Dr. John Sorenson of the University of Cincinnati College of Medicine has found during his research on anti-inflammatory drugs for arthritis, that copper chelates and complexes are potent antiulcer agents in laboratory animals.[17] Besides localized copper deficiency in the stomach lining, it has been found that ulcer patients average 23 percent less copper in their bodies.[19]

Schizophrenia

Dr. Carl Pfeiffer of the Brain Bio Center in Princeton, New Jersey, has postulated that excessive (but not toxic) copper and iron and/or zinc and manganese deficiencies are primary factors in one type of schizophrenia, called "histapenia" (low blood histamine).[20] Young schizophrenic women usually have extremely elevated blood copper levels well above normal (375 microgram percent vs. a normal level of 130). Dr. Pfeiffer also notes that histapenic schizophrenia responds to treatment which rids the body of copper. Ceruloplasmin, the copper-carrying protein, has histaminase activity which destroys histamine.

The Pill and the blues

Oral contraceptives affect metabolism in various ways. Women either pregnant or on the Pill have about a twofold rise in blood levels of copper. In healthy women not on the Pill, blood levels of copper normally averaged 130 micogram per deciliter. This normal level may rise in late pregnancy to around 250 mcg/dl. In birth control pill users, the blood level of copper ranges above 200 mcg/dl, sometimes going over 300 mcg/dl. In six women experiencing clinical side effects from the Pill, blood levels of copper were all found to be higher than 300 mcg/dl.[21-22]

Dr. Pfeiffer has suggested that since after delivery a period of two to three months is required before the original blood copper level is reached, it may be a factor in causing postpartum depression and psychosis.[10] However, more data is needed before a solid conclusion can be drawn from this interesting observation.

Aging

Copper is needed for vital cross-linking or handcuffing of molecules of protein such as collagen and elastin together to form firm tissue and blood vessels. Copper deficiency results in immature uncross-linked vessels that leak or break open.

However, excessive (but not toxic) levels of copper may lead to too many cross-linkages and thus a stiffening of tissues and blood vessels. When the skin collagen is overly cross-linked it is more like leather than supple skin. Excessive sunlight can prematurely age skin by cross-linking of skin protein, and so may excessive copper.[4]

In addition, excessive copper levels may contribute to the release of highly reactive molecular fragments called "free radicals" which in turn can produce rancid fats (lipid peroxidation) which can disrupt cell membranes. Such cellular damage, if unchecked, can accelerate aging or induce pre-cancerous changes.[4,23]

Hypothyroidism

Zinc and copper are both needed at the cell level for the conversion of thyroxin (T4) to tri-iodothyronine (T3) which is the active intracellular thyroid hormone. Copper and zinc deficiencies can therefore cause hypothyroidism, clinically at the cell level, with low basal metabolism rates, low axillary temperatures, as described in the works of Dr. Broda Barnes, even though routine blood testing of the most sophisticated type for thyroid hormone levels is normal. T4 and T3 levels can be completely normal in blood, but the T4 can still be impeded in its conversion to T3 at the cell membrane level in order to be effective in facilitating oxidative respiration in the cell itself. This also relates to lipid metabolism and risk of atherosclerosis.

Copper transport diseases

Copper deficiencies within the body can be caused by genetic defects that lead to copper absorption or transportation problems. The lack of a critical component in the body in these instances is the problem rather than the amount of copper in the diet.

Menkes' disease is a reduced ability to transfer copper across absorptive cells of the intestine. Infants having Menkes' disease absorb only about 12 percent of ingested copper in comparison to 46 percent in normal persons. In addition, most of the absorbed copper is stored in the liver for extended periods. Copper supplements and injected copper have not been measurably effective in halting the progress of the disease, which is usually fatal within the first year.

Wilson's disease is a genetic defect leading to prolonged storage and accumulation of copper in the liver, and a lack of circulating ceruloplasmin-bound copper in the blood. Hair content is not elevated in Wilson's disease. Low-copper diets and penicillamine (a drug that increases excretion of metals like copper) have been beneficial to Wilson's disease patients.

Other rarer genetic-related copper impairment diseases have been described.

Sources and needs

Copper is ubiquitous in the diet, and dietary deficiencies did not normally occur with past diets. However, concern has been expressed that depleted soils and increased reliance on highly processed foods may present an increased problem. One researcher, Dr. Carl Pfeiffer, contended in 1970 that there were still more individuals receiving too much copper in their diets than there were individuals receiving too little. We contend that copper deficiency is the more common of the two.

The Recommended Dietary Allowance for adults is 2–3 mg per day. Older surveys had indicated that most diets provided between 2 and 5 mg daily, but the accuracy of these surveys is questioned.[1] Recent surveys of a variety of diets have indicated much lower intakes, often substantially below 1 mg per day.[24] Only two of fifteen different diets had 2 mg, and some contained as little as two-tenths of a milligram. In a New Zealand survey, half of self-chosen diets provided less than 2 mg per day, and 5 percent provided less than 1 mg per day.[25]

Dr. Leslie Klevay of the U.S. Department of Agriculture's Research Service in Grand Forks, North Dakota compared the copper content of forty-seven foods purchased in 1942 with the same kinds of food bought in 1966. He found that two-thirds of the 1966 foods contained less copper than the 1942 foods.

It is not certain whether the decline represents differences in the accuracy of analysis, variation due to species differences, or variations due to soil content. The latter is the most probable.

Researchers at Rutgers University in New Jersey have found that the amount of copper in different samples of snap beans varied from 69 parts per million down to 3 ppm. Tomatoes varied from no detectable copper to 52 ppm.

In a recent four-year study by Albion Laboratories of over 4000 food samples grown in the Midwest, it was found that the copper content of corn declined 68 percent during that period.[19]

Thus it appears that we can't trust food tables, because the copper content of foods varies with the copper content of the soil they are grown in, as well as the copper content of any water used in food preparation. Table 11.1 lists several foods according to typical copper content.

TABLE 11.1 SOURCES OF COPPER

Milligrams (mg) per 100 grams edible portion (100 grams = 3½ oz.)

Oysters	13.7	Gelatin	0.4
Brazil nuts	2.3	Shrimp	0.3
Soy lecithin	2.1	Olive oil	0.3
Almonds	1.4	Clams	0.3
Hazelnuts	1.3	Carrot	0.3
Walnuts	1.3	Coconut	0.3
Pecans	1.3	Garlic	0.3
Split peas, dry	1.2	Millet	0.2
Beef liver	1.1	Whole wheat	0.2
Buckwheat	0.8	Chicken	0.2
Peanuts	0.8	Eggs	0.2
Cod liver oil	0.7	Corn oil	0.2
Lamb chops	0.7	Ginger root	0.2
Sunflower oil	0.5	Molasses	0.2
Butter	0.4	Turnips	0.2
Rye grain	0.4	Green peas	0.1
Pork loin	0.4	Papaya	0.1
Barley	0.4	Apple	0.1

Black pepper, thyme, paprika, bay leaves, and active dry yeast are also high in copper.

Source: MineraLab, Inc.

In general though, we can conclude that rich food sources of copper are oysters, nuts, liver, kidney, corn oil margarine and dried legumes. The contribution of drinking water to the total copper intake varies with the type of piping and hardness of water.[26] More will be said of this in the following section.

Toxicity

Copper is relatively non-toxic. A World Health Organization report states that no deleterious effects in man would be expected from a copper intake of 0.5 milligram per kilogram of body weight per day.[27] This represents a daily intake of 25 mg for a 110-pound person or 35 mg for a 154-pound person. The Food and Nutrition Board of the National Academy of Sciences assumes that an occasional intake of up to 10 mg is safe for adults.[1]

A U.S. Geological Survey Bulletin suggests that 2 to 5 mg per day will not change the body's copper balance, and that 250 to 500 mg per day would be toxic.[28]

Dr. Carl Pfeiffer has shown that in some suburban homes, individual water systems where the well water is unusually acid can produce copper intoxication.[20] He cites a home in Peapack, New Jersey where the well water had 0.03 parts per million copper, the upper bath had 0.32 ppm and an outside faucet had 1.62 ppm. In the house, only the upper bathroom tap had drinkable water by U.S. Public Health Service standards which set a maximum of 1 ppm copper.

Dr. Pfeiffer also cites an Australian report of copper intoxication leading to the death of a fourteen-month-old child. The well water was in the acid pH range (4 as opposed to neutral at 7) and copper plumbing was used. The water contained nine to ten times the suggested maximum copper content.

Thus the best approach seems to assure an adequate copper-content diet, without overdoing it.

Hair analysis

Elevated hair copper is clinically meaningful. Published scientific research by L.M. Klevay, in a number of medical journals, indicates a statistically significant correlation between liver copper and hair copper at the 99.9 percent confidence level.[29-31] An exception has recently been published by Epstein[32] which indicates that in primary biliary cirrhosis of the liver and perhaps in other liver diseases, hair copper does not correlate with liver copper. We must therefore, verify our hair copper evaluations by assuring that the subject has a healthy liver.

Elevated hair copper may also result from external contamination. Many swimming pools are treated with chemicals which extract copper salts from the pipes through which the water is circulated during purification and other treatments. These copper salts can be seen to cause a bluish tint in many swimming pools and a bluish contamination to the walls of the pool. If hair copper is elevated in an individual who does not normally swim in a treated swimming pool and if such an individual is determined to have normal liver function, it is very likely that that person is suffering with copper toxicity.

Elevated hair copper is increasingly being found through hair analysis. In those individuals in whom external contamination is not a cause, the increased copper is usually a result of highly corrosive drinking water coming through copper plumbing in the home. Fossil fuels are causing increasing contamination of the atmosphere with sulfuric and nitric acid residues, resulting in acid rains which are far more corrosive than in past decades. Well water and spring water are much more likely to be corrosive than city water supplies. City water is customarily treated with many chemicals to buffer the acid and to reduce the corrosiveness.

Patients found to have elevated hair copper levels caused by too much copper in their diets or in their drinking water are frequently found to have a variety of clinical symptoms which are commonly diagnosed as "neurotic." Such symptoms include fatigue, nervousness, depression, irritability, muscle and joint pain, tiredness, behavior problems, learning disabilities and mental diseases. In such patients the hair concentration of copper reflects the excess body burden and is frequently measured at levels up to six times the upper limits of normal. Ceruloplasmin, the copper-binding protein in the blood, is normal and serum copper is usually also within the normal range in these patients. The only other way to diagnose this type of copper toxicity is by measuring a 24-hour urinary copper excretion. Urinary copper output is often several times above the upper limits of normal. This is a very significant clinical observation which has been made by numerous clinicians utilizing hair analysis in their practices but which has not yet been subjected to controlled scientific studies and to our knowledge has not yet been published in the scientific literature.

It is well documented that estrogen, the female hormone contained in birth control pills, causes copper depletion from the liver. Copper moves from intracellular to extra-cellular compartments within the body. Serum or blood copper goes up while liver copper goes down. Because hair copper reflects the intracellular copper levels, such as copper within the liver, low hair copper is frequently seen in female patients utilizing oral contraceptives. Copper therapy is indicated in such patients, in combination with a physiologic ratio of other trace minerals and vitamins. Oral contraceptive tablets increase the need for vitamin B6, folic acid and other vitamins and minerals as well. You now can begin to understand how complex this problem can be.

Individuals with significant elevations of hair copper should be tested further by measuring blood levels of copper, by measuring ceruloplasmin in the blood and by measuring a 24-hour copper urinary excretion.

It has also been reported that patients with Wilson's disease, otherwise known as hepatolenticular degeneration, may have normal or low hair copper in the presence of copper toxicity within other tissues of the body. This is a disease state in which copper supplementation can be very dangerous and can increase an already existing copper toxicity, but the diagnosis can be completely missed on a hair analysis.

In the absence of external contamination, elevated hair copper has been proven to be a clinically significant screening test for copper toxicity. The scientific literature concerning evidence for the diagnosis of copper deficiency based on low hair copper concentrations is contradictory, especially in the case of Wilson's disease or other liver disease such as cirrhosis. These are but a few examples which emphasize the fact that hair analysis is only a screening test, depending on more definitive blood, urine and tissue testing to confirm a diagnosis before treatment is initiated.

Case Histories

T.M.F. was a thirty-six-year-old female attorney with symptoms of depression and wide mood swings, so severe that she had more than once attempted suicide. She had not found relief by following many traditional treatments. Other symptoms included chronic nasal stuffiness, chest pains and tightness which were related to emotional stress, cardiac palpitations and migraine headaches. She was generally just not feeling well, although she was able to function in her profession.

Hair mineral levels detected an extremely elevated copper of 300 ppm, ten times the upper limit of normal. This was confirmed to be systemic toxicity, as opposed to external contamination, by a 24-hour urine copper excretion which was 57 micrograms per 24 hours, almost twice normal. Serum amino acid fractionation revealed serine to be one-half normal, arginine to be absent and isoleucine to be approximately one-fourth of normal. Serum zinc, copper and ceruloplasmin (a copper-binding protein) were all normal. Investigation for environmental sources of copper were unrevealing, and her husband's measurements were completely normal in this regard. He shared all food, water and environmental exposures with his wife. Based on these findings, it is likely that this patient suffered with a metabolic lesion which caused selective increase in copper absorption (a variant of copper storage disease, which unlike Wilson's disease does not have abnormal ceruloplasmin).

Nutritional treatment which did not involve the use of drugs to block copper uptake, included the use of zinc and manganese in a balance of other vitamins, minerals and amino acids free from supplemental copper. All dietary and other exposure to copper were avoided to whatever extent was practical. The patient was counseled on good general nutrition and exercise conditioning. On this regiment she has improved markedly and has been outspoken in her praise for wholistic medicine.

R.T.R. was a six-year-old male child who came under treatment after having been seen and examined by a large of number of physicians, specialists, well-known medical clinics and major medical centers specializing in learning disabilities and mentally disturbed children. His family had been told

158

that he was autistic and that they simply "had to live with it." They were told that there was no treatment and that it was a hopeless case. He was poorly coordinated and repeatedly fell, becoming involved in minor accidents requiring multiple stitches. He had numerous colds, ear infections, croup and other conditions requiring antibiotics. He refused to talk and would not make eye contact. He would not cuddle and was somewhat destructive in his behavior. He definitely preferred environmental and mechanical stimuli to human contact and engaged in repetitive rocking movements. Neurological, pediatric, psychological and speech therapy consultations and evaluations had been to no avail. At six years he was still not talking. No organic cause was found for his symptoms.

On taking a careful history it was learned that this boy had improved somewhat by manipulating his diet to eliminate possible allergic foods. A hair tissue mineral analysis showed copper to be low at approximately one-half the lower limits of normal (5 percent the upper limits of normal). Zinc and chromium were also low.

Fasting plasma amino acids showed cystine to be low at approximately 10 percent the normal for his age. Cystine is normally produced by converting methionine, using other nutrients in the body, but these biochemical pathways require vitamins and minerals to proceed. Otherwise, the enzymes are not active.

The history suggested food allergy and the deficient minerals suggested impaired absorption of nutrients. He was placed on an elimination diet which excluded those foods most likely to be causing allergies. Vitamin and mineral supplementation was given to replenish his body. The amino acid cystine was supplemented. Large doses of vitamin C, B6 and other B-complex vitamins were given because of studies which have indicated benefit in autistic children. These treatments utilized only naturally occurring nutrients, with no drugs. Within a year this boy was cuddling, seeking human companionship, speaking in complete sentences, dressing himself, feeding himself and making rapid progress toward functioning at a normal level for his age. His muscular coordination was much improved.

When first seen he fit all the diagnostic criteria to be "autistic," but following a nutritional program, based in part on hair tissue mineral analysis, he has made rapid progress toward normal.

Three young women, J.H., thirty years old, M.T., thirty-three years old and K.C., thirty-one years old, were all found to be poisoned with copper and lead. These three young women lived in the same house, shared the same drinking water and environment, but were genetically unrelated. Hair mineral analysis showed all three to have elevated copper and elevated lead. J.H. had a 24-hour urine copper excretion measured to confirm that this was not external contamination on the hair but was actually a reflection of body concentrations. The urine output was more than four times the normal.

PATIENT	Hair Copper (Normal level 12–35 PPM)	Hair Lead (Safe level 0–20 PPM)	24-hour urinary copper excretion	Normal 7.5-24 mcg/24h
J.H.	120	22	204	
M.T.	200	29	—	
K.C.	395	109	—	

From the data it is clear that the relative degree of lead elevation parallels the degree of copper elevation. These three ladies lived in the country where their water was obtained from a soft-water spring. The house had copper plumbing. Copper plumbing is joined together with lead solder. This unstable, corrosive water coming through the lead and copper pipes dissolved these metals in poisonous concentrations which were then ingested by the patients.

All three had similar symptoms of extreme fatigue, irritability, multiple muscle and joint aches and recurrent headaches. After changing their water supply and taking the proper treatments to correct for these poisonous levels of copper and lead, the symptoms improved dramatically.

REFERENCES

1 National Research Council. 1980. Recommended Dietary Allowances. (9th ed.) Washington, D.C.: National Academy of Sciences, p. 151.

2 Tipton, I. H. and Cook, M. J. 1963. *Health Phys.* 9:103–145

3 Sumino, K. *et al.* 1975. *Arch. Environ. Health* 30:487–494.

4 Hochstein, P. *et al.* 1980. *Annals N. Y. Acad. Sci.* 240–248.

5 *Nutr. Rev.* 1981. 39(9) 347–349.

6 O'Dell, B. L. 1976. In: *Present Knowledge in Nutrition.* (4th ed.) New York: Nutr. Foundation, p. 305.

7 Underwood, E. J. 1971. In: *Trace Elements in Human and Animal Nutrition.* (3rd ed.) New York: Academic Press, pp. 57–115.

8 Evans, G. W. 1973. *Physiol. Rev.* 53:535–570.

9 Davis, G.K. 1980. *Annals N. Y. Acad. Sci.* 130–139.

10 Pfeiffer, C. 1975. *Mental and Elemental Nutrients.* New Canaan, CT: Keats Publishing, pp. 326–327.

11 Cartwright, G. E. and Wintrobe, M. M. 1964. *Amer. J. Clin. Nutr.* 14:224–232.

12 Waisman, J. *et al.* 1967. *Amer. J. Pathol.* 51(1):117–135.

13 Burt, Bill reported in 1978 *National Enquirer.*

14 Sorenson, J. April 1974. Spring Meeting, American Chemical Society, Los Angeles, CA.

15 Anon. April 8, 1974. *Chem. and Eng. News* 24.

16 Sorenson, J. April 1975. Spring Meeting, American Chemical Society.

17 Anon. April 25, 1975. *Chem. and Eng. News* 36–37.

18 Sorenson, J. 1976. *JAMA.*

19 Ashmead, D. November 1976. *Bestways* 68–70.

20 Pfeiffer, C. and Iliev, V. 1972. *Intern. Rev. Neurobiol.* 144–165.

21 Smith, J. C. September 1974. Trace Elements and Human Disease Symp. Detroit.

22 Anon. September 13, 1974. *Med. World News.* 32.

23 Prohaska, J. and Lukasewycz, O. 1981. *Science* 213:559.

24 Klevay, L. M. 1975. *Nutr. Rep. Int.* 11:237–242.

25 Guthrie B. E. 1973. *Proc. U Otago Med. Sch.* 51:47–49.

26 Schroeder, H. A. *et al.* 1966. *J. Chron. Dis.* 19:1007–1034.

27 Food and Agriculture Organization, WHO. 1971. Tech. Rept. No. 462.

28 Gough, L. P. *et al.* 1979. *U. S. Geol. Surv. Bull.* 1466.

29 Klevay, L. M. 1970. *Amer. J. Clin. Nutrition.* 23(3):284–289.

30 Klevay, L. M. 1970. *Amer. J. Clin. Nutrition* 23(9):1194–1202.

31 Klevay, L. M. 1973. *Archives of Environmental Health* 23:169–172.

32 Epstein, O. *et al.* 1980. *Am. J. Clin. Nutr.* 33:965–967.

12

MANGANESE

Manganese is an underrated trace element. Although it has been deemed "essential" by the Food and Nutrition Board of the National Academy of Sciences, much still remains unknown.

Adults normally contain an average 10 to 20 mg (most of which is in bone, liver and kidney) of manganese in their bodies.[1] This small amount is essential to several critical enzymes involved in energy production, bone formation and protein metabolism.[2] Manganese is involved in the metabolism of fats and in the production of cholesterol.

Manganese is incorporated into superoxide dismutase and pyruvate carboxylase enzymes and is a co-factor necessary for the activation of many different enzyme systems including glycosyltransferase enzymes which play an important role in the production of cartilage and bone. A manganese deficiency results in abnormal bone and cartilage[2] and disc degeneration due to inadequate cartilage formation in the disc.[3]

Other signs of manganese deficiency include impaired glucose intolerance, birth defects, growth retardation, reduced fertility,[4] reduced brain function and inner-ear imbalance.[3] Severe manganese deficiency produces convulsions, skipped heartbeats, weight loss, dermatitis and hair color loss.[3,5]

Manganese is involved in the building and degrading of proteins and nucleic acid, biogenic amine metabolism[5] and is necessary for RNA chain initiation.[3] Manganese is a key component of the type of superoxide dismutase found in the mitochondria (energy factories) of cells. (Zinc and copper are the trace elements present in another superoxide dismutase.) The manganese-containing superoxide dismutase is an enzyme that protects the fragile mitochondrial membrane from undesirable attack by a very reactive form of oxygen called the superoxide radical. This is perhaps manganese's most significant role.

The role of manganese that deserves further attention is its involvement in energy production. We have mentioned that manganese-containing superoxide dismutase is required to protect the "skin" of the energy factories in cells and that manganese is required for proper glucose tolerance (energy production from blood sugar). The role of manganese in glucose tolerance is not well defined, but it is believed to be due to its involvement with enzymes such as glycosyltransferase and pyruvate carboxylase. The role of manganese in diabetes, hypoglycemia and glucose tolerance will be discussed later in this chapter.

Absorption, transport and storage

Manganese is absorbed slowly and poorly throughout the length of the small intestine.[4] Most absorbed manganese is rapidly removed from circulation by the liver although a small amount becomes bound to a transporter thought to be transferrin or "transmanganin" and passed into systemic circulation.[6] The amount of manganese absorbed may not increase appreciably with dietary increases above that needed for normal nourishment, and the circulating manganese concentration varies little with changes in dietary manganese concentration.[7]

However, manganese absorption is dependent largely on the concentration of manganese already in the body.[3] Manganese absorption is also decreased by dietary calcium, zinc, phosphorus, soyprotein, iron and cobalt whereas lecithin, choline and alcohol increase intestinal and liver uptake of manganese.[9–15] Therefore, diets that may *appear* to meet the needs for manganese may not in fact do so due to the influence of other nutrients.

Most of the manganese removed by the liver is excreted into the bile. Significant amounts are resorbed. If bile flow is overloaded or blocked, then the body regulates tissue manganese levels by excretion via pancreatic juice or the intestinal walls. Thus the tissue levels of manganese are regulated at the excretory level rather than at the site of absorption. This is an efficient system that minimizes the possibility of manganese toxicity from dietary sources but allows for deficiency because excretion can continue even in deficiency.[16]

Manganese and health

The preceding discussion clearly points out how manganese deficiency may cause skeletal abnormalities, slow bone healing, backaches due to disc problems, and sore knees due to cartilage damage. However, there are some less obvious relationships between manganese deficiency and health.

Schizophrenia

Dr. Carl Pfeiffer and his colleagues at the Brain Bio Center in Princeton have been studying the role of manganese deficiency in schizophrenia and other brain disorders. They have followed leads from the late 1920s that intravenous manganese was effective in treating schizophrenia.[17,18] Dr. Pfeiffer noted that in one type of schizophrenia the problem was excessive body copper accumulation and low manganese.[19] By clinical studies, he found that zinc (80 mg daily) and manganese (4 mg daily) were very effective in eliminating the excessive copper via the urine. The two nutrients together are more effective than either alone.[3]

Epilepsy

Manganese deficiency lowers the threshold that causes seizures,[20] and some epileptic patients are found to have low manganese levels.[21] Membrane instability due to manganese deficiency could account for the lowered seizure threshold, but this has not been adequately tested.

Manganese deficiency produces reduced levels of the neurotransmitter dopamine, and it is possible that manganese is related to other mental processes. Phenothiazine tranquilizers deplete body stores of manganese.

Manganese appears to be of value in treating tardive dyskinesia (see the chapter on aluminum).

Sugar metabolism, diabetes and hypoglycemia

Chromium and zinc are important to the normal utilization of blood sugar (glucose). However, a deficiency in manganese can also lead to glucose intolerance, which can be reversed by manganese supplementation.[22] A manganese deficiency produces defective cells in the pancreas and a smaller number of pancreas islet cells which contain fewer beta cells that manufacture insulin.[23,24] The abnormalities in the pancreatic secretion of insulin caused by manganese deficiency could contribute to diabetes or at least one type of diabetes. In 1964, Dr. L. G. Konsenko found manganese levels in diabetics to be approximately half those of non-diabetics.[25]

The literature describes one diabetic patient who did not respond to insulin, but who did respond to manganese supplementation.[26] Folk remedies have suggested that alfalfa tea helps diabetics, and alfalfa tea contains considerable levels of manganese.

Cancer

Manganese deficiency has also been noted in rheumatoid arthritis and cancer. Most cancer cells are very low in or devoid of manganese-containing superoxide dismutase. An anti-cancer preparation containing manganese as an essential cell component has been described.[27]

A 1979 article in *Medical World News* alerted physicians that manganese-superoxide dismutase seems to be one key to cancer and its therapy. "A crucial bio-chemical change that all cancers seem to share and that might be their cause has been identified by researchers at the University of Iowa and Wabash College. In fifty different cancers, some triggered by viruses or chemicals, Iowa's Dr. Larry Oberly and Wabash's Dr. Garry Buettner found a breakdown in cellular defenses against superoxides—destructive free radicals formed during aerobic metabolism. All cancer cells had little or no manganese-superoxide dismutase, the enzyme that seems to protect the nucleus and mitochondria from superoxides. The fastest growing cancers proved to have the least manganese-superoxide dismutase."[28]

Heart disease

Widespread metastatic ionic or precipitated calcium salts throughout the body's intra-and extra-cellular tissues can certainly interfere with metabolism in many ways—described in unscientific terms as "sludging."

Manganese is a very specific calcium antagonist at an intracellular level, by its action on smooth muscle and elsewhere. Dietary manganese deficiencies or manganese malabsorption can enhance the toxic effects of soft tissue calcium. The Assistant Chief of the Department of Cardiology at the Wadsworth VA Hospital in Los Angeles, a faculty member at UCLA School of Medicine, who authored a lead article in *Circulation* on calcium antagonists, stated at an American Academy of Medical Preventics meeting in Los Angeles in October 1980 that manganese was just as effective as the new and much more expensive prescription calcium antagonists, Nefedipine and Verapamil (soon to be released by the FDA). Because manganese is a mineral, not patentable and not fashionable, we can be sure that manganese will seldom be used in place of these highly expensive and more toxic prescription drugs. Also, absorption problems for manganese pose clinical barriers. Manganese competes with zinc, copper and other minerals for uptake and if oral manganese is given in large amounts it can create iatrogenic deficiencies of other trace minerals. We believe that manganese (preferably as a chelate) can be given on an empty stomach at bedtime or on first arising in the morning and in that way may be absorbed without competing with other minerals taken with meals.

Sources and needs

Due to the poor absorption and rapid excretion of manganese, the relative absorption of a specific form of manganese may be an important factor in low-manganese diets. Good food sources of manganese are nuts, whole grains and legumes. The amount of manganese in each food varies with that amount of manganese available in the soil. Thus food tables are only relative indicators of manganese content. Table 12.1 lists typical values of foods grown in good soils.

TABLE 12.1 SOURCES OF MANGANESE

Milligrams (mg) per 100 grams edible portion (100 grams = 3½ oz.)

Pecans	3.5	Swiss cheese	0.13
Brazil nuts	2.8	Corn	0.13
Almonds	2.5	Cabbage	0.11
Barley	1.8	Peach	0.10
Rye	1.3	Butter	0.09
Buckwheat	1.3	Tangerine	0.06
Split peas, dry	1.3	Peas	0.06
Whole wheat	1.1	Eggs	0.05
Walnuts	0.8	Beets	0.04
Fresh spinach	0.8	Coconut	0.04
Peanuts	0.7	Apple	0.03
Oats	0.6	Orange	0.03
Raisins	0.5	Pear	0.03

SOURCES OF MANGANESE (cont.)

Milligrams (mg) per 100 grams edible portion (100 grams = 3½ oz.)

Turnip greens	0.5	Lamb chops	0.03
Rhubarb	0.5	Pork chops	0.03
Beet greens	0.4	Cantaloupe	0.03
Brussels sprouts	0.3	Tomato	0.03
Oatmeal	0.3	Whole milk	0.02
Cornmeal	0.2	Chicken breasts	0.02
Millet	0.2	Green beans	0.02
Gorgonzola cheese	0.19	Apricot	0.02
Carrots	0.16	Beef liver	0.01
Broccoli	0.15	Scallops	0.01
Brown rice	0.14	Halibut	0.01
Wholewheat bread	0.14	Cucumber	0.01

Cloves, ginger, thyme, bay leaves, and tea are also high in manganese.

Source: MineraLab, Inc.

Depleted soils and food processing rob manganese from our diet, just as is the case with many other minerals. Dr. Pfeiffer has cited lettuce as an example where the foliage of plants may be lush without manganese.[19] If lime (calcium oxide) is applied to clay soils, the more alkaline soil will retain manganese and lettuce may grow abundantly. However, the liming will lower the manganese level in the lettuce itself.

Milling removes manganese from whole grains. White flour contains less than one-tenth the manganese of whole wheat. Cornflakes contain one-tenth the manganese of whole corn, and rice cereals one-half the manganese of whole rice.

The Recommended Dietary Allowance for manganese is 2.5 to 5 mg per day. This was determined by a study that showed manganese balance at 2.5 mg per day[29] and "in order to include an extra margin of safety" the upper range was set at 5 mg per day.[1] Why this upper limit was set so low is a mystery as it follows this statement: "The toxicity of ingested manganese to animal species is low, and concentrations of more than 1000 micrograms per gram of diet must be fed to produce signs of toxicity." Since a typical American diet contains at least a pound and a quarter of caloric matter, this would be 600 mg manganese.

The poor assimilation of manganese, biochemical individuality, and increasing dependence on highly processed foods makes the advisability of such a low upper limit questionable. In studying children, the manganese requirements were found to vary between 0.02 and 0.3 mg per kilogram of body weight.[30] This would be a range of 1.4 to 21 mg per day for a 154-pound man or 1.1 to 16.5 mg per day for a 119-pound woman. Since there seems to be such a wide range according to literature reports, it is surprising that the RDA range is so narrow. After all, we need to be concerned with the amount needed for optimal health, not merely growth.

Dietary surveys have found the Japanese receive 6 to 10 mg manganese daily, Indians 6 to 12 mg and New Zealanders 1 to 7 mg.[3] One survey found U.S. diets containing 2 to 9 mg manganese per day,[4] however others have shown adult men receiving only 3.3 to 5.5 mg daily and college students, hospital patients and youngsters receiving less than 2 mg daily.[3]

Diets high in refined cereals, white bread, sugar and milk may easily contain less than 2 mg of manganese daily, if few green leafy vegetables are also eaten. If wholegrain cereals and wholegrain bread are included, the same diet could contain 9 mg manganese per day.

If for no other reason than that good healthy diets can contain 9 to 15 mg of manganese daily, the RDA should be adjusted to include this range.

Hair analysis

Hair concentrations of manganese are felt by some clinicians to be a useful guideline for determining body stores of manganese but the published scientific literature does not support such a conclusion. Manganese has been classified by the Hair Analysis Standardization Board as an element with unknown clinical significance because of the absence of published scientific data to prove otherwise.

Clinicians who have used hair analysis over a period of many years have noticed that manganese increases very slowly as patients correct their diets to eliminate processed foods and as manganese-containing supplements are prescribed.

Case histories

The normal reference ranges for manganese are considered to vary from 1 part per million to 10 ppm of hair concentration, based on large amounts of data gathered by laboratories measuring hair elements. Most Americans have levels below this reference range.

One thirty-five-year-old male patient who has had yearly hair analysis for the past ten years was initially found to have hair manganese concentrations at approximately half the lower limit of what is considered to be the normal reference range. Despite a markedly improved diet with elimination of most processed foods and daily consumption of manganese-containing supplements in the range of 10–20 mg per day, in addition to increased manganese contained in foods, the hair manganese remained below the reference range for eight years and only after ten years of dietary correction and supplementation has it approached what is considered to be the normal reference range.

Because there is no proven clinical correlation between hair manganese and body manganese stores specific case histories will not be given and we must await more published scientific data before we can make more specific statements concerning the clinic correlation between hair concentrations of manganese and the nutritional status of manganese in other body organs.

REFERENCES

1 Schroeder, H. A., Balassa, J. J. and Tipton, I. H. 1966. *J. Chron. Dis.* 19:545–571.

2 National Research Council. 1980. *Recommended Dietary Allowances.* (9th ed.) Washington, D. C.: National Academy of Sciences, p. 154.

3 Aston, B. 1980. *Orthomolecular Psy.* 9(4):237–249.

4 Underwood, E. J. 1977. *Trace Elements in Human and Animal Nutrition.* (4th ed.) New York: Academic Press.

5 Hurley, L. S. 1976. In: *Present Knowledge in Nutrition.* (4th ed.) New York: The Nutrition Foundation, Inc., chapter 34.

6 Sansom, B. F. *et al.* 1976. In: *Nuclear Tech. in Animal Prod. and Health.* Vienna: IAEA.

7 Sansom, B. F. *et al.* 1978. *Res. Vet. Sci.* 24:366–369.

8 Lassiter, J. W. *et al.* 1974. In: *Trace Element Met. in Animals,* vol. 2. Hoekstra, W. G. *et al.*, eds. Baltimore: University Park Press, p. 557.

9 Schaible, P. J. and Bandemer, S. A. 1942. *Poultry Sci.* 21:8–14.

10 Gruden, N. 1979. *Periodicum Biologorum* 81:567–570.

11 Wilgus, H. R. and Patton, A. R. 1939. *J. Nutr.* 18:35.

12 Jukes, T. H. 1941. *J. Nutr.* 20:445–458.

13 Keefer, R. C. *et al.* 1973. *Amer. J. Clin. Nutr.* 26:409.

14 Barak, A. J. *et al.* 1971. *Nutr. Rep. Int.* 3:243.

15 Davis, P. N. *et al.* 1962. *J. Nutr.* 77:217–223.

16 Britton, A. A. *et al.* 1966. *Amer. J. Physiol.* 211(1):203–206.

17 Reiter, P. J. 1927. *Z. Neur.* 108:464–480.

18 English, W. M. 1929. *Amer. J. Psychiat.* 569–580.

19 Pfeiffer, C. C. 1974. *J. Orthomolecular Psych.* 3(4):259–264.

20 Hurley, L. S. *et al.* 1963. *Proc. Soc. Exp. Biol. Med.* 106:343–346.

21 Tanaka, Y. 1977. *J. Amer. Med. Assoc.* 238:1805.

22 Rubenstein, A. H. *et al.* 1962. *Nature* 194:188–189.

23 Everson, G. J. and Shrader, R. E. 1968. *J. Nutr.* 94:89.

24 Shrader, R. E. and Everson, G. J. 1968. *J. Nutr.* 94:269.

25 Kosenko, L. G. 1964. *Klin. Med.* 42:113.

26 *Lancet.* December 29, 1962.

27 McCollester, D. L. 1979. *Biochem. Soc. Trans.* 7(5):1068–1069.

28 *Medical World News.* December 10, 1979. p. 51.

29 McLeod, B. E. and Robinson, M. F. 1972. *Br. J. Nutr.* 27:221–227.

30 Schlage, C. and Wortberg, B. 1972. *Acta Paediat. Scand.* 61:648–652.

13

IODINE

Iodine is a classic example of how a health problem due to a trace element deficiency can be corrected quickly by trace element supplementation. The story of goiter and iodine deficiency is widely known. The success of the story is due in part to the uniqueness of the goiter, an obvious enlargement in the neck resulting in many individuals living in iodine deficient areas, and is not confused with other symptoms or theories on its origin.

Unfortunately, other trace element deficiencies contribute to the disease processes of cancer, atherosclerosis, diabetes, and others but the connection with trace element deficiencies was long unknown until after other factors were accepted as the causes of these diseases. Thus we may never see mass enrichment of foods to provide adequate amounts of these trace minerals in the diet. It will be up to each individual. First, however, the individual must be informed of the problem.

It is also interesting to note that in the past there was skepticism that a trace element deficiency could cause such varied symptoms as swollen, disfigured necks, bulging eyes, rough skin, brittle nails and even an awkward walk. There continues to be skepticism that other trace element deficiencies can be involved with diseases such as heart disease, cancer, diabetes and arthritis.

Today few remnants of the endemic goiter that was a prevalent health problem in the early 1900s remain. The "goiter belt" existed in the states bordering the Great Lakes and to the northwest, where the soils had been stripped of iodine possibly by glacial action. The iodization of table salt was begun in Michigan, where the goiter rate was 47 percent, in 1924 and eventually became available nationwide by 1940.[1]

It should be emphasized that the use of iodized salt is voluntary in the United States and the United Kingdom, but other countries such as Canada, Guatemala and Colombia have compulsory iodization.[1]

Few Americans are now considered iodine deficient although 5 to 6 percent of the persons examined in Michigan and Texas are still found to have goiter.[2,3] This "residual" goiter is probably not caused by iodine deficiency, as the measure of urinary iodine excretion indicates adequate iodine stores.[4] Possibly the chemicals called goitrogens that are found in some foods such as turnips, cabbage, rutabagas, kale and rape, and in some food additives could block iodine utilization.[5]

The relationship of iodine to goiter is via the thyroid gland. Iodine is an integral part of the thyroid hormones, thyroxin and triiodothyronine, which have important metabolic roles and govern basal metabolism. Iodine deficiency leads to goiter, which is merely an enlargement of the thyroid, as a result of increases in number and size of the gland's epithelial cells.

The iodine content of thyroxin is 65 percent. The vast majority of the 20 to 30 mg iodine in the average adult body is stored in the thyroid gland as thyroxin or triiodothyronine.[6,7] Less than 1 mg iodine is found in the blood,[8] although some iodine has been found in all tissues.[9]

An iodine deficiency may cause lowered vitality, hypothyroidism and lowered basal metabolism, inability to think clearly, low resistance to infections, loss of control of the muscles of the mouth resulting in mouth contortion and droolings, defective teeth, tendency to obesity, cretinism, loss of tone of the circulatory system, and slow development of the sexual organs.[8] Iodine, in its role as a constituent of thyroid hormone, acts to stabilize and control just about every biochemical reaction in the body. It is also thought to help stabilize calcium and phosphorus metabolism and starch metabolism.[8]

Some have suggested that iodine deficiency contributes to weight gain, thus extra dietary iodine in the form of kelp should be included in weight-loss programs. This popular concept is not well documented in the scientific literature.

Absorption, storage, and excretion

Iodine is readily absorbed both in organic and inorganic forms.[1] It can be detected in the tongue and in the hand within five minutes after ingesting a capsule of radioactive inorganic iodine. Iodine can be absorbed from the stomach, but most absorption occurs in the small intestine.

The thyroid concentrates iodine by forming a complex known as thyroglobulin which consists of iodine-containing compounds such as thyroxine, monoiodotyrosine, diiodotyrosine, diiodothyronine, and triiodothyronine.[1]

Thyroxine is not the active cellular hormone, but triiodothyronine is. The thyroid gland primarily produces thyroxine and some triiodothyronine into the circulation and then the thyroxine is converted back into triiodothyronine at the cell membrane level by copper- and zinc-containing enzymes. Copper in particular, and we believe zinc as well, is marginally or frankly deficient in many individuals in this country, and is responsible for the lowered basal metabolic rate and for the low axillary temperatures found in so many patients.

Clinically we have many patients who have basal body temperatures of 96.8 to 97.5°F and core temperatures that slowly rise to 97.8 to 98.2°F during the daytime with vigorous physical activity but which never reach the normal of 98.6°F or higher during the daytime. It may be that a deficiency of essential trace minerals (such as zinc or copper) is the cause of this syndrome, rather than a frank deficiency of thyroxine production by the thyroid gland itself.

Excretion is principally via the kidneys, although lesser amounts are excreted via the intestine and in perspiration.[1] The body is fairly efficient in re-cycling iodine recovered from degradated thyroxine.

Breast cancer and breast dysplasia

Breast cancer and iodine deficiency have been linked by Dr. Bernard A. Eskin, chief of gynocologic endocrinology service at the Albert Einstein Medical Center Philadelphia, and the Medical College of Pennsylvania.[9]

Dr. Eskin had noted that the highest breast cancer mortality rates in the United States are found in the "goiter belt" bordering the Great Lakes. Increased breast cancer rates are also found in specific goiter regions of Poland, Switzerland, Australia and the Soviet Union. Mexico and Thailand have high incidences of goiter and breast cancer. Of course, these same areas are deficient in the trace mineral selenium, which is also a factor in cancer, and specific laboratory tests with animals would be required to determine if iodine deficiency plays a role.

It should also be noted that Japan and Iceland have low incidences of goiter and breast cancer, and both countries have soils relatively rich in both iodine and selenium.

Dr. Eskin has shown that a dietary iodine deficiency in laboratory rats leads to abnormal breast tissue growth called dysplasia. He has also shown that the female sex hormone estrogen hastens the development of dysplasia when iodine is lacking from the diet.

While it is generally accepted that cancer occurs four times as often in dysplastic breasts as it does in normal breasts, Dr. Eskin points out that there is still no direct evidence relating the progression of benign dysplasia to cancer.

In clinical trials with women, Dr. Eskin found that iodine supplementation could prevent breast dysplasia. He also found that the dysplasia process could be reversed by iodine supplementation. However, it should be emphasized that extension of dysplasia to cancer or linking thyroid disorders to breast cancer is controversial.

Clinically, many physicians have found that using a simple, organic iodine preparation and painting the female vagina relieves the symptoms of cystic breast disease. Iodine is very rapidly absorbed through vaginal tissues.

Dr. John Myers of Johns Hopkins Hospital in Baltimore has found that diiodotyrosine, along with magnesium, copper and manganese, relieves breast soreness and heaviness. In addition, this regimen has normalized the consistency of the vaginal mucus in the same individuals.

Dr. Myers claims that the diiodotyrosine is produced in the ovaries and helps keep cholesterol from forming, skin unwrinkled and breasts soft. Dr. Myers points out that copper has much to do with thyroid health and catalyzes the manufacture of diiodotyrosine.

Radioactive fallout

Nuclear disasters can produce radioactive iodine fallout, and radioactive iodine can cause thyroid cancer. However, normal dietary iodine can protect against the absorption of the radioactive iodine.

Inhaled radioactive iodine gas or ingested radioactive iodine salts will be rapidly excreted if the thyroid is in no need of iodine. Some have suggested keeping potassium iodide in the first-aid cabinet for immediate consumption in case of a nuclear accident that might produce fallout in your area. The important factor would be to have a high iodine intake as soon as possible to saturate your thyroid with normal iodine.

Sources and needs

As demonstrated by the iodine deficiency of foods in the goiter belt, the amount of iodine in food depends on the amount of iodine in the soil where the vegetation is grown or in the food given to farm animals. Thus food tables

TRACE ELEMENTS

are essentially useless except to offer a guide to "typical" values if produced in an iodine-adequate locality. Table 13.1 lists such typical values of iodine in food. Note that seafoods are excellent (and consistent) sources of iodine, whereas vegetables are often low in iodine. Kelp is an excellent source of organic iodine.

TABLE 13.1 SOURCES OF IODINE

Micrograms (mcg) per 100 grams edible portion (100 grams = 3½ oz.)

Clams	90	Cheddar cheese	11
Shrimp	65	Pork	10
Haddock	62	Lettuce	10
Halibut	46	Spinach	9
Oysters	50	Green peppers	9
Salmon	50	Butter	9
Sardines, canned	37	Milk	7
Beef liver	19	Cream	6
Pineapple	16	Cottage cheese	6
Tuna, canned	16	Beef	6
Eggs	14	Lamb	3
Peanuts	11	Raisins	3
Wholewheat bread	11		

Source: MineraLab, Inc.

The daily iodine requirement for prevention of goiter in adults is 50 to 75 micrograms, or approximately 1 mcg per 2 pounds of body weight.[10] The Food and Nutrition Board has set the RDA at 150 mcg for adults.[4]

Several studies have estimated typical iodine intake in the United States ranges from 64 to 680 mcg per day.[11]

However, the Food and Drug Administration was startled to find much higher amounts in their 1974 Total Diet Study.[12] Analysis of the foods sampled revealed that a 2850 calorie-per-day diet averaged 830 mcg of iodine. This figure does not include salt added at the table, which typically adds another 300 mcg iodine per day. The total of 1130 mcg is nearly eight times the official RDA. The survey found less iodine (700 mcg) in 1978.

The large iodine intake wasn't the only surprise—iodine was turning up in unexpected places. Dairy products contributed 56 percent of the iodine. Iodophors, a group of iodine-containing chemicals that kill bacteria, viruses and fungi, are widely used from the dairy farm to the dairy. However, the biggest source of iodine in milk was not the heavy use of iodophors, but that the cows were fed too much iodine in their feed as ethylenediamine dihydroiodide (EDDI). EDDI is used to prevent goiter in cows and also as an unproven preventive for foot rot.

Significant amounts of iodine are probably contributed by the food coloring, red dye No. 3 (erythrosine), which is more than 50 percent iodine.[12] The use of red dye No. 3 has more than doubled since 1976. One vitamin tablet colored with red dye No. 3 was supposed to contain 150 mcg iodine, but due to the artificial coloring, actually contained 375 mcg iodine.[12]

Table 13.2 lists the sources of iodine in the 1978 Total Diet Study by the Food and Drug Administration.

TABLE 13.2 SOURCES OF IODINE IN ADULT DIET OF 2,850 CALORIES A DAY (1978)

Food commodity	Micrograms of iodine	Percentage of total iodine intake
Dairy products	389	56.1
Meat, fish and poultry	75	10.8
Grain and cereals	111	16.1
Potatoes	2	0.4
Leafy vegetables	3	0.5
Legume vegetables	7	1.0
Root vegetables	0	0.0
Miscellaneous vegetables	1	0.2
Fruits	2	0.4
Oils, fats and shortening	5	0.7
Sugars and adjuncts	73	10.7
Beverages (including drinking water)	28	4.2
Total	**696**	

Source: FDA

Toxicity

Iodine intake at the recommended levels has no demonstrable adverse effects. An intake in adults between 50 and 1000 mcg (1 mg) iodine can be considered safe.[4] The acute toxicity of iodine has been studied by the GRAS (Generally Recognized as Safe) committee of the Food and Drug Administration.[13] Depending on the species, amounts between 200 and 500 mg/kg of body weight were required to produce death in laboratory animals. That would be a dose of 14 to 35 grams for a 154-pound man.

Some nutritionists are concerned about the increasing amounts of iodine showing up in today's diets. They recommend that the many adventitious sources of iodine such as iodophors in the dairy industry, alginates, coloring dyes and dough conditioners, be replaced wherever possible by compounds containing less or no iodine.

In spite of the increasing intake of dietary iodine, no evidence has been found of adverse reactions, such as chronic iodine toxicity or hypersensitivity.[4] Thus, it may be concluded that the present intake by the majority of the U.S. population is adequate and safe.[11]

There is concern that goiter can be induced by high dietary iodine intake, just as with iodine deficiency. This has occurred in Japan among 6 to 12 percent of the seaweed-eating fishermen consuming 10,000 to 200,000 mcg of iodine per day.[13] It is unlikely that present levels of U.S. usage would cause this effect.

One factor not considered so far in this discussion is the bioavailability of various iodine forms. Scientists are not sure yet if the iodine in red dye No. 3 is absorbed and utilized by the body.

Hair analysis

Hair analysis for iodine is not routinely performed as of this writing.

REFERENCES

1 Wilson, E. D. et al. 1965. Principles of Nutrition. (2nd ed.) New York: Wiley, p. 174.

2 Matovinovic, J. 1970. In: Iodine Nutriture in the U. S. Washington, D. C.: FNB, NAS, p. 1–5.

3 McGanity, W. In: Iodine Nutriture in the U. S., p. 5–8.

4 National Research Counsel. 1980. Recommended Dietary Allowances. Washington, D. C.: National Academy of Sciences, pp. 147–151.

5 Gaitan, E. et al. 1972. In: Trace Substances in Environmental Health, vol. 5, Hemphill, ed. Columbia, Missouri: University Missouri Press.

6 Riggs, D. S. 1952. Pharmacol. Rev. 4:284.

7 Underwood, E. J. 1962. Trace Elements. (2nd ed.) New York: Academic Press.

8 Thurston, E. W. December 1970. Nat. Health Fed. Bull. 20–23.

9 Kovaly, K. May 1970. Biomedical News 1(5):1–8.

10 Food and Nutrition Board, Nat. Res. Council. 1970. Iodine Nutriture in the United States. Washington, D. C.: National Academy of Sciences.

11 Life Sciences Research Office. 1974. Iodine in Foods. Fed. Amer. Soc. Exp. Biology, Bethesda, Maryland.

12 Taylor, F. April 1981. FDA Consumer, pp. 15–17.

13 Taylor, F. April 1981. FDA Consumer, p. 18.

Ultra-trace elements

CHROMIUM

SELENIUM

MOLYBDENUM

14

CHROMIUM

Chromium is as essential to life as are many other nutrients. However, chromium may be an especially critical factor since not only are many diets deficient in chromium but these same diets increase the excretion of chromium, thus depleting whatever chromium reserves previously exist.

Chromium has often been dismissed from concern merely because such minute amounts are required. Yet the increasing usage of processed foods, containing high proportions of refined carbohydrates such as sugar and white flour, has decreased chromium intake below even the minute amount required for optimum health. To make matters worse, sugar and white flour are quickly digested carbohydrates that rapidly increase the blood sugar level. This in turn necessitates using more chromium to help insulin control the rising blood level.

Several studies indicate that this dietary trend has resulted in lowered chromium levels (4–6 milligrams total) in modern Americans compared to those of other nations and to Americans of previous generations.[1] The net effect may be increased heart disease, diabetes, hypoglycemia and impaired protein metabolism.

When Drs. Henry Schroeder and Isabel Tipton compared the concentrations of chromium in the tissues of Americans and foreigners at all ages, they found high levels in stillborn, newborn infants and children up to ten years of age, which declined precipitously over the next two decades of life. Chromium, present in all young bodies, was not detected in tissues of from 15 to 23 percent of Americans over fifty years of age but was found in tissues from almost every foreign subject tested. (98.5 percent). Estimates based on organ weights indicated that, on the average, Africans had twice, Near Easterners 4.4 times and Orientals five times as much chromium in their bodies as Americans.[1]

Many texts will note that body chromium content decreases with age, but this is not necessarily so in all cultures and is only a reflection of chromium deficiency. The highest concentrations of chromium are in the skin, fat, adrenal, brain and muscle tissue.

Chromium is required for "glucose tolerance." This means the proper use of blood sugar (glucose) to produce energy. Without key factors such as chromium and insulin, the blood sugar can actually damage cells. This is called "glucose intolerance." The damaged eye retinas and blood vessels in many diabetics do not happen because of a lack of insulin but are due to improper reactions of glucose in various cells. These harmful reactions may be caused by a number of factors including a lack of insulin, chromium or manganese, or even defective cells.

Partial control can be achieved by avoiding an excess of refined carbohydrates (sugar and white flour) and/or insulin injections. However, complete control can be achieved only when adequate chromium and manganese are present.

Actually, it is not elemental chromium that is the critical factor, but a complex of chromium with vitamin B3 (niacin) and three amino acids. This complex is called, not surprisingly, Glucose Tolerance Factor (GTF).

In fact, the only *known* role of chromium is in the form of GTF. Normally the chromium we absorb is united with the other components to form GTF. However, some people become less efficient in forming GTF in their own bodies and diabetes or elevated blood cholesterol levels might result. Thus it is not merely a question of chromium intake, but also of GTF formation and usage.

Roles other than GTF formation have been suggested, but not confirmed as of this writing. There are indications that chromium could be involved in certain enzyme pathways and in protein synthesis.

The most interesting development concerns a recent study where investigators discovered that chromium deficiency in rats also produced decreased activity of the enzyme glycerol kinase.[2] Glycerol kinase is required to make either triglycerides or glucose out of glycerol. Thus it is possible that either chromium or another chromium factor is involved in sugar and fat metabolism, in addition to the role of chromium in GTF.

It is interesting to point out that chromium can be considered as 1) an essential trace element, 2) a vitamin in the organic complex cyancobalamin in the cobalt-containing vitamin B12 and 3) a hormone, like insulin, which is released from body stores into the bloodstream in response to a glucose load. Here we have a substance which crosses the boundaries between vitamin, element ("mineral") and hormone. The distinction between vitamins, minerals and hormones is not always as clear as the textbooks would have us believe.

Glucose tolerance factor

The research trail which led to the discovery and characterization of glucose tolerance factor began in the late 1950s with the discovery by Drs. Klaus Schwarz and Walter Mertz that rats placed on torula yeast-based semi-purified diet developed impaired glucose tolerance. Suspecting a trace element deficiency, they screened numerous compounds and found that dietary supplementation with trivalent (thrice positively charged) chromium could prevent this decline in glucose tolerance. They further found that certain chromium rich fractions from either brewer's yeast or pork kidney had a similar effect, and that this organic form of chromium was substantially more effective than inorganic chromium on a per weight basis. Spectroscopic analysis of highly purified GTF preparations indicates the likely structure of GTF: a molecule of trivalent chromium bonded with nicotinic acid (vitamin B3) and with the amino acids of glutathione.

The way GTF enhances glucose tolerance was clarified in studies demonstrating that GTF would bind both to the insulin molecule and the insulin receptor, increasing the hormonal effect of insulin up to threefold.[3] It was further found that the blood GTF activity increased in response to an insulin challenge, which indicates that GTF is stored in tissue and secreted when it is needed. Absorption studies showed that orally administered GTF is much more efficiently assimilated than are inorganic salts of trivalent chromium. However, since normal glucose tolerance can be maintained in animals fed purified diets supplemented with inorganic chromium, it is evident that inorganic chromium absorbed from the diet can sometimes be converted to GTF in some species and by some individuals. The richest known natural source of pre-formed GTF activity is brewer's yeast, whose GTF activity is tenfold higher than that of any other food.

Very significantly, it was noted that the serum and urine of maturity onset diabetics showed little or no increment of volatile chromium (a rough measure of GTF) in response to an insulin challenge. Attempts to improve glucose tolerance in maturity-onset diabetics by supplementing the diet with up to 1 milligram of inorganic chromium salts per day, have met with moderate success in about half of the patients tested. Preformed GTF, in amounts of no more than four micrograms of chromium per day, has improved glucose tolerance, reduced total blood fats and increased protective high density lipoprotein levels in several studies. Many investigators feel that maturity onset diabetics are likely to have either a defect of GTF metabolism or an increased need for GTF which will best be managed by supplementing with adequate amounts of readily absorbed and rapidly active preformed GTF.

Absorption, transport and storage

Two forms of chromium are readily found in nature. The difference is in the "oxidation state" or "valence" which concerns the number of electrons attached to the atom and how many atoms of oxygen the chromium atoms will unite with. The form having biological activity and found in food is trivalent chromium (Cr^{+3}). The form not having biological activity, but capable of causing toxicity if ingested, is hexavalent chromium (Cr^{+6}). This form would only be encountered in occupational or accidental contamination. Both trivalent chromium and hexavalent chromium can be converted to elemental chromium (Cr) which is the shining chromium metal that we are familiar with on automobile bumpers, but which is rarely found in nature.

Inorganic chromium (chromium salts) is poorly absorbed (0.5 to 0.7 percent.)[4,5] Organic complexes of chromium are more readily absorbed (10 to 20 percent.)[6,7] However, the way in which chromium is absorbed is not well understood.

Chromium appears to be transported in the blood in at least two forms. One form is GTF and the other known form is trivalent chromium bound to beta-globulin.[8] The amount of chromium transported by either may reflect nutritional status, but total blood chromium is not an indicator of nutritional status.[9] Hair analysis is a reliable indicator.[10-13] A more reliable blood indicator called the relative chromium response (RCR) has been proposed as an indicator of chromium nutritional status.

There is no known storage depot for chromium, and it has been suggested that increased needs are met by the conversion of inorganic trivalent chromium into the active GTF. Impaired conversion would result in a deficiency of GTF and damage from glucose intolerance. For people with impaired GTF production, dietary GTF would be helpful.

Excretion of chromium occurs mainly through the kidneys. However, at this time it is not known how much is excreted as inorganic or organic chromium. The determination is complicated by the very small concentrations and by the possibility of a highly volatile organic chromium fraction which may partially escape analysis.

Although prior studies had been conflicting, Drs. Victoria Liu and Steven Morris of the University of Missouri have determined that blood levels of chromium increase as the blood sugar level increases.[7] They used the relative chromium response (RCR) index to overcome the problem which had led to the conflicting results. It has been suggested that as much as 20 percent of this increase in blood chromium will be excreted. If so, this will readily explain why refined carbohydrates deplete the body of chromium.

Heart disease and longevity

There are two striking observations which researchers should make when studying the extensive scientific and medical reports on chromium. They should be amazed at the quality and quantity of studies linking chromium deficiency to heart disease and diabetes, and the fact that so few researchers and physicians are aware of the strength of this evidence. The second awareness is more subtle, but it would take a deliberate effort not to notice the frequent mention of increased longevity with chromium supplementation.

The increased longevity reports include animal studies in 1960 by Dr. Henry Schroeder of the Dartmouth Trace Mineral Laboratory when his chromium supplemented rats set "somewhat of a record for longevity." They not only lived longer, but "at death, surprisingly enough, had no atherosclerotic plaques (cholesterol deposits) in their aortas, unlike their controls of which about 20 percent of aortas had plaques."[14]

Increased longevity is also noted in populations having high incidence of heart disease. An example is a Finnish report by Dr. Punsar.[2] Finland has the highest rate of heart disease death at this writing. In a very comprehensive ten-year prospective study, Dr. Punsar found morbidity and mortality to be highest in men whose drinking water contained the lowest levels of chromium. Chromium was the only element producing this inverse relationship.

It is readily apparent to anyone seriously studying the published scientific literature that a low intake of chromium results in increased blood cholesterol levels and a build up of fatty tissues (plaques) in the aorta, thereby causing an accelerated death rate.

At a recent symposium, Dr. Wesley Canfield of the University of Colorado Medical Center remarked, "There is no doubt that when animals are fed a low-chromium diet, the blood cholesterol level rises as the blood sugar level rises and the glucose tolerance becomes impaired. It is also true that when these animals were given chromium, all of these variables returned to normal. This relationship is less well documented in man, but new information is emerging.[11]

Even a 1980 article in the conservative *American Journal of Clinical*

Nutrition noted that chromium deficiency is implicated as an important factor in the cause of atherosclerosis and coronary heart disease.[15] A quick review of some of the circumstantial evidence would include the following:

• An exceptionally marked decline in tissue chromium levels with increasing age in the United States; adult levels are found to be considerably lower than those in the Far East, Mid East and Africa.[1,16]

• The tissues of Thai have more chromium than any other group, the incidence of atherosclerosis is very low and there are few atherosclerotic complications such as heart attacks or strokes.[1,17]

• Persons dying of heart disease have virtually no chromium in their aortas, whereas those dying of accidents have aortic chromium.[18]

However, an Israeli team headed by Dr. Abraham Abraham of the Department of Medicine at Shaare Zedek Hospital in Jerusalem wanted more evidence. They investigated the effect of chromium on atherosclerosis induced in laboratory animals. They found a significant *regression* of atherosclerotic plaques.[15]

Although reversing atherosclerotic damage is not widely accepted at this time there is increasing evidence that atherosclerosis is a substantially reversible process. Regression of atherosclerotic plaque has been demonstrated in many species of laboratory animals by nutritional means[19–22] and in man by chelation therapy.[23]

Dr. Abraham's group concluded: "These experiments have shown that atherosclerosis, even when established can be *reversed* by treatment with chromium. After a relatively short treatment period of thirty weeks with chromium there was a substantial regression of the atherosclerotic lesions, both macroscopically (the aortas weighed less and were freer of plaques) and in terms of cholesterol content, as compared to the group that did not receive chromium. The difference between the extent of aortic involvement in the chromium treated and [that of] nontreated groups was significant by all the methods we used."

The link between chromium deficiency and increase in arterial plaque has been verified angiographically in man.[24] At this writing the link between increasing chromium intake and reversing the arterial plaque has been demonstrated in animals but has not been tested by scientific protocol in man. However, there is other support.

The mechanism leading to the reversal of the cholesterol deposits is not merely due to the lowering of blood cholesterol levels. The reversal most likely is due to an increase in the cholesterol carrier that scavenges cholesterol and carries it back to the liver.

There are two main carriers of cholesterol. One carrier delivers cholesterol from the liver to cells throughout the body. This carrier is called low-density lipoprotein (LDL). The other carrier, the scavenger that returns unused cholesterol to the liver, is called high-density lipoprotein (HDL). Modern research has linked the ratio of HDL to LDL as an important factor in whether or not one develops cholesterol deposits.[25–28] The higher the HDL to LDL or HDL to total cholesterol ratio, the less heart disease. In oversimplified terms, as long as you have more dump trucks (HDL) than delivery trucks (LDL), it doesn't make any difference how many trucks (total cholesterol) you have.

Thus HDL is protective against heart disease, and if you have appreciably more HDL than LDL, cholesterol deposits can be reduced in size. Good news: chromium increases the HDL level.

Dr. Rebecca Riales tested the effect of GTF on blood HDL and LDL levels by supplementing the normal diets of physicians with approximately seven grams of brewer's yeast, five days a week for six weeks. The seven grams of brewer's yeast contained 15 micrograms of organic chromium, of which 7 to 8 mcg of chromium was a part of GTF. Her experiment lacked a control group receiving an inert placebo for comparison. However, Dr. Riales noted, "the possibility of a placebo effect seemed small due to the skepticism of the physicians regarding the worth of the brewer's yeast."

After only six weeks, the physicians had a statistically significant increase of the protective HDL averaging 17.6 percent. Equally as important was the concomitant decrease in the undesirable LDL averaging 17.8 percent. Their HDL-to-LDL ratios improved from an average of 0.413 to 0.596, an improvement of 44 percent.[29]

If you are still concerned about total blood cholesterol, you can take comfort in the many studies showing that chromium lowers total blood cholesterol. Unfortunately, these studies were carried out before the importance of HDL-to-LDL ratios was widely known.

As an example, Dr. Richard Doisy of the State University of New York Upstate Medical Center in Syracuse studied the effect of GTF in 10 grams of brewer's yeast on the cholesterol levels of sixteen of his medical students over a month's time.[2,30] One-half of the students had blood cholesterol levels above 240 mg per deciliter which is the upper limit of the "normal" range. After one month of brewer's yeast supplementation, the students having elevated blood cholesterol had a decrease of an average of 56 mg/dl.

The others, who had normal blood cholesterol levels, had a lesser decrease. The average for the entire group of students was a 36 mg/dl decrease.

TABLE 14.1 CHROMIUM IN WILD AND DOMESTIC MAMMALS AND IN SUBJECTS FROM THE UNITED STATES, MEAN VALUES, WET WEIGHT

	Animals µg/g*	Human subjects µg/g*
Liver	0.16	0.02
Kidney	0.18	0.03
Heart	0.14	0.02
Lung	0.24	0.20
Spleen	0.48	0.02
Muscle	0.11	0.03
Stomach	0.04	0.03
Placenta	0.07	0.42
Mean	0.19	0.05

*Nanogram
Note: Animals included beef, lamb, pig, wild rats, squirrels, fox, beaver, woodchuck, deer; analyses by chemical methods. Placenta excluded from mean.

Source for 14.1 and 14.2: Schroeder, H. A. 1973. *The Trace Elements and Man.* Old Greenwich, CT: Devin-Adair, p. 72.

TABLE 14.2 TRACE ELEMENTS IN SEAWATER AND IN MAN, ANCIENT AND MODERN

Element	Seawater ppb	Primitive man ppm	Modern man ppm	Principal cause of difference
ESSENTIAL				
Iron	3.4	60	60	
Zinc	15	33	33	
Rubidium	120	4.6	4.6	
Strontium	8000	4.6	4.6	
Fluorine	1300	37	37	
Copper	10	1.0	1.2	Copper pipes
Boron	4600	0.3	0.7	Vegetables and fruits
Bromine	65,000	1.0	2.9	Bromides? Fuels
Iodine	50	0.1–0.5	0.2	Salt iodized
Barium	6	0.3	0.3	
Manganese	1	0.4	0.2	Refined foods?
Selenium	4	0.2	0.2	
Chromium	2	0.6	0.09	Refined sugars and grains
Molybdenum	14	0.1	0.1	
Arsenic	3	0.05	0.1	Additives, weed killers
Cobalt	0.1	0.03	0.03	
Vanadium	5	0.1	0.3	Petroleum

TRACE ELEMENTS IN SEAWATER AND IN MAN, ANCIENT AND MODERN (*cont.*)

Element	Seawater ppb	Primitive man ppm	Modern man ppm	Principal cause of difference
NON-ESSENTIAL				
Zirconium	0.02	6.0	6.7	
Lead	4	0.01	1.7	Motor vehicle exhausts
Niobium	0.01	1.7	1.7	
Aluminum	1200	0.4	0.9	Food additives
Cadmium	0.03	0.001	0.7	Refined grains, water pipes
Tellurium	?	0.001	0.4	Metallurgy
Titanium	5	0.4	0.4	
Tin	3	<0.001	0.2	Tin cans
Nickel	3	0.1	0.1	
Gold	0.004	<0.001	0.1	Ornaments
Lithium	100	0.04	0.04	
Antimony	0.2	<0.001	0.04	Enamels
Bismuth	0.02	<0.001	0.03	Drugs
Mercury	0.03	<0.001	0.19	Fungicides
Silver	0.15	<0.001	0.03	Eating utensils
Cesium	2	0.02	0.02	
Uranium	3.3	0.01	0.01	
Beryllium	?	<0.001	0.001	Fumes and smokes
Radium	0.3×10^{-10}	4×10^{-10}	4×10^{-10}	

Source: Schroeder *The Trace Elements and Man.*

Dr. Doisy also studied the effect of GTF on nine persons over the age of seventy-five and found their blood cholesterol dropped from an average of 245 milligram-percent to an average of 205 milligram-percent.[30]

Another example is the study of Dr. Ester Offenbacher of Columbia University that documents significantly improved blood cholesterol in both diabetic and non-diabetic persons receiving chromium-rich brewer's yeast.[31]

Dr. Victoria Liu found a test group with a blood cholesterol level averaging 216 milligram-percent to have a decrease of 90 milligram-percent with brewer's yeast supplementation.[32]

In 1968, Dr. Henry Schroeder found that 2 milligrams of an inorganic chromium salt, chromium acetate, lowered blood cholesterol levels by 14 to 17 percent.[33,34] Similar results have been reported by Dr. H. W. Staub.[35]

Diabetes mellitus

As chromium deficiencies are increasing, so is the incidence of diabetes. The incidence of diabetes has risen over 600 percent in little more than one generation (from 1935 to 1978).[34] An estimated one out of every twenty Americans will become diabetic. Diabetes is the third leading cause of death in the United States, accounting for 300,000 to 350,000 deaths each year. Diabetes also contributes to the development of other deadly diseases. It is estimated that one-half of those with coronary heart disease and three-quarters of the stroke victims developed their circulatory problems prematurely as a result of diabetes.[36] The common link between atherosclerosis and diabetes is a chromium deficiency.

Before the introduction of insulin as a therapeutic agent, most severe diabetics would die in diabetic coma—an episode of acute insulin insufficiency leading to massive elevations of serum glucose, circulatory hypovolemia and shock (secondary to the resulting osmotic diuresis), acidosis (due to the build-up of ketone bodies), coma and death. Diabetic coma is far less common now as a cause of death since it can be managed by sufficiently prompt insulin administration. However, many other complications of long-standing diabetes are not readily prevented by insulin therapy. Standard insulin treatments cannot prevent intermittent elevations of blood glucose which cause severe damage to filtering mechanisms of the kidney called glomeruli (with resultant high blood pressure), to the retinal arteries and the eye lens (sometimes resulting in blindness), and to the peripheral nervous system (causing pain, tingling, anesthesia, and motor defects). This damage occurs in tissues whose glucose (sugar) content tends to reflect that of the blood serum, and is thought possibly to result from osmotic damage or accumulation of the glucose metabolite, sorbitol, or even from excess blood sugar attachment to red blood cells, to the lining of blood vessels, or to the insulating material around nerve cells (myelin).[37]

Rapid increases in blood sugar resulting from the ingestion of quickly assimilated refined carbohydrate will lead to a corresponding high secretion of insulin and GTF. Much of this secreted GTF will be lost into the urine by renal filtration; thus refined diets may increase the requirement for GTF. It is also thought that peaks of glucose and insulin caused by rapid intestinal absorption may result in a reflex end-organ insensitivity to insulin.[38,39] Obesity and lack of exercise, which for unknown reasons produce a further impairment of glucose tolerance, are now much more common in our modern society.

When the diet consists of slowly absorbed, complex, fiber-rich and chromium-GTF rich carbohydrate, and when glucose tolerance is excellent, there is little need for fat as a metabolic fuel. The body's homeostatic recognition of this fact results in low serum lipid levels and a decreased incidence of atherosclerosis.

The traditional management of diabetes with a low carbohydrate diet, weight loss, anti-diabetic drugs and insulin as needed has proved less than satisfactory in many regards. Weight loss produces excellent results in many adult diabetics, but is of little value to the substantial number of diabetics who are slender. Anti-diabetic drugs which stimulate pancreatic insulin output have been found to have little effect on the long term morbidity and mortality of diabetes. Some studies suggest that they may even increase risk.[40] Insulin injections prevent diabetic coma in severe diabetes but insulin fails to prevent the dreadful complications resulting in kidney, eye and nerve damage and atherosclerosis.[38,40] The use of low-carbohydrate diets, which are usually high in fats, with the intent of preventing rises in serum glucose levels, presents a vastly different diet from the natural diets (consisting primarily of *unrefined* carbohydrates) of populations with a negligible diabetes incidence. Indeed recent clinical studies show that diets high in unrefined carbohydrates or supplementation with dietary fiber improve the glucose tolerance of maturity-onset diabetes.

The recent availability of preformed GTF will open an exciting possibility in diabetes management. Unlike exogenous insulin or anti-diabetic drugs, GTF will potentiate the action of endogenously produced insulin secreted in response to physiological needs. For this reason, the progression of end-organ insensitivity, a common flaw with standard insulin therapy, may be less likely to develop with GTF supplementation. Further clinical study will test the merit of this speculation.

Brewer's yeast has been of benefit in functional hypoglycemia, suggesting a role for GTF in the management of this problem. It seems almost paradoxical that an agent which potentiates insulin could decrease the incidence of hypoglycemia. This is because functional hypoglycemia results when, in response to a rapid rise in serum glucose due to the ingestion of refined carbohydrate, the initial increase in insulin activity is inadequate to the challenge. As a result, a roller-coaster cycle of blood sugar fluctuations begins. Hence the value of GTF. Indeed, functional hypoglycemia is frequently one of the first clinical symptoms noted during the early years of adult diabetes.

As early as 1966, Dr. Walter Mertz reported that chromium helped diabetics.[41] Since then several clinical trials have adequately confirmed the role of chromium in improving glucose tolerance in diabetics. Dr. Esther Offenbacher found that the GTF in 9 grams of brewer's yeast taken daily for two months improved glucose tolerance while decreasing insulin output in elderly patients.[31] (Chromium-poor torula yeast was also tested and found not to produce similar improvement.) Dr. Offenbacher noted that "an improvement in insulin sensitivity also occurred with brewer's yeast supplementation. This supports the thesis that elderly people may have a low level of chromium and that an effective source for chromium repletion, such as brewer's yeast, may improve their carbohydrate tolerance and blood fats.'' Elderly people are of special interest because they are more prone to diabetes (and chromium depletion). It has been estimated that 40 to 60 percent of eighty-year-olds have diabetes.

Earlier studies by Dr. Richard Doisy revealed that 150 micrograms of inorganic chromium improved glucose tolerance in 40 percent of elderly patients with glucose intolerance.[42] These findings confirmed still earlier observations by Dr. C. M. McCay.[43] GTF is a better form of supplementation because many people lose at least some of their ability to manufacture GTF out of chromium in their own bodies.

As Dr. Doisy points out:

Possibly some individuals (i.e., insulin-requiring diabetics) completely lose the ability to convert chromium to GTF. The daily dietary intake of chromium and GTF is quite variable depending on the nature of the diet selected. If it is true, as suggested, that the insulin-requiring diabetic is unable to convert chromium to GTF, then the insulin-requiring diabetic would be dependent solely on the exogenous GTF in the diet. This could explain the so-called "brittle diabetics." If GTF intake is high one day, the insulin requirement is reduced. Conversely, if GTF intake is low, then the insulin requirement is increased. By feeding brewer's yeast daily, the daily GTF intake is more constant and thus insulin dosage may remain more constant. It may be worthy of mention that a few of the insulin-requiring diabetics have reported a greater stability of blood sugar with less tendency to spill sugar in the urine and a reduced incidence of hypoglycemic reactions while on the brewer's yeast supplement.[30]

The increased effectiveness of GTF over plain trivalent chromium can be seen by the reports of Dr. Wesley Canfield in describing some of Dr. Doisy's clinical experience.[2]

In 1969, four offspring of an insulin-requiring male diabetic were available for study. The eldest had impaired glucose tolerance which became progressively worse over the next two years, by which time daily insulin injections were required. This occurred in spite of dietary therapy, daily tolbutamide (an oral medicine for diabetes) and a daily 150 mg supplement of inorganic chromium. The three younger siblings, all females, had some impairment in glucose tolerance, as determined by both glucose and insulin levels. Two received a daily supplement of brewer's yeast (10 grams), while the third served as a control for six months before receiving the supplement. After fifteen months, all three had normal glucose tolerance, without any concurrent weight loss.

Significant reductions in both blood sugar and insulin levels occurred. The third sibling had similar responses. In July 1978, Dr. Hambidge received a telephone call from one of the older girls from this family. After seven years, she was still taking brewer's yeast and not requiring insulin.

I would say just a few words about our experience with brewer's yeast supplements in insulin requiring diabetics. Doctor Doisy had five or six such subjects for whom the supplementation consisted of 10 grams of brewer's yeast daily. The yeast had been found to have high biological activity in Doctor Mertz's laboratory. Consider the progress of a representative individual who had had diabetes eight years before beginning the supplement. At that time he was taking between 58 and 60 units of insulin per day. By three months his insulin requirements had fallen to 30 units per day. Six years later, the subject is taking 34 units of insulin per day and is still taking brewer's yeast.

Studies of diabetics with insulin requirements of 60 to 130 units per day showed reductions of 20 to 45 units in their daily insulin need over a one-to-two month period.[30]

It should be stressed that the link between chromium deficiency and diabetes also can be confirmed with laboratory animals. Dr. Henry Schroeder found that chromium deficient diets produced moderate diabetes in laboratory rats. The disease was reversed when chromium was added to their drinking water.[44]

One of us, working with a strain of genetically diabetic mice, has found that GTF halted the pathology of the diabetes and greatly increased their lifespans.[45]

Another important line of evidence to consider is that Dr. Doisy found the only group of persons they studied that displayed an abnormal rate of chromium absorption were insulin-requiring diabetics.[46] During the first twenty-four hours after a single oral dose of chromium, they (in contrast to maturity-onset diabetics) absorbed two to four times more chromium than did normal persons. Parallel with this increased rate of absorption, there was an increased urinary excretion of chromium. Dr. Doisy has also noted that if insulin-requiring diabetics were given inorganic chromium intravenously, there was an increased urinary excretion of inorganic chromium (as determined by radioisotope tracing) compared to normal subjects. Dr. Doisy concludes that diabetics may be unable to utilize chromium in a normal manner, thus creating their dependence on dietary GTF.

Especially important to this line of evidence is that insulin-requiring diabetics display a markedly reduced concentration of volatile chromium in the urine as compared to normal persons.[47] This observation also suggests that diabetics have an impaired ability to convert chromium to GTF.

And one last thought on the link between chromium deficiency and diabetes— liver and hair levels of chromium are about one-third lower in diabetics.[1,10,48]

An interesting line of research is indicating that in some individuals there may be a relationship between food allergy and diabetes.

Dr. Marshall Mandell of Norwalk, Connecticut and Dr. William Philpott of Oklahoma City, Oklahoma are both reporting marked fluctuations in blood sugar with rises and falls in the ranges of 100–200 mg per deciliter by merely challenging individuals with sublingual extracts of various proteins, chemicals and other trace substances such as automobile exhaust fumes in dilutions of 1,000 to 10,000 or less. These ecologically sensitive individuals seem to have as a manifestation of their chemical or food sensitivity an ability to cause wide fluctuations in blood sugar. How this interrelates with chromium-glucose tolerance factor, insulin, polypeptide hormone, endorphins, sematostatin, and other glucose homeostatic mechanisms is yet unknown.

Sources and needs

Modern diets offer only sparse amounts of chromium; it is so poorly absorbed and rapidly excreted when highly refined-foods are consumed. Thus we feel that unrecognized chromium deficiencies may be one of the most serious nutritional problems today. This is apparent by the decrease in body levels with age and by comparison with people on less refined diets.

A study of chromium intake by Dr. Doisy's research group found that chromium consumption ranged between 5 to 115 micrograms per day with an average of 52 mcg per day per person.[49,50]

A 1979 analysis of twenty-eight American diets found that more than one-half of the higher (43 percent) fat diets and one-fourth of the lower (25 percent) fat diets contained 50 or less mcg chromium per day.[29]

Here is one daily menu containing only a total of 5 mcg chromium that might otherwise seem balanced and nutritious to the average American.

BREAKFAST Prune juice, farina, egg, toast, milk, coffee

LUNCH Clam chowder, tuna fish sandwich, white cake, tea

DINNER Creamed cod fish, mashed potato, peas, apricots, white bread

Drinking water supplies only small amounts of chromium. A typical city water supply would contain 0.4 nanograms (a nanogram is a billionth of a gram) per milliliter, although measured water supplies ranged from nondetectable to 35 nanograms per milliliter.[51]

Foods containing organified chromium are superior to simple salts of chromium. Foods rich in GTF are the most preferable of all. In terms of biological availability and activity, brewer's yeast is by far the best source. Recently, high GTF-yeasts have been developed for use as food supplements.

Dr. Walter Mertz's group has assigned relative values for various foods in terms of GTF activity. They give a rating of 45 to brewer's yeast, 4.5 to calf's liver, 1.9 to chicken leg muscle, 1.9 to haddock, 1.9 to patent flour and 1.6 to skim milk. Black pepper and other spices rank high, but their use is limited to such small quantities as to be insignificant.[52] Table 14.4 lists relative GTF content of several foods and Table 14.5 lists chromium content of foods.

TABLE 14.4 RELATIVE GTF CONTENT OF SEVERAL FOODS

Food	Relative biological value	Food	Relative biological value
Yeast, brewers (dried)	44.88	Peppers, chili (fresh)	2.27
Pepper, black	10.21	Wheat bran and middlings	2.21
Liver, calf's	4.52	Vegetarian chicken	2.16
Cheese, American	4.39	Cornmeal, white	2.09
Wheat germ	4.05	Shrimp	2.03
Bread, wholewheat	3.59	Grits	1.97
Cornflakes cereal	3.01	Lobster	1.95
Bread, white	2.99	Mushrooms	1.92
Spaghetti	2.89	Chicken leg	1.89
Beef round	2.89	Haddock	1.86
Wheat grain	2.96	Patent flour	1.86
Butter	2.81	Beer	1.77
Bread, rye	2.67	Egg white	1.77
Margarine	2.48	Chicken breast	1.75
Oysters	2.43	Vegetarian choplets	1.72
Cornmeal, yellow	2.35	Skimmed milk	1.59

Source: Toepfer, E. W. et al. 1973. J. Agr. Food Chem. 21:69–73.

TABLE 14.5 SOURCES OF CHROMIUM

Micrograms (mcg) per 100 grams edible portion (100 grams = 3½ oz.)

Food	mcg	Food	mcg
Brewer's yeast	112	Scallops	11
Beef, round	57	Swiss cheese	11
Calf's liver	55	Banana	10
Wholewheat bread	42	Spinach	10
Wheat bran	38	Pork chop	10
Rye bread	30	Carrots	9
Fresh chili	30	Navy beans, dry	8
Oysters	26	Shrimp	7
Potatoes	24	Lettuce	7
Wheat germ	23	Orange	5
Green pepper	19	Lobster tail	5
Hen's eggs	16	Blueberries	5
Chicken	15	Green beans	4
Apple	14	Cabbage	4
Butter	13	Mushrooms	4
Parsnips	13	Beer	3
Cornmeal	12	Strawberries	3
Lamb chop	12	Milk	1

Source: MineraLab, Inc.

According to *Recommended Dietary Allowances*, 9th edition, 1980, the total requirement of absorbable chromium is very small. Indeed, it is stated on page 160 of this National Academy of Science document that "the mean minimal requirement for absorbable chromium can be assumed to be near 1 mcg per day." The reason that the Food and Nutrition Board has established a much higher "safe and suitable" intake (50 to 200 mcg per day) is simply that the absorption of chromium salts is very low.

Thus, a dietary intake of 200 mcg chromium per day will provide the estimated requirement (1 mcg), even from a diet of poorest availability. Most food forms of chromium, such as grains and meat, are considerably more absorbable than chromic salts: 1 to 2 percent absorbability is commonly reported. The 50 mcg lower limit of the "safe and suitable" range is based upon a 2 percent absorption of food chromium.

The "mean minimal requirement" of 1 mcg per day of absorbed chromium is based on studies demonstrating that the average U.S. adult excretes (and thus absorbs) about 1 mcg chromium daily. (One microgram sounds like a small amount, but it represents 1.2 quadrillion atoms of chromium!) There is no evidence, however, that 1 mcg absorbed chromium daily will provide for optimal GTF function and health protection. It is probable that a truly optimal dose may be several times higher. All that can be said with certainty is that most adults who absorb 1 mcg of chromium daily do not suffer from evident chromium deficiency. (It is also true that people who get only ten milligrams of vitamin C do not suffer from scurvy.)

But a given amount of chromium absorbed as GTF is likely to be far more useful in the body than other forms of chromium. Absorbed GTF will be immediately active as an insulin potentiator, whereas other forms of chromium have no activity until biologically converted to GTF. For many people, this conversion is particularly inefficient. So the physiological equivalence between inorganic and GTF chromium is actually much greater than 10 to 1. In fact, in some people, a mere 20 mcg of GTF chromium may achieve physiological benefits which cannot be duplicated by any amount of inorganic chromium.

Dr. Mertz has tentatively suggested an intake of 10 to 30 mcg chromium per day incorporated as GTF-chromium to meet man's basic daily requirement.[53] However, it must be kept in mind that refining processes can remove a great deal of chromium. Typically refined foods contain only one-tenth the chromium of whole foods. Chromium, as is true of most trace elements, is concentrated in the bran and germ of grains which are stripped away during refining.

Toxicity

No oral toxicity has been reported for trivalent chromium. This is not surprising since chromium is poorly absorbed and rapidly excreted. It has been estimated that the therapeutic to toxic ratio for chromium is 1 to 10,000.[54]

Hair analysis

Hair analysis is considered a very reliable indicator of chromium status and correlates well with disease status. The extremly low levels of chromium found in blood and urine hinder analyses. Blood chromium is not a good indicator because it fails to differentiate between inorganic chromium and GTF chromium. Blood chromium has not been shown to reflect tissue stores.[54]

It has been well substantiated in the scientific literature that both high and low body stores of chromium are accurately reflected in hair concentrations. There are several problems, however.

Elemental hair analysis does not distinguish between the different valence states of chromium. It is not possible on hair analysis to distinguish between contamination by the hexavalent, toxic chromium and the trivalent, nutritional chromium. If we assume, as is probably the case, that except in the rare incidence of industrial poisoning, hair concentrations of chromium reflect the nutritional status of the individual's trivalent chromium, we are still faced with many problems of methodology.

Chromium levels are so low in body tissues and in hair that the instrumentation commonly used for screening analyses have difficulty detecting these low levels found in most Americans.

The normal levels of hair chromium, based on measurements made from hair taken in underdeveloped nations of the world, where refined foods are not eaten and where chromium deficiency is less prevalent, have been measured in the range of 0.5 parts per million (500 parts per billion) to 3.0 ppm. Many Americans have 1/10 or less the lower limit of this "normal" reference range. The problem encountered by many hair analysis laboratories is that the limit of detection for these very low levels of chromium is below the ambient noise level produced internally by their equipment.

The inductively coupled argon plasma method, now used by many laboratories, is insensitive at these very low levels, although it is probably accurate in the mid-to-upper normal levels of hair chromium concentration. The problem which we are faced with is in trying to compare several readings taken over a period of months or years, all of which are below the lower limits of normal and which are so low that the readings cannot be reproduced, even if the same hair specimen were tested several times on the same equipment on the same day. The readings consist mainly of spurious "noise," not of a chromium generated signal.

The most precise method for practical use in testing hair for chromium would be a flameless technique using a graphite furnace and an atomic absorption spectrophotometer. This is time-consuming and involves considerable additional expense. For that reason, accuracy at very low levels is often poor and it is often an error to try to compare one reading to another when the readings are below the lower instrumental detection limits. There are more precise techniques, involving additional expense, which can be performed by more sophisticated laboratories, but these are not readily available to clinicians who routinely use screening hair analysis in their practices.

As a result, clinical experience with large numbers of patients who have undergone hair analysis would indicate that most Americans are indeed deficient but because of technical problems with the laboratory methods most commonly used no precise conclusions may be made concerning the degree of deficiency or of comparisons from one reading to the next.

Elevated hair chromiums are rarely encountered in clinical practice and are usually the result of industrial poisoning with industrial exposures to chromium.

Because of the lack of reliability of chromium measurements at the extremely low levels so often encountered in an American population it is difficult to cite case histories with any degree of confidence.

One of us has in our files a case history of a fifty-year-old male who had a hair chromium measurement determined using the flameless, graphite furnace, atomic absorption method in 1974 at which time the hair chromium was below the lower limits of detection (below 0.04 parts per million or less than 40 parts per billion). This individual had marked glucose intolerance with dysinsulinism. A glucose tolerance test showed wide swings in blood sugar rising to 300 milligrams per deciliter at the third hour and falling to less than 50 mg/dl after the fourth hour. These rapid, wide swings in blood glucose caused extreme emotional instability, difficulty with concentration, temper outbursts and depression. Initially chromium was administered in the form of a brewer's yeast which had been analyzed and found to be very potent in the biologically active glucose tolerance factor (GTF). Because, as is the case with many hypoglycemic and dysinsulinemic individuals, this patient was quite allergic and soon became intolerant to the brewer's yeast preparation. Nevertheless, refined foods were essentially eliminated from the diet and the consumption of GTF-rich unrefined foods was greatly increased. Supplements containing 200 micrograms of organically chelated chromium were taken each day. Hair chromium slowly increased and on yearly hair analyses the hair chromium concentration showed a gradual rise into the range of detectibility and into the lower limits of normal at 0.5 ppm by 1980. Restoration of body chromium stores, in conjunction with a vastly improved diet, aerobic exercise conditioning and supplementation with numerous other vitamins and minerals, resulted in a vastly improved state of health and reversal of most symptoms which had initially caused this patient to seek medical help.

The main caution concerning hair analysis for chromium is that comparisons of one reading to another, when the readings are below the lower limits of normal, may be meaningless. The measurements may be so low that the internal noise generated by the equipment measuring the chromium is more prominent than the signal generated by the chromium itself. That is, the reports may be simply comparing one noise level to another noise level as opposed to comparing one chromium level to another. In such cases it may be possible to state that the individual is deficient in chromium, as is true of most Americans, but it is difficult, without sophisticated methodology and additional expense, to make comparisons from one reading to another when the levels are below the lower limits of normal. The same might be true even in the lower range of normal concentrations.

Thus, what occurs in the screening of hair analysis is a trade-off between excessive cost and practicality.

It has been a consistent observation by many clinicians involved in the treatment of patients with glucose intolerance that as their diabetes and hypoglycemia (glucose intolerance of various types including dysinsulinism) improves, the hair chromium concentrations do increase and come up into the normal level. This is a slow process and it frequently takes many years to replenish body stores. This should not be surprising in light of the fact that it takes a decade or more after birth to cause depletion of prenatal body chromium concentrations.

REFERENCES

1 Schroeder, H. A. *et al.* 1962. *J. Chron. Dis.* 15:941.

2 Canfield, W. 1979. In: *Chromium in Nutrition and Metabolism.* New York: Elsevier/North Holland Biomedical Press, p. 154.

3 Mertz, W. 1976. In: *Present Knowledge in Nutrition.* (4th ed.) New York: Nutrition Foundation, pp. 365–376.

4 Donaldson, R. M. and Barreras, R. F. 1966. *J. Lab. Clin. Med.* 68:484–493.

5 Doisy, R. J. *et al.* 1968. In: *Trace Substances in Environmental Health,* Hamphill, ed. vol. 11. Columbia: Univ. Missouri, p. 75.

6 Schroeder, H. A. 1967. *Amer. J. Clin. Nutr.* 21(3):247–251.

7 Mertz, W. 1969. *Physiol. Rev.* 49:163–239.

8 Hopkins, L. L. and Schwarz, K. 1964. *Biochim. Biophys. Acta* 90:484–491.

9 Liu, V. J. K. and Morris, J. S. 1978. *Amer. J. Clin. Nutr.* 31(6):972–976.

10 Hambidge, K. M. *et al.* 1968. *Diabetes* 17:517–519.

11 Hambidge, K. M. *et al.* 1972. *Amer. J. Clin. Nutr.* 25(4):376–389.

12 Hambidge, K. M. 1974. *Amer. J. Clin. Nutr.* 27:505.

13 Davison, I. W. F. and Secrest, W. L. 1972. *Anal. Chem.* 44:1801.

14 Schroeder, H. A. 1973. *The Trace Elements in Man.* Old Greenwich, CT: Devin-Adair, p. 72.

15 Abraham, A. S. *et al.* 1980. *Amer. J. Clin. Nutr.* 33:2294–2298.

16 Tipton, I. H. and Cook, N. J. 1963. *Health Phys.* 9:103.

17 Schroeder, H. A. 1958. *J. Chron. Dis.* p. 287.

18 Schroeder, H. A. *et al.* 1970. *J. Chron. Dis.* 23:123.

19 Daoud, A. S. *et al.* 1976. *Arch. Pathol. Lab. Med.* 100:372.

20 Wissler, R. W. 1978. *Advan. Exptl. Med. Biol.* 104:77.

21 Malinow, M. R. *et al.* 1978. *Atherosclerosis* 30:27.

22 Malinow, M. R. *et al.* 1978. *Atherosclerosis* 31:185.

23 Casdorph, H. R. *et al.* 1981. *J. Holistic Medicine* 3(1):53–59.

24 Newman, H. A. *et al.* 1978. *Clin. Chem.* 24:541.

25 Gordon, T. *et al.* 1977. In: *Hyperlipidemia: Diagnosis and Therapy*, Rifkind and Levy, eds. Grune and Stratton, p. 71.

26 Hulley, S. B. *et al.* 1977. *J. Amer. Med. Assoc.* 238:2269.

27 Carew, T. E. *et al.* 1976. *Lancet* 1315.

28 Passwater, R. A. 1977. *Supernutrition for Healthy Hearts.* New York: Dial Press, pp. 37–38.

29 Riales, R. 1979. *Chromium in Nutrition and Metabolism.* Elsevier/North-Holland Biomedical Press, pp. 199–212.

30 Doisy, R. J. *et al.* 1976. In: *Trace Elements in Human Health and Disease*, vol. 11, Prard and Oberleas, eds. New York: Academic Press.

31 Offenbecher, E. and Pi-Sunyer, F. X. 1980. *Diabetes* 29:919–925.

32 Liu, V. J. K. and Morris, J. S. 1978. *Amer. J. Clin. Nutr.* 31:972–976.

33 Schroeder, H. A. 1968. *Amer. J. Clin. Nutr.* 21(3):230–244.

34 Schroeder, H. A. and Balassa, J. J. 1965. *Amer. J. Physiol.* 209:433–437.

35 Steub, H. W. *et al.* 1968. *Science* 166:746–747.

36 Official Report, National Diabetes Commission, and National Diabetes Data Group, National Institutes of Health.

37 Kolata, G. B. March 16, 1979. *Science* 203:1098–1099.

38 *Science News* 182 (3/24/70).

39 *Science News* 116:104 (8/11/79).

40 University Group Diabetes Program, *J. Amer. Med. Assoc.* July 1978. Also see Kolata, G. B. March 9, 1979. *Science* 203(9):986–990.

41 Glinsmann, W. and Mertz, W. 1966. *Metabolism* 15:510.

42 Levine, R. A. *et al.* 1968. *Metabolism* 17(2):114–125.

43 McCay, C. M. 1952. In: *Cowdry's Problems of Aging*, Lansing, ed. Baltimore, MD: Williams Wilkens.

44 Schroeder, H. A. 1965. *Life Sci.* 4:2057–2062.

45 Passwater, R. A. (work in progress).

46 Doisy, R. J. *et al.* 1971. In: *Newer Trace Elements in Nutrition*, Mertz and Cornatzer, eds. New York: Dekker.

47 Canfield, W. K. and Doisy, R. J. 1975. *Diabetes* 24(2):406.

48 Morgan, J. M. 1972. *Metab. Clin. Exp.* 21:313–316.

49 Levine, R. A. *et al.* 1968. *Metab. Clin. Exp.* 17:114–125.

50 Kumpulainen, J. T. *et al.* 1979. *J. Agric. Food Chem.* 27(3):490.

51 Dufor, C. N. and Becker, E. 1962. *Geological Survey Water Supply* paper 1812. Washington, D. C.: U. S. Govt. Printing Office.

52 Toepfer, E. W., *et al.* 1978. *J. Agr. Food Chem.* 21:69–73.

53 Mertz, W. 1971. *Ann. N. Y. Acad. Sci.* 199:191–199.

54 Mertz, W. 1969. *Physiol. Rev.* 49:163–239.

15

SELENIUM

Selenium is an essential trace element[1] that is a vital concern today because the amount of selenium in typical diets has decreased alarmingly. Selenium is required to maintain resistance to many diseases, yet selenium-deficient soils, modern fertilization practices and the spread of acid rains has reduced the amount of selenium in our foods. We regard selenium as the major micronutrient problem facing Americans, followed by chromium and manganese. Most of the pioneering work on selenium and health was performed by Dr. Klaus Schwarz.[2]

The total-body content of selenium in an average adult is less than a milligram with major portions of that concentrated in the liver, kidney and pancreas.[3,4] The normal blood level of selenium is 21 to 23 micrograms per 100 milliliters, mostly transported via the alpha- and beta-globulins.[5]

The absorption of selenium seems to be efficient (44–70 percent), but the mechanism is unknown.[6] Excretion is principally in urine although a small fraction is excreted in the feces, and a trace is lost in the breath.[7] Homeostasis is achieved by the regulation of urinary selenium excretion. Selenium absorption and fecal excretion are not regulated.

At the present time the only known function in man for selenium is as a component of the antioxidant enzyme, glutathione peroxidase.[8] Glutathione peroxidase protects vital components of the cell against oxidative damage.

Although no human disease has been shown to be due to a selenium deficiency, the role of selenium (as glutathione peroxidase and otherwise) is quite extensive. In protecting each of our body's 60 trillion or so cells, selenium prevents the decay of cellular function.

Cancer

Current evidence suggests that improved selenium nutrition can reduce cancer risk. In recent studies, moderate amounts of selenium were added to the normal diets of animals who had been treated with cancer-causing substances, or who had evidenced a high, spontaneous incidence of cancer. In almost every case, selenium supplementation substantially reduced the incidence of cancer.[9–16]

One particularly striking study by Dr. Gerhard Schrauzer of the University of California at San Diego included a control group of mice of a type that normally develops breast cancer spontaneously.[17] Among the group that did not receive extra selenium, 83 percent developed breast cancer, while those mice whose diets were supplemented by selenium throughout their lives lived longer and cancer developed in only 10 percent of the animals. This finding is supported by the fact that in selenium-poor New Zealand the incidence of intestinal cancer in sheep dropped sharply after the sheep received selenium supplements.

At the human level, there is equally impressive evidence that increased selenium intake can protect people, too. In those cases where regional nutritional selenium consumption has been effectively measured, a negative correlation between selenium intake and the incidence of many types of cancer—including breast, colon, ovary, pancreas, prostate, lung and bladder—has consistently resulted. In other words, the more selenium consumed, the lower the incidence of cancer.[18–28]

Additional details may be found in *Selenium as Food and Medicine*.[29]

Heart disease

Studies conducted by such researchers in cardiovascular diseases as Dr. Raymond Shamberger of the Cleveland Clinic and Dr. Johan Bjorksten of the Bjorksten Research Foundation suggest that selenium is an important protective factor in high blood pressure, stroke, heart attack and hypertensive kidney damage.[29–34] Inhabitants of areas low in selenium have high rates of heart disease, while those with high selenium intake experience low rates of heart disease.

This protective role of selenium may be the result of several different mechanisms. For one, selenium is necessary for the health of the heart muscle itself.[35] It can, for example, improve the function of mitochondria (the energy-producing units of cells) by protecting them from lack of oxygen. This may account for the fact that selenium supplementation is effective in the treatment of chest pains associated with heart disease (angina pectoris).[36,37] Selenium is also required for the production of a specific type of hormone-like substance called prostaglandin, which helps regulate blood pressure.[37,38] And selenium detoxifies cadmium, a pollutant which produces high blood pressure.

Chinese physicians recently reported that a serious heart disease—Keshan disease, one that affected children especially—was prevalent throughout vast areas of rural China.[39] Since this land is known to be low in selenium, the physicians set up a controlled study.

The study of the effect of selenium supplements on Keshan disease was initiated in 1974. In Mianning county, selenium supplements were given to 4,510 children selected at random, while 3,985 others made up the control group receiving the placebo. The following year these two groups were increased to 6,709 and 5,445, respectively. The results were so dramatic that the control group was abolished in 1976 and all children (who now numbered 12,579) were given selenium supplements. Thus, 99 percent of the children aged one to nine in four communes in the county participated in the clinical trial.

As reported in the *Chinese Medical Journal* and *Lancet*:

In 1974, of the 3,985 children in the control group, there were fifty-four cases of Keshan disease (1.35 percent), while only ten of the 4,510 selenium supplemented children fell ill (0.22 percent). The difference in morbidity rate between the two groups was highly significant:

Again a significant difference was shown in the 1975 figures with fifty-two of 5,445 children in the control group (0.95 percent) and only seven of the 6,767 in the treated group (0.1 percent).

As a result of these two years [showing] that oral administration of selenium had positive effects in the prevention of Keshan disease, all the children were given selenium supplements from 1976 on. In consequence, only four cases occurred out of the 12,579 children in 1976, further lowering the rate to .03 percent. In 1977 there were no fresh cases among the 12,747 treated children.[39]

The Chinese are seriously considering adding selenium to table salt as a protective measure. We added iodine to salt to prevent goiter but as yet have not decided to add selenium as a routine preventive. Of course, people should always be able to choose between supplemented or not supplemented products.

Soon after the Chinese findings became known in the United States, alert physicians noticed the disease here (it had been here all along, but simply mis-diagnosed as congestive heart failure due to some other cause such as a virus).

The first recognized case published in a major U.S. medical journal was that of a forty-three-year-old man who had been on parenteral alimentation (fed by solution into a vein in a manner similar to, but more advanced than older types of intravenous feeding) for two years.[40] The same issue of *The New England Journal of Medicine* also carried an editorial explaining the essentiality of selenium in man to the medical profession.[41]

The following week that journal described a two-year-old girl on Long Island who had the typical features of Keshan disease. "She was admitted to the hospital with dyspnea, cardiomegaly, and congestive heart failure. Five days before admission increasing dyspnea, cough, and weakness developed. She had tachycardia, cardiomegaly, and bilateral rales; there was no heart murmur. Her liver was enlarged and palpable."[42]

The report also described her hair analysis and diet: "The zinc concentration in her hair was 80 micrograms per gram (normal: 130), and the urinary zinc was 2825 mcg/g creatinine (normal 450). The copper concentration in her hair was 66 mcg/g (normal 70). After four weeks of selenium supplementation . . . the serum selenium concentration rose to 0.15 from 0.04 micrograms per milliliter. . . . She improved steadily at home. . . . Her diet before the onset of this illness had consisted of grits, sausage, and beans for breakfast, a frankfurter and beans at lunch, and pork and beans with rice for supper. Her only beverage was water or Kool-Aid. Her estimated selenium intake was 10 micrograms per day and her zinc intake 1 to 2 mg."

Another article in *The New England Journal of Medicine* reported that oral selenium supplementation reversed the biochemical evidence of another patient's selenium deficiency.[43]

Immune system

Strengthening your immune system means increasing your resistance to disease. Selenium has improved the protective level of the immune system by as much as twenty to thirty times.

In 1972, Soviet Researcher Dr. T. F. Berenshtein discovered that supplements of selenium plus vitamin E produced more antibodies when a vaccine was given than when the vaccine was given alone. Dr. Berenshtein found that selenium alone was less effective than the combination, and vitamin E alone had no effect on antibody formation. Dr. Berenshtein measured the antibodies produced during the immunization of rabbits with typhoid vaccine.[44]

In 1973, studies indicated a similar stimulation of the immune response in mice by selenium. Drs. John Martin and Julian Spallholz and their colleagues at Colorado State University found that dietary supplementation with selenium at levels above those recommended as nutritional requirements enhanced the primary immune responses.[45] (Drs. Spallholz and Martin are now at Texas Tech University.) The Colorado State University researchers measured the number of antibody-forming cells and the levels of antibodies in sheep. The stimulatory effect of selenium was independent of vitamin E levels.

Selenium promoted the increased number of immunoglobin-M-producing cells and immunoglobin-M antibodies. Diets at 0.7 parts per million and 2.8 ppm produced respectively sevenfold and thirtyfold more antibodies.

In a later symposium, the researchers also reported enhanced secondary antibody response to tetanus toxoid. Their experiments showed selenium enhanced the immune response in guinea pigs. They attributed selenium's role in stimulating the immune response to provoked inflammation, increased ubiquinone production and depressed cyclic AMP (adenosine monophosphate, a nucleotide) formation.[46] They concluded: "Clearly, dietary selenium enhances both primary and secondary immune response. There is an increased production of both immunoglobin-M and immunoglobin-G."

In 1978 experiments with dogs confirmed the earlier observations (in mice, sheep and guinea pigs) that selenium enhanced the immune response. Drs. B. Sheffy and R. Schultz found that antibody production in response to canine distemper-infectious hepatitis virus vaccine was dependent upon both selenium and vitamin E status of the dog.[47]

In 1980, scientists started taking advantage of the immune enhancement property of selenium and used selenium supplements to strengthen the protective effect of a malaria vaccine.[48]

Sources and needs

The selenium content of plants varies with the selenium content and *availability* in the soil. The selenium content of animal products varies with the selenium content of the diet fed the animals. Thus the foods vary markedly from region to region in their selenium content, and food tables (such as Table 15.1) are unreliable. Good selenium foods are seafood, whole grains, organ meats, garlic, onion, and yeast. The best approach is a varied diet. If blood or hair analysis indicates a selenium deficiency, selenium supplements are available.

The Food and Nutrition Board has recommended a dietary intake of 50 to 200 micrograms of selenium per day.[1] We feel that a range of 100 to 300 mcg may be more optimal. This can readily be achieved by eating a varied diet and taking a moderate selenium supplement.

Toxicity may begin at 1000 micrograms (1 milligram) per day of inorganic selenium, and 2000 to 3000 micrograms per day of organic selenium.

Hair analysis

Because of technical difficulties with the methodologies used to measure selenium, routine selenium measurements on hair analysis have not been especially reliable until very recently.

Hair measurements of selenium are further complicated by the fact that anti-dandruff shampoos contain high concentrations of selenium which becomes tightly bound to hair. Hair which has been shampooed with a selenium-containing compound retains artificially elevated levels of selenium on hair analysis. The fact that selenium-containing shampoos, when used only on the scalp, cause a clearing of seborrheic dermatitis (a form of dandruff) in the eyebrows and on the chest, in areas remote from the scalp, would indicate that selenium is absorbed through the skin and is an effective treatment for seborrheic dermatitis. Therefore, an individual using a selenium-containing shampoo for dandruff may well be treating a selenium deficiency. Elevated hair selenium may therefore indirectly cause clinical suspicion for a selenium deficiency.

In those areas of China where Keshan heart disease was epidemic, caused by selenium-deficient diets, hair concentrations of selenium were found to average less than 0.12 parts per million. Keshan disease was not found in any child with a hair selenium concentration greater than 0.12 ppm. Individuals living in areas where adequate selenium was consumed were found to have hair selenium levels ranging from 0.25 to 0.6 ppm. These figures were reported in the English-language journal *Lancet* and were translated from the *Chinese Journal of Medicine*.

Selenium measurements taken with atomic absorption techniques are sometimes quite different from measurements obtained from the same specimen using argon plasma emission. For that reason, clinical significance has not been attributed by the authors to hair selenium measurements available from commercial laboratories in the United States unless the hair selenium was so high as to indicate the use of an anti-dandruff shampoo. In those cases selenium deficiency was suspected but could not be proven without blood or serum selenium measurements.

Because hair selenium has not yet been completely proven to have clinical significance, at least by techniques commonly available to health-care practitioners, no specific case histories will be given. Rapid progress is being made to refine and to improve the accuracy of selenium measurements and in the near future it is felt that reliable selenium measurements will be available on screening tests at a reasonable cost.

TABLE 15.1 SOURCES OF SELENIUM

Micrograms (mcg) per 100 grams edible portion (100 grams = 3½ oz.)

Butter	146	Garlic	25
Smoked herring	141	Barley	24
Smelt	123	Orange juice	19
Wheat germ	111	Gelatin	19
Brazil nuts	103	Beer	19
Apple cider vinegar	89	Beef liver	18
Scallops	77	Lamb chop	18
Barley	66	Egg yolk	18
Wholewheat bread	66	Mushrooms	12
Lobster	65	Chicken	12
Bran	63	Swiss cheese	10
Shrimp	59	Cottage cheese	5
Red swiss chard	57	Wine	5
Oats	56	Radishes	4
Clams	55	Grape juice	4
King crab	51	Pecans	3
Oysters	49	Hazelnuts	2
Milk	48	Almonds	2
Cod	43	Green beans	2
Brown rice	39	Kidney beans	2
Top round steak	34	Onion	2
Lamb	30	Carrots	2
Turnips	27	Cabbage	2
Molasses	26	Orange	1

Source: MineraLab, Inc.

REFERENCES

1 National Research Council. 1980. *Recommended Dietary Allowances*. Washington, D. C.: National Academy of Sciences, pp. 162–163.

2 Schwarz, K. and Foltz, C. M. 1957. *J. Amer. Chem. Soc.* 79:3292–3293.

3 Lathrop, K. A. *et al.* 1972. *J. Nucl. Med.* 13(56):7–30.

4 Wenzel, M. *et al.* 1971. *Int. J. Appl. Radiat. Isotop.* 22:361–369.

5 Dickson, R. C. and Tomlinson, R. H. 1967. *Clin. Chim. Acta* 16:311–321.

6 Thomson, C. D. and Stewart, R. D. 1972. *Proc. V. Otago Med. Sch.* 50:63–64.

7 Burk, R. F. *et al.* 1972. *J. Nutr.* 102:1049–1056.

8 Hoekstra, W. G. 1974. In: *Trace Element Metabolism in Animals*. Baltimore, MD: University Park Press, pp. 61–77.

9 Medina, D. October 2, 1981. *J. Amer. Med. Assoc.* 246(14):1510.

10 Harr, J., Exon, J., Whanger, P. and Weswig, P. 1972. *Clinical Toxicology* 5(2):187–194.

11 Passwater, R. 1973. *American Laboratory* 5(6):10–22. (Also U. S. Pat. appl. 39140, 97011, 271655, 398596, 481788.)

12 Wattenberg, L. 1972. *Journal of the National Cancer Institute* 48:1425–1431.

13 Jacobs, M. and Griffin, C. 1977. *Cancer Letters* 2:133–138.

14 Griffin, C. and Jacobs, M. 1977. *Cancer Letters* 3:177–181.

15 Schrauzer, G. and Ishmael, D. 1974. *Annals of Clinical Laboratory Science* 4:441–447.

16 Whanger, P., Tinsley, I., Schmitz, J. and Exon, J. May 1980. Second International Symposium on Selenium in Biology and Medicine, Texas Tech University, Lubbock, Texas.

17 Schrauzer, G. 1978. *Inorganic and Nutritional Aspects of Cancer*. New York: Plenum Press, p. 330.

18 Schrauzer, G. 1978. *Inorganic and Nutritional Aspects of Cancer*. New York: Plenum Press, p. 336.

19 Schrauzer, G. and Rhead, W. I. 1971. *Experientic* 27:1069–1071.

20 Schrauzer, G., Rhead, W. and Evans, G. 1973. *Bioinorganic Chemistry* 2:329–340.

21 Shamberger, R. and Frost, D. 1969. *Canadian Medical Association Journal* 100:682.

22 Shamberger, R. and Willis, C. 1970. *Journal of the National Cancer Institute* 44:931.

23 Shamberger, R. and Willis, C. June 1971. *Critical Reviews in Clinical Laboratory Sciences*, pp. 211–221.

24 *Chemical and Engineering News.* January 17, 1977. p. 35.

25 Schrauzer, G. 1978. *Inorganic and Nutritional Aspects of Cancer*. New York: Plenum Press, p. 334.

26 Schrauzer, G., White, D. and Schneider, C. 1977. *Bioinorganic Chemistry* 7:36.

27 *Critical Reviews in Clinical Laboratory Science* 2:211–221.

28 Wedderburn, J. 1972. *New Zealand Veterinarian Journal* 20:56.

29 Passwater, R. A. 1980. *Selenium As Food & Medicine*. New Canaan, CT: Keats Publishing, Inc.

30 Frost, D. March 1980. *CRC Critical Review of Toxicology* 15(6).

31 Private communication, Executive Health Report, 1980 and May 3, 1976. *Chemical and Engineering News*, p. 25.

32 Bjorksten, J. 1979. *Rejuvenation* 7(3):61–66.

33 *Chemical and Engineering News.* September 24, 1979. p. 24.

34 Vincent, J. 1970. *Prostaglandins* 8(4):339–340.

35 Folkers, K. 1970. *Feedstuffs*. Also see 1965. Kummerow, F., ed. *Metabolism of Lipids*. Springfield, IL: Charles C. Thomas, p. 262.

36 *Wall Street Journal*. March 13, 1973.

37 Willalon, J. 1974. Thesis, Univ. Michoacana de Dan Nicolas de Hidalgo, Morelia, Mexico.

38 Perry, H. *et al.* 1974. In: *Trace Substances in Environmental Health Proceedings*, D. Hemphill, ed. Univ. of Missouri 8:51.

39 *Chinese Medical Journal*. 1979. 92(7):471–476. Also see October 27, 1979. *Lancet*, p. 890.

40 Johnson, R. A. *et al.* 1981. *N. Eng. J. Med.* 304(20):1210–1212.

41 Young, V. R. 1981. *N. Eng. J. Med.* 304(20):1228–1230.

42 Collipp, P. J. and Chen, S. Y. 1981. *N. Eng. J. Med.* 304(21):1304–1305.

43 King, W. W. *et al.* 1981. *N. Eng. J. Med.* 304(21):1305.

44 Berenshtein, T. 1972. *Zdravookh. Belorussia* 18(10):34–36. C. A. 78:24162.

45 Spallholz, J. *et al.* 1973. *Proceedings of the Society of Experimental Biological Medicine* 143:685–698.

46 Martin, J. and Spallholz, J. 1976. *Proceedings of the Symposium on Selenium-Tellurium in the Environment*. Pittsburgh, PA: Industrial Health Foundation, pp. 204–225.

47 Sheffy, B. and Schultz, R. 1978. *Cornell Veterinarian* 68(Suppl. 7): 48–61.

48 Desowitz, R. and Barnwell, J. 1980. *Infection and Immunity* 27(1):87–89.

16

MOLYBDENUM

Molybdenum is an essential trace mineral for man and other mammals. It is a key component of three important enzymes in our bodies: xanthine oxidase, aldehyde oxidase and sulfite oxidase. These enzymes are involved with fat oxidation and purine metabolism. The average adult has about 9 milligrams of molybdenum concentrated mostly in the liver, kidney, adrenal gland, bones and skin.

Molybdenum deficiencies are becoming a concern to nutritionists because of modern diets consisting largely of refined foods. Soil depletion often restricts plant growth, especially crops depending on nitrogen fixing bacteria, such as peas and beans. The best food sources of molybdenum are beans, whole grains and organ meats. However, we strip the grain to make white flour, and half of the molybdenum remains in the bran.[1] Beans can lose molybdenum during preparation, and few organ meats find their way into modern menus. Therefore, most molybdenum deficiencies stem from poor food selection rather than poor soils.

Molybdenum deficiencies are now being associated with cancer of the esophagus, sexual impotency and tooth decay.

Some crops can be low in molybdenum. Crops in the Transeki region of South Africa have become molybdenum deficient, and cancer of the esophagus there is increasing rapidly. In the United States, areas deficient in molybdenum have high rates of cancer of the esophagus.[2] However, it has been found recently in China that where there is low molybdenum in the soil, there is a high nitrogen content which leads to the formation of nitrosomines in the soil, which in turn affects the plants. This seems to be the factor influencing the cancer rate rather than the direct influence of molybdenum itself.

A diet relatively rich in molybdenum was believed to have been responsible for a surprisingly low incidence of tooth decay among U.S. Navy recruits from Ohio.[3] More research is required to confirm this possible link.

There is a suggestion that a molybdenum deficiency may be a factor in some cases of gouty arthritis.[4]

Molybdenum's unique functions appear to be related to its ability to catalyze chemical reactions that require the simultaneous exchange of two electrons and two protons. Enzymes containing molybdenum give up two electrons at one end of the molecule, changing the attraction for other atoms, and causing protons to be given up at the other end. Thus, molybdenum containing molecules act much like a battery with chemical reduction (gain of electrons) taking place at the "anode" end of the molecule, and oxidation at the "cathode" end.

Molybdenum and copper seem to have a "balancing" relationship where they may interact or even share or compete for common enzyme systems. High copper intakes increase molybdenum excretion. A great deal needs to be learned of the possible reactions and interactions of molybdenum and other nutrients.

The RDA range for molybdenum is 150 to 500 micrograms daily for adults. The best food sources of molybdenum are buckwheat, oatmeal, wheat germ, sorghum, lima beans, soybeans, navy beans, liver, peas, sunflower seeds and lentils. Table 16.1 lists molybdenum content of some typical foods.

No toxic effects have been reported.

Hair analysis

The clinical significance of hair concentrations of molybdenum are unknown at this time. Much more research must be done.

TABLE 16.1 SOURCES OF MOLYBDENUM

Micrograms (mcg) per 100 grams edible portion (100 grams = 3½ oz.)

Lentils	155	Cottage cheese	31
Beef liver	135	Beef	30
Split peas	130	Potatoes	30
Cauliflower	120	Onions	25
Green peas	110	Peanuts	25
Brewer's yeast	109	Coconut	25
Wheat germ	100	Pork	25
Spinach	100	Lamb	24
Beef kidney	77	Green beans	21
Brown rice	75	Crab	19
Garlic	70	Molasses	19
Oats	60	Cantaloupe	16
Eggs	53	Apricots	14
Rye bread	50	Raisins	10
Corn	45	Butter	10
Barley	42	Strawberries	7
Fish	40	Carrots	5
Whole wheat	36	Cabbage	5
Wholewheat bread	32	Whole milk	3
Chicken	32	Goat milk	1

Source: MineraLab, Inc.

REFERENCES

1 Schroeder, H. J. 1973. *Trace Elements and Man*. Old Greenwich, CT: Devin-Adair.

2 Schroeder, H. J. 1970. *J. Chron. Dis*. 23:481.

3 *Caries Research*. 1969. 3(1).

4 *Nutr. Rev*. 1974. 32:120–122.

Research trace elements

SILICON

VANADIUM

NICKEL

TIN

LITHIUM

RUBIDIUM

STRONTIUM

SULFUR

COBALT

Introduction

Another group of trace elements are under investigation as possibly essential to man. However, trace element research is difficult and sufficient information is lacking to establish their essentiality unequivocally.

The National Research Board has noted that the following trace elements have been established in animals other than man: silicon, vanadium, nickel, and tin. Cobalt has also been postulated as being essential in some laboratory animals aside from its role as a component of vitamin B12.

Still other researchers are studying trace elements such as germanium, lithium and strontium to determine if they are essential or even health-improving.

Of the research trace elements listed above, silicon, vanadium and nickel seem to be the closest to being determined "essential." Deficiencies of these three trace elements have been produced in two or more animal species and independently confirmed. Deficiencies of tin have been produced but as yet studies have not been independently confirmed by other researchers.

17

SILICON

Silicon is a "research trace mineral" but the term "trace" may or may not be applied appropriately. The main problems in silicon research are that there is more silicon in the environment than any other element except oxygen and that the diseases possibly associated with silicon deficiency are considered to be caused by other factors by most researchers.

With silicon so abundant in our environment and any silicon requirement too small to be readily noticed, it is not especially logical to expect silicon to be lacking in our diets. Yet there is important evidence to suspect that this is the case.

Silicon is very similar to carbon. Carbon is the main structural element in the molecules of plants and animals. Carbon is the element of life, and chemists refer to most carbon-containing molecules as "organic" molecules.

Silicon can form long complex molecules in the same manner as carbon. However, chemical bonds involving silicon atoms are stronger than bonds involving carbon atoms. As a result, silicon-containing molecules are relatively stable and structurally strong. There is evidence that some complex molecules in plants and animals are either linked together by silicon or have silicon substituting for one of the carbon atoms at regular intervals or at least inserted periodically in the complex molecules. It may be that silicon is used to provide strength or "architectural" rigidity wherever certain structural molecules are used extensively, such as in bone and organ tissue.

The stony skeletal structures of diatoms (one-celled brown algae), radiolarians (shelled protozoa related to amebas), and some sponges contain silica. Until recently, biologists believed that silicon was not essential in any other animals. However, certain animal tissues—such as arteries, tendons, skin, connective tissue, cornea and sclera (white of the eye)—have recently been found to contain large amounts of silicon, up to several hundred micrograms of silicon per 100 milligrams of tissue. Other tissues, such as liver, kidney and blood, contain very little. Collagen, the "glue" that holds us together, contains silicon in silanolate form. While vitamin C functions only as a catalyst in the formation of collagen, silicon is actually a structural part of collagen. Silicon-containing substances are found in all cartilage, and in the material binding body cells together.

Silicon is also present in a variety of plant fibers, including sugar-beet and sugar-cane pulp, oat and rice hulls, oat, rice and wheat straw, and alfalfa. This silicon may occur in organic or inorganic form. Silicon is also present in certain complex polysaccharides purified from plants, including alginic acid from horsetail kelp, and pectin from citrus fruit.

The silicon content of plant fibers is not related to their cellulose content, and, in fact, cellulose contains very little silicon. Starch and glycogen also contain practically no silicon, and refined flour and soybean products are also low in this element. Bran is not a reliable source of silicon and "high fiber" bread made with cellulose contains practically none.

Silicon is concentrated in sites of active calcification in the bones of young birds and mammals including humans.[1,2] Calcium and silicon are probably concurrently necessary for bone formation.

The nutritional essentiality of silicon in animals was discovered in 1972 in a series of brilliant experiments by Dr. Klaus Schwarz and Dr. Edith Carlisle of the School of Public Health at the University of California at Los Angeles.[3–5]

Young rats fed a silicon-free amino acid diet showed retarded growth. The bone structures surrounding their eye sockets were distorted, and their incisors (front teeth) were not normally pigmented, indicating abnormal tooth-enamel development. The skeletal alterations involved the cartilage matrix.[6] Rats fed the same diet with silicon grew 25–34 percent faster and had teeth which appeared normal. When atherosclerosis was induced in rabbits by injection with adrenalin, or by a high cholesterol diet, the silicon content of their aortas declined up to 20 percent. When sodium silicate or lysine silicate was injected intravenously into these rabbits or added to their diet, the silicon content of their aortas returned to normal, and their aortas contained only mild or no atherosclerotic deposits.[7,8]

The elasticity of mouse skin is increased more than fourfold when mice are injected under the skin with 2.9 mg silicon dioxide per day over an eight-to-fourteen-day period, or when pieces of skin are immersed in a 0.25 percent solution of silicon dioxide. Perhaps silicon-containing foods can help to maintain youthful skin. They may even reverse skin changes accompanying aging.

Since several components of collagen (structural polysaccharides such as chondroitin sulfate and hyaluronic acid) contain 300 to 550 parts per million of bound silicon, this silicon may be cross-linking these molecules, increasing their size and stability.[9] As a result, the structural stability of such tissues as skin and arterial and stomach linings could be improved by silicon. Arterial linings which have been stabilized by this chemical cross-linking may be less susceptible to small injuries that can initiate atherosclerosis. The silicon content of arteries declines by more than half over the first forty years of age or in atherosclerosis, even though the chondroitin sulfate content does not.[10,11]

Several studies have shown that wherever atherosclerotic plaque is found in human arteries, there is a considerable decrease in silicon in that artery in comparison to arteries without plaque.[12-14] One study of persons over sixty years of age determined the difference. There was fourteen times as much silicon in disease-free arteries as in atherosclerotic arteries.[15] There was also a significant difference in the amount of silicon in the blood.

Trace mineral researcher Herbert H. Boynton points out:

The biological mechanisms by which chondroitin sulfate and other silicon compounds alleviate cardiovascular disease are not well known at this time. It may be that they architecturally strengthen the walls of the arteries and render them resistant to fatty infiltration, and it may be that they inhibit the synthesis of an enzyme called hyaluronidase. Hyaluronidase causes the degradation of the collagen-like, silicon-containing material which forms the interior of the blood vessels.

Mr. Boynton further emphasizes:

There is a clear and almost invariable relationship between the amount of silicon in the aorta (the chief artery) and the degree of atherosclerotic deposits in the aorta: If silicon is high, the arteries are clear. If silicon is moderate, there is moderate atherosclerosis. If silicon is low, atherosclerosis is severe. It would seem, then, that adding biologically available silicon to the diet might well be helpful in preventing or alleviating atherosclerosis. Experimental evidence confirms that this is true.

In a number of clinical trials, Dr. L. M. Morrison and B. H. Ershoff of the Institute for Arteriosclerosis Research at Loma Linda University have shown that chondroitin sulfate, a natural collagenlike substance rich in silicon, has been dramatically successful in reducing the symptoms of heart disease associated with atherosclerosis. Similar experiments have been conducted with equally impressive results by a team of Japanese physicians headed by Dr. Kenjiro Izuka. Chondroitin sulfate greatly lessens the chest pains associated with heart disease and also reduces serum cholesterol levels. Jacqueline Loeper, a French researcher, duplicated Morrison, Ershoff and Izuka's tests with the same results. However, she used inorganic compounds of silicon rather than chondroitin sulfate.[16]

Heart disease deaths are lowest in the regions of England and Finland where silicon concentrations in drinking water are highest.[17]

Dr. Tom Bassler, former president of the American Medical Joggers Association and Advisor to the Pritikin Research Institute in Santa Monica, California, is a strong proponent of a high-fiber diet and exercise. He believes the dramatic improvement that results in most cases suggests that the fiber itself is replenishing the silicon which is needed for the prevention of both arthritis and atherosclerosis.[18]

Dr. Bassler points out that patients who develop musculoskeletal injuries during training have low levels (4 ppm) of silicon in their hair, whereas those who endure training to become marathoners have normal levels (over 20 ppm). A secondary effect of silicon deficiency may be to limit the physical activity that is protective against heart disease.

Dr. Bassler notes that patients supplementing their diets with bran and alfalfa have extremely high levels (up to 100 ppm) of silicon in their hair.[19] These patients are able to train sufficiently to halt the progression of their disease or possibly even to promote regression of their disease.[20,21]

The dietary intakes of silicon-containing plant fiber products such as pectin, but not silicon-free products such as most bran, can reduce blood fats and cholesterol in rats, chicks, rabbits, pigs, monkeys and humans.[22] The silicon-containing products can bind bile acids in the test tube. Perhaps in the intestine, dietary silicon forms relatively insoluble complexes with cholesterol and related substances (bile acids and cholesterol are chemically related). These complexes, if unbound to silicon, may enter the bloodstream with difficulty. The cholesterol they contain would tend to be eliminated rather than absorbed on a high silicon-fiber diet.

Research by Dr. T. Robinson has also indicated that silicon may be of use against gastric ulcers.[23] Also the fact that silicon is a component of both connective tissue and the fluid that lubricates our joints implies that silicon should be studied for possible involvement with arthritis. Silicon could help determine the viscosity of this lubricating fluid.

Dr. Robinson also notes that the normal blood level of silicon may be twice as high as that of calcium, and there is evidence that the parathyroid hormone exerts a regulatory influence on the blood silicon level.[23]

Dr. A. Charnot, Head of Medical Research in Morocco, experimented over many years on a large number of elderly patients suffering from recalcitrant and painful musculoskeletal disorders such as rheumatoid and osteoarthritis, Paget's disease and intractable sciatica of undetermined origin.[24] In three to six months, he achieved a dramatic increase in articular mobility and marked lessening of pain in the majority of the cases. Furthermore, Dr. Charnot found that with silica supplementation, sclerotic areas tended to disappear while decalcified areas tended to recalcify, a frequent finding on X rays. This calcium regulating function has been observed by others.

In the 1960s, Dr. J. Randoin obtained spectacular results using silicon supplements in experiments with fractured femurs in two groups of young rats.[25] Ten days after fracturing, X rays revealed that rats on the silicon supplemented diet showed advanced healing. By the seventeenth day, X rays showed a complete cure. In the control group on the seventeenth day, there was still no evidence of fusion! Certainly the possible role of silicon in stemming osteoporosis should be investigated.

There is also suggestion that hair, skin, and nails would be healthier, particularly in the aging, with more organic silicon in the diet.

"Dietary fiber" is poorly defined chemically. It designates constituents of food which are resistant to digestion. This comprises not only cellulose but also hemicelluloses, pectins, other polyuronides, gums, mucilages and lignin. Many studies have been published on the effects of these products on blood cholesterol and lipid levels and on experimental models of atherosclerosis. Cellulose, alone, was without influence on serum-cholesterol in all tests except one. Indeed, in some of these studies cellulose functioned as a filler or placebo. Since only certain types of fiber are effective under various experimental conditions, it seems inappropriate to speak about "fiber" in general as a cholesterol-lowering agent.[22]

Dr. Klaus Schwarz has analyzed a variety of products belonging to the category of dietary fiber.[22] See Table 17.1. The results indicate that an exceptionally high amount of silicon is a common denominator of seemingly unrelated components of dietary fiber and other products which have been reported to be effective in lowering cholesterol and lipid levels, preventing experimental atherosclerosis, or binding bile acids.

Dr. Schwarz points out: "Different kinds of dietary fiber might affect chronic diseases through a variety of mechanisms. Fiber might change fatty-acid absorption, bacterial flora, formation of volatile fatty acids, intestinal-transit time, and consistency of feces. It also counteracts toxic effects. Its mode of action in atherosclerosis could clearly be different from the mechanisms which have been invoked in the prevention of other diseases—e.g., diverticulitis and cancer of the colon."[22]

Besides hard water and pectin, food sources of silicon include alfalfa, cabbages, lettuce, onions, dark greens, "horsetail" plants (Equisetaceae), kelp, comfrey, nettles and milk.

One dietary study showed that a typical English diet contained 1.2 grams (1200 milligrams) of silicon. Thus silicon should be considered a "macro"-element, rather than a "trace" element.[26]

It seems like the same old story. As with many other important minerals and trace elements, silicon is processed out of common foods but never restored. Milled flour contains only 2 percent of the silicon originally present. Can it be possible that a deficiency of the second most abundant of all elements is degrading the health of Americans?

TABLE 17.1 SILICON IN DIETARY FIBER

Sample	Silicon (ppm of dry weight)	Sample	Silicon (ppm of dry weight)
Cellulose powder	6	Wheat flour (65% extraction)	21
Cellulose Whatman F-11	6	Soybean meal	1680
Filter paper, Whatman No. 1	50	Soya fluff	80
Cotton, pure, sterile	116	Nutrisoy flour	93
Sugar beet pulp	23,110	Citrus pectin	1130
Sugar cane pulp	11,270	Lemon pectinin	1100
Alfalfa	12,740	Na-polypectate	1040
Rice straw	27,300	Na-pectate, enzymatically de-esterified	1100
Rice hulls	22,500	Guar gum	1420
Oat hulls	16,910	Curry powder	1800
Oat straw	7140	Chondroitin-4-sulphate	1175
Wheat straw	12,240		
Wheat bran	229-1720		

Source: Schwarz, K. Feb. 26, 1977. *Lancet* 454–457.

Hair analysis

Adequate scientific data has not yet been accumulated to prove or disprove the clinical significance of hair concentrations of silicon in relation to concentrations in other organs. Despite this lack of published scientific data, as has been related earlier in this chapter, there is a common opinion among clinicians who measure hair silicon that those patients with higher hair silicon are more resistant to injury and generally exhibit better health for their age than patients with lower hair silicon. At this time, the evidence is anecdotal and of unproven scientific significance.

The methodology for measuring silicon is somewhat more complicated than that used for other elements and hair silicon therefore adds a considerable additional cost to the usual elements measured on a screening panel. It is possible to obtain hair silicon but it is not possible to state with any scientific certainty that the measurement is meaningful in terms of health or susceptibility to disease.

REFERENCES

1 Carlisle, E. M. 1970. *Science* 167:279.

2 Carlisle, E. M. 1971. *Fed. Proc.* 30:462.

3 Carlisle, E. M. 1972. *Fed. Proc.* 31:700.

4 Carlisle, E. M. 1972. *Science* 178:619.

5 Schwarz, K. and Milne, D. B. 1972. *Nature* 239:333.

6 Carlisle, E. M. 1973. *Fed. Proc.* 32:930.

7 Loeper, J. and Loeper, J. April 26, 1958. *Soc. Biologie* 563–565.

8 Gollan, F. 1961. *Proc. Soc. Exp. Biol. Med.* 107:442.

9 Schwarz, K. 1973. *Proc. Nat. Acad. Sci.* 70:1608–1612.

10 Charnot, Y. and Peres, G. 1971. *Ann. Endocrinol.* 32:397.

11 Leslie, J. G. *et al.* 1962. *Fed. Proc.* 110:218–220.

12 Loeper, J. *et al.* 1966. *Giornale di Clinica Medica* 47(7):595–605.

13 Loeper, J. *et al.* April 2, 1966. *Presse Medicale.*

14 Loeper, J. and Loeper, J. March 11, 1961. *Soc. Biologie* 468–470.

15 Mars, G. *et al.* 1970. *Cattedra di Gerontologia e Geriatria dell'Università de Pavia* 18:645–659.

16 Boynton, H. H. March 1977. *Let's Live* 24–30.

17 *Lancet.* May 1980. pp. 1324–1325.

18 Bassler, T. J. July 1978. *Current Prescribing* 60.

19 Bassler, T. J. 1978. *Brit. Med. J.* 1:919.

20 Bassler, T. J. 1977. *Ann. N. Y. Acad. Sci.* 301–579.

21 Bassler, T. J. 1978. *Ann. Intern. Med.* 88:134.

22 Schwarz, K. February 26, 1977. *Lancet* 454–457.

23 Robinson, T. and Robinson, W. 1965. *Military Medicine* 130:1082–1085.

24 Charnot, A. March 1952. *Maroc Medical* 337, 32.

25 Randoin, J. 1961. *Laboratoire de la Société Scientifique d'Hygiène Alimentaire.* Paris.

26 Underwood. E. J. 1977. In: *Trace Elements in Human and Animal Nutrition.* New York: Academic Press.

18

VANADIUM

Vanadium is most likely an essential trace mineral for man, and a deficiency may increase one's susceptibility to the killer diseases such as heart disease and cancer. Evidence from four different laboratories, and on two different species, has established that vanadium is an essential nutrient for higher animals.[1-6]

The total amount of vanadium in the average adult's body may be in the range of 17 to 43 milligrams.[7] Vanadium is essential for growth[1-6] and is involved in fat metabolism.[3,5,6,8,9] A vanadium deficiency results in increased blood cholesterol and triglyceride levels.[3,5,6,8,9] A vanadium deficiency also produces impaired reproductive performance in laboratory animals that does not show up until fourth generation animals are mated.[9] Vanadium deficiency also retards bone formation.[8]

In addition to increased blood cholesterol and triglyceride levels in vanadium deficiency states, it has been found that pharmacological levels of administered vanadium can affect tissue cholesterol levels.[10] One has to wonder about all the commotion over a small reduction in blood cholesterol achieved only by a very large percentage change in dietary intake of certain polyunsaturated fatty acids, when a large percentage reduction of blood and tissue cholesterol can be achieved with only a few extra milligrams of vanadium or a few micrograms of chromium.

222

The altered levels of blood and tissue cholesterol have been related to vanadium inhibition of the microsomal enzyme system known as squalene synthetase, and to the vanadium stimulation of the enzyme, acetoacetyl-CoA deacylase in liver mitochondria.[10,11] This enzyme is important to the conversion of fat into coenzyme A.

Little is known about the dietary intakes of vanadium in various populations, but it is enlightening to compare the heart disease rates of people living near large vanadium deposits to those of people eating diets consisting largely of refined foods.

One interesting comparison is that the heart disease death rate of the vanadium (and selenium) rich New Mexico population is much lower than that in the New England states.[12] In 1955, this was 94 per 100,000 population compared to 341 per 100,000. In 1977, this was 267 per 100,000 population compared to 413 per 100,000.

South Africa also has large deposits of vanadium. Diseases of the heart and circulatory system are practically unknown among the Bantu tribes in that area. Diseases of the heart are practically unheard of in an area of a South American province having large vanadium deposits.[12]

Of course, such observations do not prove a thing since many other factors may be involved. However, it is also interesting to note that the 1932 edition of *Dorland's* (an illustrated medical dictionary) edited by the staff of the American Medical Association recommended vanadium in the treatment of several diseases including neurasthenia, diabetes, and in conjunction with selenium in cancer. The 1957 reprint included the same recommendation. Vanadium was also recommended for treating atherosclerosis in the April 1958 edition of *American Medical Association's Archives of Internal Medicine* (101:685–689).

Why haven't trace minerals been pursued with more vigor? Is the work too hard or are there more funds available for fat and cholesterol research because it is in favor by the heads of the funding institutions?

It is also believed that vanadium functions as an oxidation-reduction catalyst,[13,16] and in bone and tooth formation.[17,18] There is abnormal bone growth in vanadium deficiency, and when radioactive vanadium is used to trace the travel of vanadium in the bodies of laboratory animals, the highest uptake of vanadium is found to be in tooth dentine and bone.[17] The zones of mineralization show the greatest vanadium uptake.[18]

The human requirement for vanadium is not known, and dietary intake data are meager. Typical intakes have been estimated at 2 milligrams daily,[7] but calculations have shown that diets consisting exclusively of milk, meat, and certain vegetables could contain less than one-tenth milligram.[11]

Table 18.1 lists the typical vanadium content of some foods, but keep in mind that the vanadium content of food varies with the vanadium content of the soil.

Toxicity

Vanadium may have a role in manic-depressive patients. These patients have an imbalanced sodium transport through the cellular membranes, which may be caused or at least influenced by vanadium.

Several methods were used to study the effects of vanadium. A double-blind, placebo-controlled crossover trial of a single 3-gram dose of ascorbic acid was carried out in a group of manic and depressed patients. These patients showed significant improvement from ascorbate therapy after the two day trial. In a ten-day double-blind crossover trial, oral vanadium was compared with oral EDTA on mania and depression. (Both ascorbic acid and EDTA are successful treatments for vanadium poisoning.) In this trial, eleven of the thirteen patients were less ill when on EDTA than on vanadium.[19-24] There is evidence that excess vanadium in respect to chromium may contribute to cataract development, but this may be more of a problem of chromium (and selenium) deficiency than vanadium excess.[25]

Hair analysis

The vanadium content in hair correlates with tissue vanadium content in toxic states.[26] Vanadium disappears from the blood and is involved in skeletal tissue mineralization. Radioactive vanadium used as a tracer disappears from blood after twenty days.

The clinical significance of hair vanadium concentrations in other than toxic elevations is not known. If hair vanadium is elevated, further studies must be done on blood, urine or biopsy specimens of other tissues to eliminate the possibility of external contamination.

The clinical significance of low hair vanadium has not yet been proven.

TABLE 18.1 SOURCES OF VANADIUM

Micrograms (mcg) per 100 grams edible portion (100 grams = 3½ oz.)

Buckwheat	100	Carrots	10
Parsley	80	Cabbage	10
Soybeans	70	Garlic	10
Safflower oil	64	Tomatoes	6
Eggs	42	Radishes	5
Sunflower seed oil	41	Onions	5
Oats	35	Whole wheat	5

SOURCES OF VANADIUM (*cont.*)

Micrograms (mcg) per 100 grams edible portion (100 grams = 3½ oz.)

Olive oil	30	Lobster	4
Rice	26	Beets	4
Sunflower seeds	15	Apples	3
Corn	15	Plums	2
Green beans	14	Lettuce	2
Corn oil	12	Millet	2
Oysters	11	Liver, fish and meat	<1
Peanut oil	11	Peas, pears and milk	<0.01

Source: MineraLab, Inc.

REFERENCES

1 Schwarz, K. and Milne, D. B. 1971. *Science* 174:426–428.

2 Hopkins, L. L. and Mohr, H. E. 1971. In: *Newer Trace Elements in Nutrition*, Mertz and Cornatzer, eds. New York: Dekker, pp. 195–213.

3 Hopkins, L. L. and Mohr, H. E. 1971. *Fed. Proc.* 30:462.

4 Strasia, C. A. 1971. Thesis, Univ. Microfilms, Ann Arbor, MI.

5 Nielsen, F. H. 1971. In: *Newer Trace Elements in Nutrition*, Mertz and Cornatzer, eds. New York: Dekker, pp. 215–253.

6 Nielsen, F. H. January 1974. *Food Technology* 38–39.

7 Schwarz, K. 1974. *Fed. Proc.* 33:1748–1757.

8 Nielsen, F. H. and Ollerich, D. A. 1973. *Fed. Proc.* 32:929.

9 Hopkins, L. L. and Mohr, H. E. 1973. *Fed. Proc.* 33:1773–1775.

10 Curran, G. L. and Burch, R. E. 1967. In: *Trace Substances in Environmental Health*, Hemphill, ed. vol. 1. Columbia, MO: Univ. Missouri Press, pp. 93–102.

11 Nielsen, F. H. 1976. In: *Trace Elements in Human Health and Disease*, Prasad, ed. vol. 2. New York: Academic Press, pp. 390–394.

12 Gross, R. H. Personal Communication, May 11, 1959.

13 Schwarz, K. 1974. *Fed. Proceed.* 33:1748–1757.

14 Schroeder, H. *et al.* 1963. *J. Chronic Dis.* 16:1047–1071.

15 Underwood, E. J. 1971. In: *Trace Elements in Human and Animal Nutrition*. (3rd ed.) Underwood, ed. New York: Academic Press, pp. 369 and 416.

16 Bernheim, F. and Bernheim, M. L. C. 1939. *J. Biol. Chem.* 75:789–794.

17 Soremark, R. *et al.* 1962. *Acta Odontol. Scand.* 20:225–232.

18 Soremark, R. and Ullberg, S. 1962. In: *Use of Radioisotopes in Animal Biology and the Medical Sciences*, Fried, ed. New York: Academic Press, pp. 103–114.

19 Naylor, G. J. 1981. *Neuropharm.* 19:1233.

20 *Lancet*. 1981. 8245:511–512.

21 Dick, D.A.T. *et al*. 1981. *J. Physiol*. 310, 27.

22 Naylor, G. J. *et al*. 1981. *Psychol. Med*. 11:249–256.

23 Witkowska, D. and Brzezinski, J. 1979. *Pol. J. Pharmacol. Pharm*. 31:393–398.

24 Anon., 1982. *Nutr. Rev*. (40)10 293–295.

25 Lane, B.C. Private communication. 1982. Dec. 3, 1982.

26 Strain, A. 1964. *J. Nuc. Med*. 5:664.

19

NICKEL

Nickel has long been suspected as having an essential role in human health, but the research has been confusing. Early studies suggesting that low-nickel diets resulted in reduced growth rate of laboratory animals were flawed because the control diets used also produced sub-optimal growth.[1-6] In 1974, Dr. F. Nielsen produced convincing evidence that the growth rate may not be appreciably effected by a low-nickel diet, but in chickens, at least, nickel deficiency results in shorter and thicker legs, and less pigmentation of their shank skin.[7] Blood abnormalities such as decreased hematocrits and abnormal blood cholesterol were also observed. Thus substantial direct evidence exists that indicates nickel is essential.

In laboratory rats, a nickel shortage appears to reduce their normal activity and produces a less-than-healthy appearance characterized by rough hair. During the periods of rapid growth and greatest RNA/DNA turnover, nickel deficient animals have higher death rates than nickel-adequate animals. Dr. Nielsen found that 17 percent of nickel-deficient laboratory rat pups died during the last few days of the suckling period compared to no deaths in the nickel-adequate control group. After weaning, the appearance, activity and growth of the nickel-deficient animals improved. In another experiment involving the second generation, nickel-deficient animals had twice as many pup deaths as the nickel-sufficient.

The biological role of nickel may be in the metabolism or in the structure of cell membranes.[8] Evidence suggests that nickel may also have a role in RNA, DNA and/or protein structure or function. Significant amounts of nickel are present in RNA and DNA. The aforementioned experiment[9-11] with nursing laboratory rats along with other evidence suggests that nickel may have some role in prolactin regulation via an influence on hormonal control.[12] Nickel can activate several enzymes in test tube experiments, but this hasn't been confirmed in animal tests.

Nickel deficiency is not known to be a dietary problem. Grains and vegetables are comparatively rich in nickel,[13] whereas meats, eggs, milk, butter and white bread are very low in nickel.[14] The dietary requirement, if nickel is essential, may be somewhere near 50 to 75 micrograms per day.[15] Table 19.1 lists typical nickel levels in selected foods.

Dietary nickel has not been shown to be toxic, but nickel dusts and gases, such as nickel carbonyl, have been shown to cause skin ailments and lung cancer. Dr. Harvey Ashmead has argued persuasively that the nickel in tobacco contributes to the development of lung cancer.[16] Dr. Ashmead cites the accumulation of nickel in the lungs of cancer patients (as opposed to no accumulation with age in any other organ so far examined) and the formation of the carcinogen nickel carbonyl gas in burning tobacco.

Hair analysis

Nickel is proven to be clinically significant when elevated in hair as evidence of nickel toxicity. External contamination of hair must be eliminated as a cause of hair elevation by blood, urine or organ biopsy studies. The significance of low hair nickel is not known.

TABLE 19.1 SOURCE OF NICKEL

Micrograms (mcg) per 100 grams edible portion (100 grams = 3½ oz.)

Soybeans, dry	700	Carrots	25
Beans, dry	500	Eggs	24
Soy flour	410	Cabbage	22
Lentils	310	Tomatoes	20
Split peas	250	Onions	20
Green peas	175	Potatoes	18
Green beans	153	Beef	16
Oats	150	Apricots	16
Walnuts	132	Oranges	16
Hazelnuts	122	Cheese	15

SOURCE OF NICKEL (*cont.*)

Micrograms (mcg) per 100 grams edible portion (100 grams = 3½ oz.)

Buckwheat	100	Watermelon	15
Barley	90	Lettuce	14
Corn	90	Apples	13
Parsley	90	Wholewheat bread	12
Whole wheat	38	Beets	12
Spinach	35	Pears	12
Fish	30	Grapes	8
Cucumber	27	Radishes	8
Liver	26	Pine nuts	6
Rye bread	25	Lamb	6
Pork	25	Milk	3

Source: MineraLab, Inc.

REFERENCES

1 Nielsen, F. H. and Sauberlich, H. E. 1970. *Proc. Soc. Exp. Biol. Med.* 134:845–849.

2 Nielsen, F. H. 1971. In: *Newer Trace Elements in Nutrition*, Mertz and Cornatzer, eds. New York: Dekker, pp. 215–253.

3 Nielsen, F. H. and Higgs, D. J. 1971. In: *Trace Substances in Environmental Health*, Hemphill, ed. vol. 4. Columbia, MO: Univ. Missouri Press, pp. 241–246.

4 Nielsen, F. H. and Ollerich, D. A. 1974. *Fed. Proceed.* 33:1767–1772.

5 Nielsen, F. H. *et al.* 1974. In: *Advan. Exp. Med. Biol.*, Friedman, ed. vol. 48. New York: Plenum Press, pp. 389–403.

6 Sunderman, F. W. *et al.* 1972. *J. Nutr.* 102:259–267.

7 Nielsen, F. H. 1974. In: *Trace Element Metabolism in Animals*, Hoekstra *et al.*, eds. vol. 2. Baltimore, MD: Univ. Park Press, pp. 381–395.

8 Nielsen, F. H. 1976. *Trace Elements in Human Health and Disease*, Prased, ed. New York: Academic Press, pp. 380–387.

9 Wacker, W. E. and Vallee, B. L. 1959. *J. Biol. Chem.* 234:3257–3262.

10 Eichhorn, G. L. 1962. *Nature* 194:474–475.

11 Sunderman, F. W. 1965. *Amer. J. Clin. Pathol.* 44:182–188.

12 LaBella, F. S. *et al.* 1973. *Nature* 245:330–332.

13 Tiffin, L. O. 1971. *Plant Physiol.* 48:273–277.

14 Schroeder, H. A. *et al.* 1962. *J. Chronic Dis.* 15:51–65.

15 Nielsen, F. H. January 1974. *Food Technology* 39–40.

16 Ashmead, H. Intern. Assoc. Cancer Victims & Friends, 10th Annual Cancer Convention, Los Angeles (September 1–3, 1973).

20

TIN

The essentiality of tin to the rat was established by Dr. Klaus Schwarz who showed that a lack of tin produced a 35 percent growth deficit.[1] Previously, tin had been discounted as a possible essential trace element.

Tin does form interesting organic compounds that have chemical properties in harmony with the view of a biochemical role for tin. Tin has a strong tendency to form coordination complexes and easily bonds covalently with carbon. Furthermore, tin readily participates in oxidation-reduction reactions with an electronic potential similar to that of the flavine enzymes.

The estimated dietary intake of tin seems to vary between 2 and 20 milligrams per day.[2] Tin is present in trace amounts in many tissues, but does not appear to accumulate with age in any organ.

The clinical significance of hair tin concentrations is unknown at this time.

REFERENCES

1 Schwarz, K., *et al.* 1970. *Biochem. Biophys. Res. Commun.* 40:22–29.

2 Schwarz, K. 1971. In: *Newer Trace Elements in Nutrition.* Mertz and Cornatzer, eds. New York: Dekker, pp. 215–253.

21

LITHIUM

Lithium is best known for its pharmacological action against psychiatric disorders, although there is a line of evidence suggesting lithium may be an essential trace element. Lithium may be required as a modulator in the conversion of essential fatty acids into prostaglandins preventing both over-production and underproduction.[1,2]

If lithium proves to be essential, the daily requirements would probably be 2–3 milligrams.

Although isolated information is available on the action of lithium in the body, the specific physiological basis for its action remains obscure.[3] Lithium may stabilize serotonin neurotransmission.[4] Research on behavior has been hampered because the effects of lithium seem to depend greatly on experimental variables such as the route of administration, the dose, the concentration injected and the time of injection.

One of the pioneers in establishing the effectiveness of lithium treatment in both acute mania and depression is Dr. William Bunney, chief of the Adult Psychiatry Branch of the National Institute of Mental Health. Dr. Bunney documented that lithium decreases manic symptoms and that some patients have a recurrence of manic symptoms when lithium is discontinued for only twenty-four hours.

Not all depressed patients obtain relief with lithium. Drs. J. Mendels and

A. Frazer of the Veterans Administration Hospital in Philadelphia found that the depressed patients who were helped by lithium also experienced an uptake of sodium through their cell membranes; whereas, depressed patients who did not get relief did not show much uptake of sodium.[5] This suggests that some depressed patients have cell membranes that do not allow the right mineral ions (particularly sodium) to penetrate, but that lithium can get these ions through and reverse depression.

Drs. Alan Pestronk and Daniel Drachman of the Department of Neurology at Johns Hopkins University School of Medicine suggest that lithium prevents recurrent manic-depressive episodes by regulating receptors on cell membrane surfaces. They found that lithium inhibits the increase in the number of acetylcholine receptors.[6]

Lithium also seems to increase lymphocyte (white blood cell) proliferation and inhibits suppressor cell activity.[7] If so, this suggests a role for lithium in the modulation of cyclic AMP in lymphocytes, which could also be due to the general effect of lithium on cell membranes.

While treating cancer patients, Dr. Paul Calabresi of Brown University noted that lithium not only boosted white blood cell counts of patients on chemotherapy, but it increased the growth rate of cultured cells (in test tubes) from patients with leukemia and lymphoma. This has not been confirmed in the body.

If this should also be found to occur in cancer patients, it is still not clear whether the effect is beneficial or harmful, but Dr. Calabresi urges caution in the meantime. "Lithium's influence on malignant cells suggests its use for cancer patients requires close scrutiny."[8]

Some researchers believe that adequate lithium in the diet or drinking water helps keep people cheerful and having a tranquil outlook on life,[9] but the role of lithium on "non-depressed" persons is not known. As shown by Drs. Mendels and Frazer, lithium may only help those few with defect transport across cell membranes.[5] Dr. Frederick Goodwin of the National Institute of Mental Health agrees that lithium calms down manic depressives but believes it has no discernible calming effect on normal people, and he warns that lithium can be harmful to schizophrenics.[10] Dr. Goodwin notes, "Lithium calms down schizophrenics but it also disorganizes their thoughts and makes them more psychotic."[5]

Recent evidence hints that lithium may help "unipolar" depressed patients in addition to manic-depressives.[11,12] Depression is said to be unipolar when it exists alone and bipolar when it alternates with mania, as in manic-depressive disorders.

Lithium has also been used in the treatment of alcoholics because it can produce a taste aversion to alcohol.[13] In addition, it may benefit Ménière's disease, Huntington's chorea and tardive dyskinesia.

Toxicity

Excess lithium disturbs mineral transport across cell membranes and fluid balance. It can produce nausea, vomiting, tremors, thirst, excessive urination, thyroid swelling, weight gain, drowsiness, confusion, disorientation, delirium, skin eruptions, and even seizures, coma or death.[14-17]

Some cases of irreversible kidney damage have been reported in patients on long term therapeutic doses of lithium for manic depressive illness.

Hair analysis

At this time there is no scientific evidence in the literature to substantiate a conclusion concerning dietary or body lithium content from a measurment of hair lithium.

REFERENCES

1 Horrobin, D. 1981. *Lithium Research Review Series,* vol. 1. New York: Human Sciences Press.

2 Horrobin, D. 1981. *Med. Hypothesis* 7:891–905.

3 Smith, D. F. 1981. *Lithium and Animal Behavior,* vol. 2. New York: Human Sciences Press.

4 *Science.* 1981. 213:1529.

5 Mendels, J. and Frazer, A. November 1980. *Amer. J. Psy.*

6 Pestronk, A. and Drachman, D. B. 1980. *Science* 210:342–343.

7 Gelfand, E. W. *et al.* 1979. *Science* 203:366–367.

8 Anon. July 20, 1981. *Med. World News.*

9 Dawson, E. B., American Medical Associations Western Hemisphere Nutrition Congress (August 31, 1971).

10 Associated Press, Miami Beach, FL (September 1, 1971).

11 Fieve, R. R. *et al.* 1976. *Arch. Gen. Psychiatry* 32:1541–1546.

12 Kiev, A. April 1977. *Drug Therapy.*

13 Revusky, S. March 1981. *Behavioral Research and Therapy.*

14 *Science News.* May 26, 1979, p. 345.

15 *Science News.* August 4, 1979, p. 89.

16 West, A. P. *et al.* July 1979. *Amer. J. Psy.*

17 Bakris, G. L. *et al.* 1980–1981. *Internat. J. Psy. Med.* 10(4):327–331.

22

RUBIDIUM

Rubidium is not yet considered to be an essential trace element, but it may have a role in mineral transport across defective cell membranes as in the case of cancer. Like lithium, which appears to have a role as a mineral transporter across defective membranes in depressed persons, rubidium may have a similar role but in a different membrane defect, one that occurs with cancer.

Research by one of the authors has shown that rubidium decreased the number of tumors and average tumor weight in laboratory animals fed carcinogens or receiving transplanted tumors.[1] This was confirmed by researchers at the Biology Department of American University.[2]

Tumors were transplanted in the abdomen of mice and allowed to grow for eight days. The mice were then divided into two groups. The control group was continued on conventional mouse chow. The test group, in addition to the mouse chow, was force fed 1.1 milligrams per day rubidium carbonate dissolved in distilled water. At the end of thirteen more days the tumors in the control mice had grown to a very large size and all the mice were sacrificed. The tumors were then removed and weighed. The tumors in the rubidium-treated animals weighed only one-eleventh the weight of the tumors in the untreated mice. In addition the treated animals showed no adverse effects from the cancers. The probability that this marked difference in tumor size could have come about by pure chance is exceedingly small.

234

Rubidium may reduce the glucose carried into cancer cells by potassium, by a process in which rubidium replaces potassium. Rubidium is above potassium in the Hofmeister electromotive series (4.16 vs. 4.318 v) and is more readily transported into the cell while at the same time rubidium carries fewer molecules in with it in piggyback fashion, as is the case with potassium. (See the Appendix to this chapter.)

Regardless of the postulated mechanism, it is important for researchers to take note of the reduced number of tumors and reduced tumor weights in laboratory animals given chemical carcinogens or transplanted tumors when fed supplemental rubidium. It is also interesting to note that populations inhabiting countries with low cancer rates also tend to have higher rubidium concentrations in their diets.[3] In the United States, vegetables and fruits typically contain 35 parts per million of rubidium. We do not know what the optimal dietary amount would be if rubidium does prove to play a vital role in health.

For the benefit of researchers interested in our research on the possible role of rubidium and tumor inhibition, the following brief discussion is offered.

By utilizing phosphorescence decay patterns we were able to study the potential distribution of a variety of substances over the membrane surfaces peculiar to individual cells.[4,5]

We observed that carcinogens covered the cell membrane with a blanket of absorbed molecules permanently attached at random points.[6] This "blanket" altered sodium and calcium transport through the membrane, which also reduced oxygen transport into the cell. Dr. Otto Warburg had pointed out over forty years ago that cancer cells are deprived of their oxygen supply.[7] Potassium ions along with associated water and glucose (blood sugar) continued to enter the cell as their electronic potential propelled them through the membrane, independent of membrane excitation (which is stopped by the carcinogen blanket). The glucose, no longer oxidized to carbon dioxide because of oxygen deficiency, is converted to lactic acid instead.

The direct consequence of this effect is that the cell pH drops drastically into the acid range from the normal of 7.35 to 6.0 or lower.[8,9] The low pH and altered transport of large molecules into the cell combined to produce a distinct change in cell metabolism. The acids formed in this low pH medium reacted directly with DNA and thus destroyed its ability to act as a template. Details of this mechanism are given in References.[6,10–13]

This investigation was undertaken to determine the effects of rubidium on tumor growth. Studies of isotope transport through membranes and fluorescence decay patterns indicate that rubidium and cesium ions should be taken up by cancer membranes even more readily than potassium which is the main cation in cancer tissue. Ions below potassium in the Electromotive Series are not readily taken up by cancer tissues due to the adsorption of carcinogenic molecules on the membrane. As a consequence, the concentrations of cations

RESEARCH TRACE ELEMENTS

such as calcium are reduced to essentially one percent in cancer cells as compared to the concentration of normal cells.[14,15]

Because rubidium ions and cesium ions readily attach to cancer membranes they may possess two distinct therapeutic properties: 1) they raise the pH of the cell, and 2) they transport only water into the cell, in contrast to potassium which can transport glucose in addition to water.

The possibility exists that rubidium or cesium ions may not only neutralize toxic enzymes but may also lead to the death of cancer cells. This idea is supported by the fact that diets are high in rubidium in geographic areas where the incidence of cancer is very low.[3]

The research reported here lends further support to the idea that rubidium can markedly retard cancer cell growth. The results indicate that rubidium, if given in larger doses and for longer periods of time, would completely repress cancer growth and eventually result in the death of the cancer cell.

The clinical significance of hair concentrations of rubidium is unknown at this time.

TABLE 22.1 COMPARISON OF TUMOR AND BODY WEIGHTS BETWEEN RUBIDIUM TREATED AND CONTROL ANIMALS

Treatment	Number	Tumor Weight (g)	Body Weight (g)
Rubidium carbonate (0.06 mg/g body wt.)	8	0.275[1]	17.13[2]
Control	6	2.90	18.55

1 = probability that the difference in means is due to chance is < .005
2 = probability that the difference in means is due to chance is < .025

Source for 22.1 and 22.2: Brewer, A. K., Clarke, B. J., Greenberg, M. and Rothkopf, N. 1979. *Cytobios* 24, 99–101.

TABLE 22.2 ORGAN WEIGHTS FROM RUBIDIUM TREATED AND CONTROL ANIMALS

Treatment	Number	Spleen	Kidney
TUMOR-BEARING			
Rubidium carbonate (0.06 mg/g body wt.)	8	113.18[1]	128.42
Distilled water	6	121.72[2]	143.025
WITHOUT TUMOR			
Rubidium carbonate (0.06 mg/g body wt.)	15	83.53[1]	121.75
Distilled water	8	71.95[2]	120.15

1 = probability that the difference in means is due to chance is < .05
2 = probability that the difference in means is due to chance is < .005

Appendix to rubidium discussion

In the unexcited state of the membrane the electron donor capacity is capable of adsorbing cation electron acceptors only down as far as K in the Hofmeister displacement series. In this series, the cations line up as follows:

$$Cs^+ > Rb^+ > K^+ > NH_4^+ > Ba^{++} > Na^+ > Ca^{++} > Li^+ > Mg^{++}$$

The instant a K^+ ion becomes adsorbed on the phosphate $(P=O)$ radical of the membrane it finds itself in a negative potential gradient of some 10^5 v/cm, which is capable of accelerating it across the membrane in the order of 10^{-8} sec.

In the unexcited state only, cations in the plasma mediated by the potassium ion (K^+) of the Hofmeister series are able to enter and pass through the membrane. This accounts for the fact that in cold-blooded animals the ratio of K to Na in the cytoplasm is close to 125:1. In warm-blooded animals it is close to 25:1. In embryonic and cancer tissues, the potassium content is much higher than in normal tissues. In the blood serum, in contrast, the ratio of Na^+ to K^+ is 15.8:1. From this it will be seen that even in warm-blooded animals the preferential selectivity for K^+ over Na^+ is close to 400 to 1, whereas in cold-blooded animals it is almost 2000 to 1. These values do not give the true selectivity, since they involve the return of Na^+ to the plasma. In warm-blooded animals the membrane is excited much more frequently than in cold-blooded animals; hence the return of Na^+ is not as complete. The maximum value for selectivity is certainly materially above the ratios observed.

In our research on the separation of K isotopes by membrane dialysis, it was observed that all cations were associated with polar molecules within the solvent, and that they tended to carry these associated molecules into the membrane with them when there was any degree of mutual compatibility between the molecules in solution and the membrane substance. The fact that K^+ and Rb^+ ions are only lightly associated indicates that they are not the prime contributors to molecular transport. It is possible, however, that they may transport some light polar molecules such as simple sugars and peroxidase.

REFERENCES

1 Brewer, A. K. and Passwater, R. A. 1976. *Amer. Lab.* 8(4):80.

2 Brewer, A. K., Clarke, B. J., Greenberg, M. and Rothkopf, N. 1979. *Cytobios* 24, 99–101.

3 Calloway, D. H. *et al.* 1974. *Ecology of Food and Nutr.* 3:203.

4 Brewer, A. K., U.S. Patent 3,470,373.

5 Adelman, S. L. *et al.* 1967. *Nature* 213:718.

6 Brewer, A. K. and Passwater, R. A. 1976. *Amer. Lab* 8(4):39–47.

7 Warburg, O. 1969. *Konrad Kriltsch.*

8 Von Ardenne, M. 1972. *Adv. Pharmacol. Chemother.* 10.

9 Von Ardenne, M. 1969. *Z. Naturforsch.* B24:1610.

10 Brewer, K. and Passwater, R. A. 1974. *Amer. Lab.* 6(4):59.

11 *Ibid.* 6(6):19.

12 *Ibid.* 6(11):49.

13 *Ibid.* 7(1):41.

14 Lasnitzki, A. and Brewer, A. K. 1942. *Nature* 149:257.

15 Lasnitzki, A. and Brewer, A. K. 1942. *Cancer Research* 2:404. Also see Kandutsch, A. A. *et al.* 1978. *Science* 201:500 and Chen, H. W. *et al.* 1978. *J. Biol. Chem.* 253:3180.

23

STRONTIUM

Strontium has long been associated with strong teeth and bones. There is a strong suggestion that the improved resistance to dental decay claimed for certain high-mineral waters was due more to the strontium, molybdenum and phosphorus content than the fluoride content.[1] Investigations are currently underway to see if strontium will be useful in treating osteoporosis. It is not known whether the increased bone and tooth strength is due to strontium entering into the structure or because strontium increases the utilization of calcium.[2]

There is also a suggestion that strontium improves cell structures. Dr. S. C. Skoryna of McGill University in Montreal has found that after exhaustive exercise the cell structure of animals receiving diets supplemented with strontium was superior to that of animals receiving strontium-deficient diets.

Research also suggests that energy levels may be improved by optimizing the dietary strontium intake.

If strontium is ever confirmed to be an essential nutrient for man, the dietary needs will probably be met by one milligram of strontium per day.

The clinical significance of hair concentrations of strontium is unknown at this time.

REFERENCES

1 U. S. Dept. Interior Geological Survey Paper 1312. 1964.

2 1969. *Caries Research* 3:1.

24

SULFUR

Sulfur is essential to human life, but elemental sulfur is not known to be utilized by man. Ruminant animals can make organic sulfur compounds out of sulfate, but we are dependent on plants and other animals to incorporate sulfur into amino acids, such as methionine, cysteine, cystine and taurine. Methionine is an essential dietary nutrient.

Sulfur-containing amino acids are vital to many enzymes and structural proteins. Evidence indicates that people tend to consume proportionally lower dietary amounts of sulfur-containing amino acids as they age, and as a result, aging people may have less than optimal amounts of sulfur-containing amino acids in their bodies. Vegetarians may also have low sulfur-containing amino acid intakes, especially if they avoid eggs.

Good food sources of sulfur-containing amino acids are eggs, beans, brussels sprouts, onions, garlic and cabbage.

25

COBALT

According to the Food and Nutrition Board, the only known function of cobalt is that of an integral part of vitamin B12.[1] Ruminant animals can utilize inorganic cobalt to produce vitamin B12, but nonruminant species, including man, must meet their cobalt requirements through their vitamin B12 intake.[2] A requirement for inorganic cobalt in laboratory animals has been postulated but not confirmed.[3] A requirement for man has not been established, other than the cobalt contained in vitamin B12 (cyanocobalamin).

REFERENCES

1 National Research Council. 1980. *Recommended Dietary Allowances*. (9th ed.) Washington, D. C.: National Academy of Sciences.

2 Underwood, E. J. 1977. In: *Trace Elements in Human and Animal Nutrition*. (4th ed.) New York: Academic Press.

3 Novikova, E. P. 1963. *Fed. Proc*. 23:T459–460.

Toxic elements

LEAD

CADMIUM

MERCURY

ALUMINUM

ARSENIC

Introduction

The distinction between nutritive and toxic elements is sometimes arbitrary. Even nutritive elements can become toxic at some level, just as water and oxygen can. *Dosis sola facit venenum*—only the dose makes the poison.

There are indications that arsenic may be essential, but it is better known as a poison. Selenium is essential but definitely toxic at high dosages. Copper is essential, but detrimental at high dosages. There may be more elements now recognized as poisons which may have an essential function. All essential elements follow a pattern wherein very low levels produce death from frank deficiency to higher levels that maintain life but produce deficiency diseases, to higher levels that produce average health, to higher levels that produce optimal health, to yet higher levels that produce toxicity signs, to still higher levels that produce death due to excessive toxicity.

The following are classified as toxic elements because essentiality has not been conclusively established—and in most cases, not even suspected—and they *are* known for their toxicity.

The detection of unsuspected toxic elements is the area of usefulness in which hair analysis provides its greatest service.

26

LEAD

Lead is considered the worst pollutant element. Arsenic and other elements may be more toxic poisons, but lead is more dangerous because it is so widespread in our environment. Many have heard how lead poisoning may have contributed to the fall of Rome, and made the Hatter Mad, and they hear of lead poisoning when children eat certain paint chips. Lead poisoning is an insidious health problem that has been detected in many children as a result of an active lead poisoning screening program. Dr. William Strain, director of the trace element laboratory at Cleveland Metropolitan General Hospital, calls lead pollution ". . . the greatest neurotoxin (nerve damaging substance) threat to all mankind. It is a damn epidemic."[1]

We know that ancient man encountered little lead, but once smelting was invented, civilization has encountered lead from many sources. Analysis of annual layers of polar ice has shown that airborne lead levels have increased 200-fold in the past 3000 years.[2,3] The lead content of the oceans has increased tenfold since prehistoric times. Sediment dredged from the bottom of lakes in the United States contains twenty times more lead than it did a century ago.

Dr. Clair Patterson, a geochemist at the California Institute of Technology has calculated that the typical American has more than 100 times as much lead in his blood (15 to 25 micrograms per deciliter) as the typical man did before smelting.[4] The bone content is 500 to 2000 times higher. The lead content of the bones of ancient Peruvians and Nubians is 500-fold lower than present-day Americans.[5,6] Inhabitants of remote areas, such as in the foothills of the Himalayas in Nepal or the Yanomama Indians, have only one-fifth or one-sixth the amount of lead in their blood as does the typical inhabitant of industrialized nations.[7, 8]

Two thousand years ago, the Roman Empire became the first civilized society on earth to use a soft, malleable metal, lead, in its plumbing and in the lining of its wine casks. Even as the first airborne lead began drifting down onto the remote glaciers of Greenland's ice cap, Pliny was warning his contemporaries about the hazards of breathing fumes from the lead smelters of ancient Rome. Some scientists are convinced that the lower birth rates and the mental decline of the ruling class that contributed to the fall of the Roman Empire may have been triggered, in part, by the increased intake of lead from Rome's wine and water.

The typical person today has more lead in his or her body than is compatible with health. More than 400,000 tons of industrial lead now pour into the atmosphere every year. As it settles back to earth, it covers the surface of all exposed soils, plants and window sills. Slowly, but insidiously, it works its way into the body—and the brain—of modern man.

Lead contamination is now so widespread that scientists are having trouble gauging the effect that it has on man. It is too difficult to find anyone who hasn't been exposed to it.

Scientists at the American Association for the Advancement of Science meeting in 1981 agreed there is a growing body of evidence to suggest that modern civilization—at least in a clinical sense—may be slowly going the way of the Roman Empire.

In the laboratories of the U.S. National Institutes of Health, Dr. Ellen K. Silbergeld has found that even extremely low levels of lead have a measurable, detrimental effect on the brains of rats. Once it works its way into the brain, lead clings tenaciously to nerve cells, where it disrupts the communication link between them.

"We know that lead is one of the most ubiquitous and persistent neurotoxins in the environment," Dr. Silbergeld told scientists at the meeting. "The laboratory evidence shows that adverse effects occur at very low levels, but the biochemical bases of lead toxicity do not support the notion that there is any safe threshold for lead exposure. They also raise the disturbing possibility that the effects are irreversible as long as any lead is present in the brain."[9]

Hair analysis studies of 35,504 people by Dr. Emanuel Cheraskin, professor emeritus of the University of Alabama, and Dr. Gary Gordon, chairman of the board of the American Academy of Medical Preventics, found that over 38 million Americans are being slowly poisoned by lead.[1,50]

Early signs of lead poisoning are usually missed because the complaints are vague or associated with other problems. The early symptoms include head-aches, fatigue, muscle pains, indigestion, tremors, constipation, vomiting, anemia, pallor, vertigo and poor coordination. Low-level lead poisoning decreases intelligence, impairs one's ability to pay attention, and affects language function and memory. It can trigger mental problems such as hyperactivity, retardation and senility. Lead pollution has been linked to increased numbers of stillbirths and cancer. The action of lead in the body seems to be to interfere with certain enzymes.

Moderate lead levels can cause kidney damage and suppress the immune system, thus increasing one's susceptibility to many diseases including cancer. Definite signs of heavy lead poisoning are shortened life-span and death, and we are talking about levels well below that of the type of "lead poisoning" referred to in classical "Westerns."

Twenty to twenty-five percent of American men and 10 percent of American women suffer to some extent from lead poisoning.[1] Those persons especially at risk are urban children who eat leaded paint chips or lead-laden dust and soil, adults exposed to lead in their workplace, and pregnant women. Hair analysis and other screening techniques indicate that 40 percent and more of all children in large cities in America have health problems due to lead poisoning.[1] Children are particularly sensitive to lead as they absorb 30–50 percent of that ingested, whereas adults absorb only 5–10 percent.

Dr. Herbert L. Needleman, Professor of Pediatrics at Harvard Medical School, correlated lead levels in the teeth of children with yes or no answers to eleven questions by the teachers of those children. Deciduous or baby teeth were collected as they spontaneously fell out in a population of 2,146 elementary school children. The questions dealt with distractibility, persistence with a task, independent work, ability to organize, hyperactivity, excitability and impulsiveness, frustration tolerance, daydreaming, ability to follow simple directions or sequences and, in general, the ability to function as well in the classroom as other children of the same age. He then plotted in graphic form the lead concentration of these 2,146 children in the city of Philadelphia according to percentage of yes answers to these questions. There were eleven questions and there was a direct, straight-line, linear correlation between the percentage of adverse answers reported by teachers concerning each one of these areas of behavior or learning.

There was no cut-off point. That is, there was no level of lead in which the percentage of yes answers leveled off. The percentage increased linearly from the lowest lead concentration to the highest. This would mean that either the lowest level of lead measured was the threshold, above which increasing lead correlated with behavioral and learning impairment, or more likely, that every child was affected and that the threshold had long since been exceeded by all children. More studies must be done to determine which is the correct interpretation. This one was reported in the *New England Journal of Medicine* in 1979 (300:689–695).

Blood is not a good indicator of lead poisoning because lead quickly departs from the bloodstream and enters the skeletal tissues and hair. Hidden in the skeletal tissue, lead interferes with red blood cell production. A clever technique for detecting occult lead is by measurement of the accumulation of a hemoglobin precursor called zinc protoporphyrin. A better technique of screening for lead is hair analysis.

Environmental contamination

Chemical and Engineering News reports the following industrial uses for lead and resulting sources of lead contamination:

Today, U.S. industry consumes 1.3 million tons of lead annually to make such products as batteries, pigments, solders, pottery, and the antiknock agent in leaded gasoline. Smelting and fabricating lead for these products and burning leaded gasoline to drive our mobile societies can expose workers to high lead levels, and send more than 600,000 tons of lead into the atmosphere to be inhaled or—after deposition on food crops, in fresh water, and on soils and streets—to be ingested by the general population.

Food also can be contaminated by lead from the solder in tin cans, pesticide sprays, and cooking utensils. In older homes where the plumbing consists of lead pipes, and the water is acidic and low in mineral content, lead may leach into the water supplies. Weathering of lead-laden paint and putty in older homes contaminates dust with lead, which can be inhaled or ingested; chipping, peeling, and flaking paint in these homes may offer a child a tempting but dangerous morsel.[9]

The average American daily intake of lead may be 350 to 400 micrograms per day, of which 5 to 10 percent is absorbed by the average adult.[10] The typical adult can excrete 30 milligrams of lead per day.

In 1971, the U.S. Congress passed the Lead-based Paint Poisoning Prevention Act because paint chips were thought to be the major source of ingested lead in children. Studies by Dr. Irwin Billick of U.S. Department of Housing and Urban Development indicate that airborne lead is the bigger problem.[9] However, no one should question that urban children receive most of their lead from dust and soil contaminated by paint chips and/or lead from automobile exhaust.

The Food and Drug Administration was able to toughen the Lead Paint Act and after December 31, 1973, no paint was allowed in interstate commerce that was intended for home use and contained more than 0.06 percent of lead.

Unfortunately, the Lead Paint Act will not appreciably help urban children for many years to come. Although few exterior surfaces are still coated with lead-based paints (up to 50 percent lead), the paint that has flaked off the walls over the years has accumulated in the soil and remains immobile for decades. Lead and other metallic pollutants do not degrade. The natural lead content of soil is 10 to 20 parts per million, but soils near buildings often contain as much as 10,000 ppm of lead.[11]

In older homes, many surfaces have been painted with multiple layers of lead paints, which can chip off even when coated with non-lead paints. If a paint chip contained only 2 percent lead, a child would need only 5 milligrams of paint—a small flake or two—each day to be at risk.[11]

Data obtained in the late 1970s in a random sample of housing in Pittsburgh by the National Bureau of Standards show that more than 40 percent of houses built before 1940 have some surfaces with more than 5 mg per square centimeter of lead in paint, and 13 percent of homes built after 1960 have 2 mg of lead per square centimeter on painted walls.[11]

Titanium dioxide based paints have better color, better hiding, last longer, and fail by chalking, thus do not have to be "burned off" before repainting. The demands of the marketplace are probably more effective than the law regarding exterior paints, but the "Lead Paint Act of 1971" is needed to prevent lead chromates from being used as coloring agents in interior paints. Substitutes have not been as well received by the marketplace for the lead chromate deep yellow.

The U.S. Environmental Protection Agency next ruled that after 1974 at least one grade of low-lead gasoline must be made available throughout the United States. More than 90 percent of the lead in the air in most cities was thought to be from automobile exhausts in the early 1970s. However, it is not clear if the EPA wanted low-lead gasoline because they were concerned about lead pollution or because low-lead gasoline was required because catalytic converters to reduce carbon monoxide emission on cars built after 1974 could be ruined by leaded gasoline.

Lead-containing compounds are used in gasoline as a quick and cheap means of raising octane levels (anti-knock compounds).

This ruling caused an appreciable reduction in airborne-lead. In 1975, 359 million pounds of lead were used by automobiles, but by 1981, the consumption was down to an estimated 118 million pounds (see Table 26.1). At this writing, pressure is being exerted to revoke the ruling which would double the usage according to EPA's Robert Weissman.[12]

Still the danger is not past because of the lead-coating and impregnation of our city streets and highway roadsides. Lead pollution hangs onto the environment just as tenaciously as it hangs onto our bone marrow and causes nerve and mental problems in our children.

TOXIC ELEMENTS

Dietary lead

Adults receive most of their 60–90 micrograms or so of ingested lead from food, not dirt. Most of the dietary lead comes from contamination from soldered tin cans. This problem became apparent in 1972 when canned evaporated milk which is widely used in infants' "formulas" was found to contain one to three parts per million of lead.[13,14]

Just how much lead we get in typical diets seems to vary with the region in which one lives. In 1974, the Food and Drug Administration found an average of 90 micrograms of lead in typical (market basket survey) diets, but the amount varied between averages of 70 to 106 mcg per day in six different regions (see Table 26.2).[15] The year before the FDA found 60 mcg lead per day as the typical adult intake.[16]

Dr. Robert Schaffner of the FDA adds, "while 100 to 150 micrograms per day of lead intake was once thought safe, it is now suspected to be too high. The lead content of many children's diets exceeds that amount. We simply still do not know. What, if any, is the safe level of dietary lead, particularly for children?"[17]

Some scientists contend that the FDA's goal of reducing lead exposure of children to less than 100 micrograms per day is not adequate for health protection. A safe maximum exposure range, the consumer's group argues, is from 0.6 to 10 mcg per day for infants and young children, and from 10 to 78 mcg per day for pregnant women, the two most vulnerable groups.[9]

In 1979, the FDA announced a goal to reduce lead intake 50 percent in five years from lead soldered cans, the only source of lead the FDA believes it can control.[18]

TABLE 26.1 AIRBORNE LEAD FROM GASOLINE

	Average lead content of all gasoline (grams per gallon)	Total pounds of lead used by U.S. cars (millions of pounds per year)
1975	1.60	359
1976	1.62	383
1977	1.46	354
1978	1.32	330
1979	1.16	276
1980	0.71	158
1981 (est.)	0.55	118

Source: Groth, E. March 9, 1981. *Chemical Engineering News* 2–3, and the Ethyl Corp.

Dr. Clair Patterson pointed out that the FDA has really missed the boat in assessing just how much lead is added by lead-soldered cans. The FDA analyses were not performed in lead-free trace element laboratories, thus the fresh food samples were contaminated. Even though the FDA showed considerable lead contamination from lead-soldered cans, the FDA understated the degree of contamination by several orders of magnitude.[19]

In 1978, Dr. Patterson's research group found that the National Marine Fisheries service had made a similar error. The NMFS reported canned tuna had nearly twice as much lead as fresh tuna (700 nanograms per gram of tuna flesh versus 400 nanograms), but more accurate analysis showed that canned tuna acquires over 10,000 times as much lead compared to fresh tuna.[20]

At this writing (1982), the standard three-piece tin-plate can, sealed with a solder that is 97 percent lead, remains the mainstay of the industry.[11] Varnish or no-varnish, the lead content of foods in lead-soldered cans has consistently been found to be significantly higher than the lead content of the same foods in fresh or frozen forms.[11] (FDA says two to three times; Patterson says several orders of magnitude more.)

Dr. Patterson explains how to recognize lead-soldered cans:

Usually, lead-soldered cans are made of tin-plated steel. Aluminum cans, plastic-paper cans and flexible pouch cans are not soldered with lead. The way to tell whether a can contains lead solder is first to see whether it is made of metal, or plastic paper, or is a flexible metal pouch. Don't worry about the latter two kinds. They are not soldered. If the can is metal, look where the side joins the bottom. If the sides of the can flow continuously without a break around the bottom edge onto the bottom of the can, sometimes with a forged ridge, so that it looks like one continuous piece of metal, then it is probably lead-free, since most of these kinds of cans are not soldered. Don't worry about this type of can. Most of these kinds of cans have been forged from sheets of aluminum, but some have been forged from sheets of steel.

The kinds of cans to worry about are those which have a break in the metal where the side joins the bottom. That is, running around the bottom edge is a circular crimp holding the bottom piece to the sides. You can actually see a circular crack at the edge of this crimp separating the side from the bottom. Such cans have a vertical seam running up and down the side from top to bottom and it is this seam that is usually soldered with lead. It is not the circular seam around the bottom edge that is usually soldered. The vertical seam is the potentially dangerous one to be checked.

This type of seam is sealed by pouring hot, molten lead solder on the outside of the seam and then brushing it into the seam as it cools and solidifies. The solder makes an air-tight seal, but it comes in contact with the food on the inside of the can, where very tiny amounts of lead are transferred to the food. Although the actual amounts of lead involved in the transfer are small, lead is so poisonous and the natural concentrations of it in foods are so extremely low that the lead added from the solder contaminates the food by such enormous amounts it makes the food hazardous to eat.

To check for lead solder on the vertical seam, rotate the can in your hand looking at the gap between the top or bottom of the label and the top or bottom circular crimp until you can see the seam. Usually the gap is large enough to allow you to see whether lead solder has been applied to the outside of the seam. If you cannot tell, pull the label away from the seam for a small distance, about a quarter of an inch. The applied lead solder looks like someone has brushed heavy aluminum paint onto it and it has dried as an unsightly, rough patch of silvery, greyish metal of different color and texture than the smooth, shiny, tinned surface of the can. If you see this, the can is soldered. Many such vertical seams are soldered with lead. However, some are not. Those that are not soldered may have a painted label which rolls smoothly and continuously over the vertical seam. Sometimes these non-lead soldered vertical seams are covered with paper labels and in such cases, the shiny sides of the can come together into a smooth, neat vertical crack which is not smeared and discolored.

Alternatives to lead-soldered cans described above are forged steel cans, aluminum cans, glass containers, plastic-paper cans, and flexible metal pouches which contain "canned foods."[21]

Lead enters our food in ways other than environmental pollution of migration from soldered cans. Lead can be leached from improperly glazed dinnerware or lead-based decorations on glassware such as coffee mugs. Acid foods extract lead and cadmium from such improperly glazed utensils. A family of five was poisoned over a three-year period by using an earthenware pitcher for orange juice and an eighteen-month boy in Philadelphia died of lead poisoning due to grape juice being stored in an earthenware pitcher.[22,23]

Food supplements can also contain lead and other pollutants, depending upon the origin and treatment of the supplement. As an example, bone meal, a popular supplement of calcium, can come from the bones of relatively young cattle from Argentina where little traffic exists or from old U.S. horses sent to glue factories. The latter source may be high in lead because of the environmental contamination and the age-dependent accumulation of lead in bones. The former can be virtually lead-free (less than one or two parts per million) as in the former source or extremely high (up to 190 parts per million) as in the latter source. Label directions could cause consumers to ingest 70 to 230 micrograms of lead daily in the latter case. (See the example given under "Case Histories.")

We do not recommend bone meal because of its phosphorus content and suggest chelated calcium, calcium lactate or other calcium salt as a source of calcium. Dolomite is also widely used, but we feel that other calcium and magnesium compounds are easier to digest and assimilate. Occasionally, a brand of dolomite is reported to be contaminated with lead.[24] This may be so, but in 1981 *Prevention* magazine obtained a representative number of dolomite samples from health food stores and mail order sources and had them analyzed by three independent laboratories. Their results showed no dolomite sample had more than three parts per million of lead, which would equal seven micrograms in three average-sized dolomite tablets.[25]

The Food and Drug Administration incorporated heavy-metal contamination of such products into their compliance programs beginning in their 1978 fiscal year.

Other sources of lead contamination

Industrial sources such as smelters and battery plants are obvious sources, but several less-obvious occupational exposures are listed in Table 26.4.

Personal-use sources of lead can include drinking water from solder in plumbing pipes and even hair-color restorers. The Food and Drug Administration has approved lead acetate for use as a color additive in hair dyes.[26] Lead acetate, the ingredient in some dyes that progressively darken gray hair, has been on the list of color additives "provisionally" approved by the agency.

A petition to approve lead acetate, a white lead crystalline compound, had been pending since 1973. Tests were undertaken to resolve the most important safety issue—whether a significant amount of lead acetate is absorbed through the skin when it is used as a hair dye.

The tests showed that about 0.5 micrograms of lead acetate (one half of a millionth of a gram) are absorbed per application. This is a minuscule amount when compared to the 100 to 500 mcg lead that adults receive from food sources each day, and the 20 to 400 mcg lead received from air sources every day.

TABLE 26.2 DIETARY INTAKES OF THE SIX HEAVY METALS BY GEOGRAPHIC REGION IN THE U.S.

Geographic region	Number of samples	Lead (μg/day)	Cadmium (μg/day)	Zinc (mg/day)	As_2O_3 (μg/day)	Selenium (μg/day)	Mercury (μg/day)
Northeast	10	105.5	32.1	19.2	31.3	146.9	2.39
Southeast	7	75.7	24.1	18.7	11.4	154.1	3.84
Central	6	105.5	35.5	18.3	4.4	197.8	3.59
West	7	69.7	43.3	17.7	28.6	190.5	1.85
Average Intake		90.2	33.5	18.6	20.7	168.9	2.84

Source: Cohn, J. Dec. 4, 1972. *Washington Post.*

The tests on which FDA based approval were conducted under the sponsorship of Combe, Inc., the maker of Grecian Formula, and the Committee of the Progressive Hair Dye Industry.[27,28]

Reducing lead toxicity

There is a simple way to combat lead poisoning—include adequate fiber in your diet and take vitamin and mineral supplements.[1] Calcium,[29] copper,[30-32] zinc,[31,32,34] iron,[30,31,33] chromium,[35] vitamin C,[34] and the B-complex vitamins,[36-43] all protect against the toxic effects of lead. Most of the nutrients work by decreasing the absorption of lead, while others work by blocking lead from enzymes or reduce tissue buildup.

Dr. Gerald Bratton, of the University of Tennessee found that megadoses of vitamin B1 reduced symptoms of lead poisoning and tissue buildup of lead.[43]

A mistaken diagnosis first led him to try the vitamin. Lead poisoning in cattle and thiamine deficiency are clinical look-alikes, he points out. "I saw a sick animal so close to a textbook description of thiamine deficiency that I began treatment with the vitamin." Two weeks later, the animal was sick again, and a workup showed lead poisoning. The animal was again treated with thiamine, the source of contamination found and removed, and it recovered completely.

Dr. Bratton treated a few more animals before launching a controlled study of calves fed lead and either treated with thiamine for twenty days or not treated at all. Only untreated animals showed clinical signs of illness: truncal ataxia, pharyngeal paresis, scoliosis, and, eventually blindness. Tissue levels of lead in the treated animals, while not normal, were a tiny fraction of controls.[43]

Dr. Bratton is now investigating the benefits of combining chelation therapy with EDTA along with vitamin B1 injections as a better treatment for lead poisoning.

TABLE 26.3 ESTIMATED DIETARY INTAKES OF HEAVY METALS BY FOOD CLASS

		Lead		Cadmium		Mercury		Arsenic	
		μg/day	% of total	μg/day	% of total	μg/day	% of total	μg/day	% of total
I	Dairy products	0.0	0.0	3.94	7.7	0.0	0.0	2.34	23.1
II	Meat, fish, and poultry	4.00	6.6	2.49	4.9	2.89	100.0	5.64	55.6
III	Grain and cereal	4.16	6.9	11.66	22.8	0.0	0.0	1.35	13.7
IV	Potatoes	0.70	1.2	9.11	17.8	0.0	0.0	0.64	6.3
V	Leafy vegetables	3.03	5.0	3.18	6.2	0.0	0.0	0.0	0.0
VI	Legume vegetables	18.80	31.1	0.42	0.8	0.0	0.0	0.0	0.0
VII	Root vegetables	3.83	6.4	0.76	1.5	0.0	0.0	0.0	0.0
VIII	Garden fruits	11.36	18.8	1.71	3.4	0.0	0.0	0.0	0.0

ESTIMATED DIETARY INTAKES OF HEAVY METALS BY FOOD CLASS (*cont.*)

	Lead		Cadmium		Mercury		Arsenic	
	μg/day	% of total	μg/day	% of total	μg/day	% of total	μg/day	% of total
IX Fruits	9.49	15.7	9.38	18.3	0.0	0.0	0.0	0.0
X Oil and fats	0.67	1.1	1.36	2.7	0.0	0.0	0.17	1.7
XI Sugars and adjuncts	0.55	0.9	0.68	1.3	0.0	0.0	0.0	0.0
XII Beverages	3.81	6.3	6.49	12.7	0.0	0.0	0.0	0.0
Totals	60.4		51.2		2.89		10.1	

Source: FDA. Jan. 21, 1977. FY 1974 *Total Diet Studies* (7320.98)

TABLE 26.4 OCCUPATIONAL SOURCES OF LEAD CONTAMINATION

Acid finishers
Actors
Babiters
Battery makers
Blacksmiths
Bookbinders
Bottle cap makers
Brass founders
Brass polishers
Braziers
Brick burners
Brick makers
Bronzers
Brushmakers
Cable makers
Cable splicers
Canners
Cartridge makers
Chemical equipment makers
Chlorinated Paraffin makers
Chippers
Cigar makers
Crop dusters
Cutlery makers
Decorators (pottery)
Demolition workers
Dental technicians
Diamond polishers
Dye makers
Dyers
Electronic device makers
Electroplaters
Electrotypers
Embroidery workers
Emery wheel makers
Enamel burners
Enamelers
Enamel makers

Explosives makers
Farmers
File cutters
Firemen
Flower makers (artificial)
Foundry workers
Galvanizers
Garage mechanic
Glass makers
Glass polishers
Glost kiln workers
Gold refiners
Gun barrel browners
Incandescent lamp makers
Ink makers
Insecticide makers
Insecticide users
Japan makers
Japaners
Jewellers
Junk metal refiners
Labelers (paint can)
Lacquer makers
Lead burners
Lead counterweight makers
Lead flooring makers
Lead foil makers
Lead mill workers
Lead miners
Lead pipe makers
Lead salt makers
Lead shield makers
Lead smelters
Lead stearate makers
Lead workers
Linoleum makers
Linotypers
Linseed oil boilers

TABLE 26.4 OCCUPATIONAL SOURCES OF LEAD CONTAMINATION

Lithotransfer workers	Rubber buffers
Match makers	Rubber makers
Metal burners	Rubber reclaimers
Metal cutters	Scrap metal workers
Metal grinders	Semiconductor workers
Metal polishers	Service station attendants
Metal refiners	Sheet metal workers
Metal refinishers	Shellac makers
Metallizers	Ship dismantlers
Mirror silverers	Shoe stainers
Musical instrument makers	Shot makers
Nitric acid workers	Silk weighters
Nitroglycerin makers	Slushers (porcelain enameling)
Painters	Solderers
Paint makers	Solder makers
Paint pigment makers	Steel engravers
Paper hangers	Stereotypers
Patent leather makers	Tannery workers
Pearl makers (imitation)	Television picture tube makers
Pharmaceutical makers	Temperers
Photography workers	Textile makers
Pipe fitters	Tile makers
Plastic workers	Tinners
Plumbers	Type founders
Printers	Typesetters
Policemen	Vanadium compound makers
Pottery glaze mixers	Varnish makers
Pottery glaze dippers	Vehicle tunnel attendants
Pottery workers	Wallpaper printers
Putty makers	Welders
Pyroxylin-plastic workers	Wood stainers
Riveters	Zinc mill workers
Roofers	Zinc smelter chargers

Source: MineraLab, Inc.

Pectin and algin are effective forms of fiber that decrease lead absorption and show evidence of possibly increasing lead excretion.[44,45] A two-part treatment with EDTA and dimercapto-1-propanol has been found to be an effective means of inactivating lead.[46]

Hair analysis

Hair analysis is the method of choice for uncovering lead poisoning. The fluorometric method for zinc protoporphryn content is a second choice for screenings. However, blood lead levels are inadequate as a measure of lead content because blood rapidly deposits lead into the skeletal tissue and hair.[47–49]

Several investigators have confirmed that hair analyses indicate ingested levels and body stores of lead.[50-56] An analysis indicating significant levels of lead in the hair should be confirmed by other methods.

Case histories

One case history is reported in the medical literature where a physician had prescribed 50 to 60 grams of powdered bone meal daily for a forty-year-old Hollywood "bit-role" actress.[57] The bone meal was from a glue factory in England and it did contain 190 parts per million of lead. Thus, she was ingesting 10 to 11 milligrams (9,500 to 11,400 micrograms) daily and probably accumulating more than 500 milligrams of lead per year. She took the contaminated bone meal and became weaker and weaker. She did indeed have lead poisoning.

"Over the next several years, her health progressively deteriorated. She lost weight. Her auburn hair turned dark brown, then black, and began to fall out. Muscular weakness became profound, and her right arm became paralyzed with wrist-drop, obvious in retrospect. Her skin became sensitive to sunlight, blotching brown or red. Formication of her extremities became a troublesome symptom, as did a sensation of oppressiveness within the bridge of her nose, a sensation that she likened to a 'gnawing of termites.' Abdominal pain with bursts of colic, constipation, and a persistent metallic taste, with ptyalism also developed."[57]

Her acting career ended when she became unable to walk without a cane. The following year she was hospitalized because of a fever, but no one properly diagnosed the lead poisoning. It's a shame that all patients aren't given a routine hair analysis. During the years of progressive illness, she consulted twenty-two California physicians, all of whom failed to find the cause of her illness.

Many diagnoses were considered: tuberculosis, toxoplasmosis, leukemia, lupus erythematosus, rheumatoid arthritis, and time after time, psychoneurosis. The repetitiousness of the diagnostic studies is reflected in her personal tally of more than 340 roentgenographic examinations. The patient wrote an account of her experience and her ultimate reaction to a physician's recommendation, "You must learn to live with it."

The patient relates, "As I finally came to see it, I had three options: 1) commit suicide; 2) go to a psychiatrist to attempt to learn to live with the pain, accepting the fact doctors couldn't diagnose it; or 3) find the answer myself."[57]

She had her friends carry her to the medical library at UCLA and diagnosed herself as having a metallic poisoning. She was able to consult with Dr. Klaus

Schwarz (1914–1978), then at the Veterans Hospital in Long Beach, and after a thorough interview he suspected the bone meal and analyzed it. Urine analysis confirmed the heavy lead poisoning. Two years after she stopped taking the lead-contaminated bone meal, her urinary excretion of lead was 0.25 milligrams per day which is ten times higher than the normal amount.

After discontinuing the lead-contaminated material, her strength gradually improved, but her immune system remained depressed. She died of leukemia. Lead is known to increase the risk of cancer.

W.D., a forty-five-year-old male patient with chronic myologenous leukemia was found to have a hair analysis showing elevated lead of sixty parts per million (usually less than 20 ppm) and a very low zinc. Lead is a known contributing cause of cancer and lead is more toxic in the presence of zinc deficiency.

Following supplementation with zinc and a variety of other vitamins and minerals, this patient's leukemia became much easier to control and his doses of chemotherapy, necessary to keep his white blood count at acceptable levels, were far less than had previously been the case. His general sense of wellbeing and his ability to perform his usual occupation were restored. It is impossible to say how much his lead burden contributed to his malignancy. There was no doubt clinically that supplementation with those minerals which lead displaces brought about a marked improvement in his symptoms and facilitated other treatments which were already in progress.

C.T., a thirty-three-year-old physician, became mentally ill with a diagnosis of paranoid schizophrenia. He was alcoholic and consuming large quantities of both drugs and alcohol while practicing medicine prior to entering a mental hospital. He responded poorly to treatment until a patient came to him asking for hair analysis. He had no prior knowledge of hair analysis and after looking into the matter ordered a hair analysis not only for his patient but for himself. He discovered very high levels of lead in his own hair four times the upper limit of what is considered to be acceptable in our culture and also elevated levels of cadmium, mercury and copper. The lead concentration was by far the highest into the toxic range.

Following intravenous EDTA chelation therapy and treatment with a variety of nutritional and supplement therapies his condition improved dramatically and his symptoms of mental illness reverted to normal. EDTA provocative testing proved the diagnosis of lead toxicity. He lost his craving for alcohol and had no further need for psychoactive drugs. This is a case which might have gone on indefinitely, with the loss of his license to practice medicine and with the loss to society of a competent physician, had a hair analysis not been done to make the diagnosis which had been missed by many other forms of testing.

Two very important studies were performed by Dr. Oliver J. David, a child psychiatrist in New York City, correlating lead and hyperactive behavior in children. In 1972, Dr. David and his associates at the State University of New York Medical School measured blood lead levels before and urinary lead levels after challenge with a single dose of an oral chelating agent, penicillamine. Hyperactive children had significantly higher values on both measures than did non-hyperactive children. Sixty percent of the post-penicillamine urine levels were in the "toxic" range. Dr. David concluded that there was a correlation between body lead burden and hyperactivity in children.[59] In 1976, Dr. David and his associates performed another study in which lead chelating medication was used to treat thirteen hyperactive, learning-disabled school children whose blood and urine lead levels were in a "non-toxic" range, but in the upper ranges of normal. Children thus treated who had no known brain damage or other organic cause for their hyperactivity or learning disability showed marked improvement following treatment to remove lead from their bodies. Dr. David concluded that lead-chelating agents may have a major place in the treatment of hyperactivity.[60]

In another study the blood lead concentrations of twenty-six healthy medical students were compared with the activity of a zinc-dependent enzyme, delta-aminolevulinic acid dehydrogenase. The blood levels of lead were found to be in the low range of what was considered to be the safe or normal, from 5 to 35 micrograms per deciliter. At that time 80 mcg/dl was considered the upper limit of normal. Most of the students' blood lead measurements ranged from five to 15 mcg/dl. Despite these very low levels of blood lead the activity of the enzyme correlated in a linear fashion with lead concentration. There was therefore evidence that these otherwise healthy young subjects had diminished or poisoning of activity of at least one enzyme as a result of environmental lead contamination, which was probably at a level of close to that in every person alive. The authors, Hernberg and Nikkanen, concluded that "even the comparatively low exposure to lead, prevailing today, interferes with metabolism."[61]

REFERENCES

1 Blosser, J. October 13, 1981. *National Engineer* 16.

2 Murozumi, M. *et al.* 1969. *Geochim Cosmochim. Acta* 33:1247.

3 Settle, D. M. and Patterson, C. C. 1980. *Science* 207:1167.

4 Patterson, C. C. 1965. *Arch. Environ. Health* 11:334.

5 Erickson, E. J. *et al.* 1979. *N. Engl. J. Med.* 300:946.

6 Grandjean, P. *et al.* 1979. *J. Environ. Pathol. Toxical.* 2:781.

7 Hecker, L. *et al.* 1974. *Arch. Environ. Health* 29:181.

8 Piomell, S. *et al.* 1980. *Science* 210:1135–1137.

9 Knight-Ridder News Service, January 25, 1981.

10 Ember, L. R. June 23, 1980. *Chem. Eng. News* 28–35.

11 Schwarz, K. 1977. *J. Amer. Med. Assoc.* 288:2262.

12 Groth, E. March 9, 1981. *Chem. Eng. News* 2–3.

13 *Washington Post,* A-11, October 5, 1981.

14 Anon. November 6, 1972. *N. Y. Times*

15 Cohn, J. December 4, 1972. *Washington Post.*

16 Food and Drug Admin. FY 1974. *Total Diet Studies* (7320.98) January 21, 1977.

17 Food and Drug Admin. FY 1973. *Total Diet Studies* 1974.

18 *Prevention.* July 1981, p. 160.

19 *Federal Register,* August 31, 1979. 44:51233.

20 Chow, T., Patterson, C. and Settle, D. 1974. *Nature.*

21 Patterson, C. and Settle, D. 1980. *Science* 207:1167–1176.

22 Cooney, M. October 1980. *Let's Live* 108–110.

23 *Good Housekeeping.* November 1969, pp. 215–217.

24 *Let's Live* May 1971, p. 2.

25 Roberts, J. 1981. *N. Engl. J. Med.* vol. 305(7):423.

26 *Prevention* July 1981, p. 14.

27 *Federal Register.* October 31, 1980.

28 FED News Release, Dept. Human Health Services. October 31, 1980. p. 51–80.

29 Marzulli, F. N. *et al.* 1978. *Curr. Probl. Dermatol.* 7:196–204.

30 Johnson, N. July 1977. *Trace Element Metabolism in Man and Animals.* Bavaria, Germany.

31 Klauder, D. S. and Petering, H. G. 1975. *Environ. Health Pers.* 12:77–80.

32 Petering, H. G. 1978. *Environ. Health Pers.* 25:141–145.

33 Tsuchiya, K. and Lwao, S. 1978. *Environ. Health Pers.* 25:119–124.

34 *Science News* 1981. 118:136.

35 Papauiabbiym, R. *et al.* 1978. *J. Orthomol. Psychiatry* 7(2):94–106.

36 Aldanazarov, A. and Sabdeova, S. 1961. *Chem. Abst.* 55:26204g.

37 Caccuri, S. and Cesaro, A. 1946. *Chem. Abst.* 40:3532.

38 Pecora, L. 1966. *Panminerua Med.* 8:284.

39 Acocella, G. 1967. *Chem. Abst.* 66:8425.

40 Pokotilenko, G. 1964. *Chem. Abst.* 60:15038h.

41 Herada, A. 1955. *Jap. J. Nat. Health* 24:143.

42 Saita, G. 1955. *Med. Lav.* 46:404.

43 Garminati, G. 1959. *Chem. Abst.* 53:15359b.

44 Bratton, G. R. May 25, 1981. *Med. World News*, p. 3.

45 Koshcheev, A. K. *et al.* 1970. *Gig. Tr. Prov. Zabol* 14(1):52–54.

46 Goyer, R. 1972. *Env. Health Pers.* 2:73.

47 *Chem. Eng. News* January 22, 1973, p. 22.

48 Vitale, L. F. *et al.* 1975. *J. Occup. Med.* 17(3)155–156.

49 Habercam, J. W. *et al.* 1974. *J. Dent. Res.* 53(5):1160–1163.

50 Bushnell, P. J. *et al.* 1979. *Bull. Environm. Contam. Toxicol.* 22:819–826.

51 Cheraskin, E. and Ringsdorf, W. M. 1979. *J. Orthomol. Psych.* 8(2):82–83.

52 Kopito, L. *et al.* 1967. *N. Engl. J. Med.* 276(17):949–953.

53 Kopito, L. *et al.* 1969. *J. Amer. Med. Assoc.* 209(2);243–248.

54 Suzuki, Y. *et al.* 1958. *Tokushima J. Exptl. Med.* 5:111–119.

55 Hasegawa, N. *et al.* 1971. *Ann. Rept. Res. Inst. Envirn. Med. Nagoya Univ.* 18:1–5.

56 Chattopadhyay, A. *et al.* 1977. *Arch. Environ. Health* 32:226–236.

57 Baumslay, N. *et al.* 1974. *Arch. Environ. Health* 29:186–191.

58 Crosby, W. H. 1977. *J. Amer. Med. Assoc.* 237(24):2627–2629.

59 David, O. *et al.* 1972. *Lancet* 2:900–903.

60 David, O. *et al.* 1976. *Amer. J. Psychiatry* 133:1155–1158.

61 Hernberg, S. and Nikkanen, J. January 10, 1970. *Lancet* 63–64.

27

CADMIUM

Cadmium is a pollutant that is fast becoming a more serious health problem than lead. Cadmium can produce high blood pressure, kidney and liver damage, anemia and a host of symptoms due to its inhibition of enzymes and nutrient utilization.

There are no known biological functions of cadmium, except that of interference, inhibition and toxicity. However, the 1980 Recommended Dietary Allowances includes deficiency of cadmium, along with tin and arsenic, as involved in reduction of growth, reproduction or pathologic changes in several animal species.[1] Such reports are still awaiting confirmation by independent investigators before an essential function for these three elements can be established. If an essential role for cadmium in humans can ever be confirmed, many of us will be greatly surprised.

Cadmium concentrates in the kidney and causes damage ranging from kidney failure to high blood pressure (which can be caused by kidney damage). The kidney damage may be due to the fact that cadmium competes with zinc for binding sites in various enzymes and other proteins. The kidney is rich in zinc-containing enzymes; thus cadmium may inhibit these enzymes and interfere with kidney function. Very severe cadmium toxicity can cause the reverse with a decrease in blood pressure with increasing toxicity.

High calcium intake can partially protect against cadmium assimilation.[2,3]

Zinc, selenium, copper, iron and vitamin C can also reduce cadmium uptake and increase cadmium excretion.[4-10] A high-protein diet reduces cadmium retention.[11] Pectin may also decrease cadmium absorption.

Unsuspected chronic cadmium intoxication may be leading to various symptoms that are attributed to other causes. Hair analysis is a useful screen for cadmium toxicity, and even "healthy" adults should have a hair analysis every few years as a screen to detect such suspected toxic minerals. Mild toxicity can become severe with continued exposure.

The most dramatic instance of cadmium poisoning occurred in a fishing village in Japan, along the Jintsu River.[12,13] At first, it was nothing more than excessive lower back pains among the older—aged fifty to sixty—women.

As the pain got progressively worse, the women—those who could walk—would shriek "Itai! Itai!" (the Japanese expression for "ouch!") with every step. Soon, the very few who could move around at all were reduced to an agonizing waddle. Their bones were breaking for no detectable reason, and half of the victims died.

Japanese doctors eventually discovered the cause of what came to be called Itai-Itai or "ouch-ouch" disease: they discovered excessive amounts of cadmium in the urine of the victims, which was traced to a cadmium mine upstream. It was dumping its wastes into the village's drinking and irrigation water.

The severe disease symptoms are attributed to impaired calcium metabolism and impaired regulation of the calcium and phosphorus balance in the body.[14-17] The dietary intake of cadmium was estimated to be 300 to 600 micrograms per day.

Normally streams and reservoirs have low cadmium levels, but drinking water in areas of soft acid water pick up cadmium from water mains, pipes, fittings and solder. Many metallic parts are coated with cadmium to prevent corrosion. Years ago, certain ice cube trays supplied with refrigerators were plated with cadmium. Some people still contain residues of toxic cadmium from past exposures.

Less severe symptoms of cadmium poisoning include protein and sugar in the urine brought on by injury to the kidney and high blood pressure.[13]

It seems that women are particularly at risk of cadmium toxicity. Older women often have osteoporosis and/or have experienced loss of bone minerals in connection with pregnancy and lactation. Women are often iron deficient which increases calcium requirements,[16] and they are also quite often deficient in calcium and vitamin D.

Tests with laboratory animals indicate that pregnant and nursing women may accumulate cadmium at a rate two to three times higher than normal.[19,20] Fortunately for babies, a protective barrier in breast tissue screens out nearly all cadmium from mother's milk. If cadmium enters the diet of infants in appreciable quantities, it is believed to drastically decrease verbal intelligence.[21]

The Environmental Protection Agency (EPA) has recognized the need for limiting the amount of cadmium that enters food as a result of chemical dump runoffs or the use of sewage sludge. On September 13, 1979, the EPA published guidelines for sludge management in the *Federal Register* that established an "acceptable" maximum increase of 30 micrograms of cadmium per day from foods grown on sludge-fertilized soil.[18] This is based on a theoretical maximum acceptable dietary intake of 70 mcg cadmium per day, and a Food and Drug Administration estimate of cadmium in the "average" American diet of 39 mcg per day.

The Joint FAO/WHO Export Committee on Food Additives published guidelines of 57 to 71 mcg cadmium as a maximum limit in 1972.[22]

Inhaled cadmium is more effectively absorbed than ingested cadmium. In heavy smokers, cigarette smoke is a significant source of cadmium. Studies at Tufts University, conducted by Drs. George P. Lewis, Manis Nandi, Hershel Jick, Dennis Slone and Samuel Shapiro, have revealed that 70 percent of the cadmium content of a cigarette passes into smoke.[23]

Animal experiments have shown that the chronic inhalation of cadmium fumes can produce pulmonary emphysema. One pack of cigarettes contains 23 micrograms of cadmium. Chronic inhalation of cigarette smoke would obviously lead to an enhanced cadmium intake, Tufts investigators point out.

Using six different brands of cigarettes smoked by a simple smoking machine, they found the cadmium content in the ash of smoked cigarettes to be 15 to 20 percent of that in unsmoked cigarettes. The filters of smoked cigarettes contained a further 15 to 20 percent. The results indicated that the major part of a cigarette's cadmium content passes out in smoke.

Shortly before coming to Tufts University School of Medicine, Dr. Lewis assayed the cadmium, copper and iron levels in sixty human liver specimens after death. Those patients dying with mention of chronic bronchitis and/or emphysema were found to have a mean cadmium level greater than three times higher than the rest.

Others have confirmed the accumulation of cadmium in the kidneys of heavy smokers. Cigarette smoking results in the absorption of an average of 2 micrograms per pack.[24]

High blood pressure

Cadmium has been implicated as a cause of some forms of high blood pressure by several researchers. High cadmium to zinc ratios in the kidney have been linked to high blood pressure in various populations around the world.[25]

Patients dying from high blood pressure related effects have a high cadmium to zinc ratio in their kidneys.[26] A direct relationship between environmental cadmium and the death rates due to high blood pressure has been shown for several American cities.[27] The damage observed to the kidneys of many high blood pressure patients resembles that in laboratory animals fed cadmium.[28-31]

Elevated blood pressure in laboratory animals occurs when the cadmium-to-zinc ratio exceeds 0.35.[32] Increased renin activity is observed for as long as a month after an oral dose of cadmium is given to laboratory animals.[33] Further studies have uncovered more details of this mechanism.[34]

Cadmium-caused high blood pressure can be reversed by injecting 2-diaminocyclohexane disodium zinc tetraacetate, which chelates cadmium and adds zinc to the kidney and liver.[32]

A dietary approach would be to optimize the selenium, zinc and calcium intake, while avoiding cadmium.

Cadmium in the environment

Cadmium is ubiquitously present in food, water and air. Volatilized by factories, by the burning of wastes and by fertilizing, cadmium first appears in the air, from where some of it is inhaled, but most of which settles into the soil and water.

Cities characteristically have higher atmospheric concentrations of cadmium than rural areas. There is a great deal of variation among cities, depending on their degree of industrialization. Among twenty-eight major American cities, Chicago, a heavily-industrial city, had the highest atmospheric cadmium level, 0.062 micrograms per cubic meter, as opposed to Las Vegas, an isolated non-industrial metropolis, which had the lowest, 0.000. Most of the remaining cities had reported values between 0.005 and 0.020 mcg per cubic meter. These values were an average for the period 1960 to 1961. The rate of industrial consumption of cadmium has more than doubled since then, so one would expect current values to be considerably higher.

Since the average adult inhales about 20 cubic meters of air daily, exposure to cadmium is actually much greater than indicated above. In 1960–61, cities with 0.005 and 0.020 mcg per cubic meter had inhabitants inhaling 0.1 and 0.4 mcg daily, and these figures have also probably increased considerably since then.

Water may be contaminated with cadmium by the settling of airborne cadmium or by effluents from mines, certain factories and smelters. In areas not known to be polluted by cadmium, the reported concentration of cadmium in the water has ranged from less than 1 ppb to 10 ppb. The higher values may result from the use of metal or plastic pipes for distribution. Much higher levels of contamination have been reported in areas downstream from smelters or mines. Assuming an average daily intake or 2 liters of water in unpolluted areas having one to 10 ppb cadmium, daily intake of cadmium in water would be 2 to 20 mcg.

Scientists at Oak Ridge National Laboratory have found a connection between lead and cadmium, which exist in small amounts in soft water, and the development of atherosclerosis. In studies supported by the Department of Energy and EPA, the scientists found that pigeons whose drinking water contained lead, cadmium, or both were more likely to develop cardiovascular disease. However, the effects of cadmium could be reduced significantly by adding calcium to the water, and the effects of lead by adding calcium and magnesium. A three-year study to determine the level of calcium required to eliminate the effects of lead and cadmium has begun.[35]

The trace concentration of cadmium in the soil is being increased daily by the settling of airborne cadmium, by irrigation with cadmium-containing water and particularly by high phosphate fertilizers and sewage sludge, which are heavily contaminated with cadmium. Some plants (wheat and rice) seem to concentrate this mineral. Tomatoes and potatoes also have higher than average cadmium levels. Animal products, particularly liver and kidney, also contribute cadmium to the diet.

Fish and crustaceans are also heavily contaminated with cadmium. In unpolluted areas, shellfish have been reported to have concentrations of 50 ppb. Large ocean fish (cod, tuna, flounder and haddock), which are high on the food chain, have been known to accumulate high levels of cadmium.

According to Dr. Spivey Fox of the Food and Drug Administration:

"In the U.S., man is exposed to cadmium daily via air, food and water. The 'average' intake from these three sources is 0.02, 50 and 10 micrograms of cadmium per day, respectively. If a person elects to smoke twenty cigarettes per day, the intake of cadmium is significantly increased, by approximately 20 micrograms/day. The amount of cadmium that actually enters the body is generally considered to be greater for inhaled cadmium, compared with ingested cadmium, provided the particle size is sufficiently small."[36]

The concentrations of cadmium in foods by twelve classes have been determined by the FDA for several years.[36] Foods were collected in five geographic areas of the U.S., cooked by a dietitian according to local custom and assayed by food class composite. For samples collected between June 1968 and April 1970, the concentrations in most foods ranged between 0.01 and 0.03 micrograms/gram.[37] Cadmium could not be detected in many samples. The highest concentrations for individual composites, 0.08 and 0.07 mcg/g occurred in potatoes and leafy vegetables, respectively.

An estimate of total daily intake was calculated from the concentrations found in the food classes.[38] Grains and cereals contributed the largest amount of cadmium, 14 micrograms. Intermediate amounts of cadmium, 4–7 mcg, were contributed by dairy products; meat, fish and poultry; potatoes; leafy vegetables; fruits; and beverages. Only 1 or 2 mcg cadmium were contributed by legume vegetables, root vegetables, garden fruits, oils, fats and shortening, sugars and adjuncts.

A few specific foods have long been known to contain amounts of cadmium that are higher than the above values. These include oysters, clams, liver and kidney. The only one of these foods included in the diet composites studied by FDA was liver. Oysters contain offsetting high zinc concentrations.

Cadmium interrelationships

Dr. Fox has constructed a simplified table (see Table 27.1) that shows the relationship between cadmium and certain nutrients.[36]

The relationships are considered from the point of view of required nutrients. The question is whether or not cadmium affects the metabolism or function of the required nutrient under "normal" conditions of dietary intake. "Normal" is used in a very imprecise way. Ideally it should refer to experiments in which each required nutrient was present at exactly or only slightly above the requirement level for the particular species. Rather, the studies were carried out with various adequate purified and stock diets which had varying levels of nutrients. A question mark indicates ambiguous findings or lack of studies. Without exception, the data for this table were obtained from studies involving the toxic effects or levels of cadmium in excess of the average man's daily intake.

Hair analysis

Even when high dietary cadmium is fed, the blood level of cadmium remains extremely low. Even intravenously injected cadmium rapidly disappears from blood. Consequently, cadmium data from blood have little diagnostic value.[13,38–40]

The fact that the cadmium level in the hair has statistically significant correlations with respective levels in the kidney ($r = 0.52$) and liver ($r = 0.36$) and that hair sampling can distinguish occupational from non-occupational exposure ($t_{28} = 4.88$) argues well for the use of hair as an indicator of cadmium accumulation.

TABLE 27.1 RELATIONSHIPS BETWEEN CADMIUM AND ESSENTIAL NUTRIENTS

Nutrient	Dietary intake of individual nutrients		
	Normal[a]	Deficiency[b]	Excess[c]
Zinc	+	+	+
Iron	+	+	+(Fe^{2+})
Manganese	+	?	?
Copper	+	+	+
Selenium	+	?	+
Calcium	+	+	?
Ascorbic acid	?	?	+
Vitamin D	?	+	?
Protein	?	+	+

[a] + Cadmium affects metabolism and/or function of the nutrient; ? No relationship has been established.
[b] + A deficiency of the nutrient increases the severity of cadmium toxicity.
[c] + An excess of the nutrient decreases the toxicity of cadmium.

Source: See reference 35.

Case histories

Mrs. H.N. was a sixty-nine-year-old female patient who for decades was afflicted with periods of severe muscular and skeletal pain. She had frequent disabling headaches. At one point in her middle years she was bedridden for approximately twelve months with a mysterious disease which was never diagnosed. The symptoms consisted of muscular weakness and pain.

Hair analysis on this patient revealed cadmium to be 12 parts per million which is approximately twelve times the upper limit of what is considered to be acceptable by most laboratories in this country. This was confirmed by repeat testing. Zinc and chromium were quite low in hair tissue. Zinc is known to be an antidote for cadmium toxicity. Cadmium is much more toxic in the presence of zinc deficiency.

Following EDTA chelation therapy and supplementation with a variety of vitamins and minerals this patient became much more able to enjoy a normal life, with much less pain and many fewer headaches.

Following six months of treatment hair cadmium had increased from 12 to 16 ppm despite clinical improvement. This was interpreted as an indication of mobilization of cadmium from tissue stores throughout the body and increased excretion, using hair as one route of excretion. Her symptoms of angina and cardiovascular disease diminished simultaneously with her improvement of pain. As described earlier in this chapter, the Japanese name for cadmium toxicity translates as the "ouch" disease.

D.P., a sixty-year-old male patient, was first seen for evaluation of high blood pressure in 1979. His blood pressure at that time was 144 systolic and 108 diastolic. He also had a history of maturity-onset diabetes.

A hair analysis initially showed lead of 55 ppm (acceptable less than 20), cadmium 1.4 ppm (acceptable less than 1) and zinc was recorded at 90 ppm (normal 160 to 240), which was low. Both lead and cadmium are more toxic in zinc deficiency states.

This patient was employed at a local foundry where he was daily exposed to lead, cadmium and a variety of other metals and metal fumes. It was suggested that he be treated for his elevated toxic metal levels, but he did not want his employer to find out that he had even had a mineral analysis done because he was afraid he might lose his job. He did agree to a nutritional detoxification program with high-dosage vitamin C.

His blood pressure did not improve and a repeat hair analysis in September, 1980, showed lead at 34 ppm (some improvement), but cadmium had risen significantly to 4.5 ppm. Cadmium is known to cause high blood pressure and it was felt that both cadmium and lead were responsible for the patient's lack of improvement. His blood pressure was treated with increasing doses of routine medications and he is still employed at the foundry.

This represents a documented case of hypertension with increasing severity as cadmium increased in the hair. It is unfortunate that the patient would not agree to more aggressive detoxification therapy.

C.F., a ten-month-old child, was seen with symptoms of spells lasting several seconds and which appeared to be like "seizures." The child grimaced and would become rigid. These spells occurred every five to ten minutes. The child was evaluated fully by a neurologist with brain scans, electroencephalograms and complete neurological evaluation, all of which were completely normal.

Hair mineral analysis initially showed 29 ppm lead (acceptable less than 20) and 0.96 ppm cadmium which was at the upper limits of the acceptable range. This child was treated by her parents with small doses of vitamin C in hopes of neutralizing the lead.

Follow-up hair analysis one year later showed that lead had diminished from 29 to 14 ppm but cadmium had risen markedly from 0.96 to 3.5 ppm. This would be considered a toxic range. At that time the seizure-like episodes were continuing and had progressed to episodes—the patient suddenly dropped on her knees and sometimes made uncontrollable verbal sounds. There were also shaking spells.

An intensive study was done to determine cadmium and lead levels in the environment. Initially lead and cadmium were measured using a DPTA extraction procedure on soil samples and drinking water. The soil lead using this technique was found to be 16 ppm and soil cadmium was 0.2 ppm. Garden plants were found to contain 45 ppm of lead and 0.6 ppm of cadmium. Tap water was found to contain insignificant amounts of lead and cadmium. To further evaluate these results specimens were also sent to a more sophisticated reference laboratory which repeated the determinations using a whole specimen digestate rather than an extraction procedure to see how much lead and cadmium were totally present in the soil, food and water. Using this technique the garden soil was found to contain 44 mg per gm of lead (46,000 ppm) and 380 ppm of cadmium. Leaves of garden vegetables had 14,000 ppm of lead and 780 ppm of cadmium. Again, negligible amounts of lead and cadmium were found in the drinking water.

It became obvious that this patient's source of cadmium and lead contamination was from the garden soil. The family was very nutrition conscious and this child had been raised on breast feeding and organic foods from their own garden since birth. The mother was eating foods from this garden while nursing. Unfortunately, it did not become known that the soil on which their "organic" garden was grown was contaminated until their child became ill. Routine types of medical testing had shown nothing. This is a case which was initially diagnosed by hair analysis and confirmed by other sophisticated follow-up tests.

REFERENCES

1 National Research Council. 1980. *Recommended Dietary Allowances*. Washington, D.C.: National Academy of Sciences.

2 Washo, P. W. *et al*. 1974. *Nutr. Rep. Int*. 10(3):139–149.

3 Pond, W. G. *et al*. 1975. *Proc. Soc. Exp. Biol. Med*. 148(3):665–668.

4 Hill, C. H. *et al*. 1963. *J. Nutr*. 80(3):227–235.

5 Banis, R. J. *et al*. 1969. *Proc. Soc. Exp. Biol. Med*. 130(3):802–806.

6 Ohkata, K. 1972. *Nichidai Lyaku Zasshi* 31(2):105–124.

7 Mason, K. *et al*. 1964. *Anat. Rec*. 148(2):309.

8 Powell, G. W. *et al*. 1964. *J. Nutr*. 84(3):205–214.

9 Lucis, O. J. *et al*. 1969. *Arch. Environ. Health* 19(3):334–336.

10 Maji, T. *et al*. 1974. *Nutr. Rep. Int*. 10(3):139–149.

11 Suzuki, S. *et al*. 1969. *Ind. Health* 7(3/4):155–162.

12 O'Neill, T. 1976. *Nat. Bull*. 15(21):2.

13 Friberg, L. *et al*. 1971. In: *Cadmium in the Environment*. Cleveland, OH: CRC Press.

14 Kazantis, G. 1979. *Environ. Health Pers*. 28:155–159.

15 Fox, M. R. S. 1979. *Environ. Health Pers*. 29:95–104.

16 Nordberg, G. F. 1974. *AMBIO* 3(2):55–66.

17 Bingham, F. T. *et al.* 1975. *J. Environ. Qual.* 4:207.

18 *Federal Register* 1979. 44(179):53438–53468.

19 Bhattacharyya, M. H.and Whelton, B. D. FASEB Meeting, Anaheim, CA (April 1980).

20 Anon. 1980. *Science News* 117:262.

21 Thatcher, R. 1980. Applied Neuroscience Institute of the University of Maryland Eastern Shore, Dept. of Human Health Services release.

22 World Health Organization Tech. Rept. no. 505, p. 32.

23 Anon. May 1970. *Biomedical News* 8.

24 Ellis, K. J., *et al.* July 20 1979 *Science.* 205:323–324.

25 Schroeder, H. A., 1965. *J. Chronic Dis.* 18:647.

26 Schroeder, H. A., 1964. *J. Amer. Med. Assoc.* 187:358.

27 Carroll, R. E., 1968. *J. Amer. Med. Assoc.* 195:267.

28 Schroeder, H. A. and Vinton, W. H. 1962. *Amer. J. Physiol.* 202:515.

29 Perry, H. M., et al. 1961. *J. Chronic Dis.* 14:259.

30 Kenisawa, M. and Schroeder, H. A. 1969. *Exp. Mol. Path.* 10:81.

31 Axelsson, B. *et al.* 1968. *Arch. Environ. Health* 17:24.

32 Schroeder, H. A., *et al.* 1968. *Amer. J. Physiol.* 214–796.

33 Perry, H. M. and Erlanger, M. W. 1973. *J. Lab. Clin. Med.* 83:399.

34 Kopp, S.J. *et al.* 1982. *Science* 217, 837–839.

35 Fox, S. 1974. *J. Food Sci.* 39(2) 321–324.

36 Corneliussen, P. E. 1972. *Pest. Monitor J.* 5:313.

37 Duggan, R. E. and Corneliussen, P. E. 1972. *Pest. Monitor J.* 5:331.

38 Neathery, M. W. and Miller, W. J. 1975. *J. Dairy Sci.* 58 (12) 1767–1781.

39 Miller, W. J., *et al.* 1968. *J. Dairy Sci.* 51:1836.

40 Neathery, M. W., *et al.* 1974. *J. Dairy Sci.* 57:1177.

28

MERCURY

Today, high school chemistry courses often teach of the hazards of mercury by using the example of the "mad hatters." Evidence suggests that some "hatters" became poisoned by the mercury used in the process of making felt hats. Insanity is a typical sign of severe mercury poisoning.

Early scientists frequently used mercury in their experiments because they were fascinated by the intriguing physical and chemical properties of this "quicksilver." Some scientists have suggested that Sir Isaac Newton went mad for a short period in the middle of his otherwise brilliant scientific career because of mercury poisoning.[1,2] How do they know? By hair analysis! Doctors P. Spargo and C. Pounds obtained several locks of Sir Isaac Newton's hair and analyzed them by two methods. Newton's hair contained 197 parts per million mercury (as well as high lead) compared to 5 ppm mercury in "normal" hair.

In 1692, shortly before his irrational behavior, Newton entered in his laboratory notebook, "After I had stirred the mercury and salt together, I put it in the fire to evaporate." At the conclusion of another mercury experiment, Newton noted that the product tasted "strong, sourish, ungrateful." He joked in his later years that his hair turned gray at the age of thirty because of his many experiments with quicksilver.[1]

After Newton became a recluse and ceased experimenting with heavy metals, the effects of the mercury wore off. In 1696, he gave up his reclusive ways to become President of the Royal Society but he never again showed his earlier brilliance. However, there is no evidence of the typical mercury toxicity tremor. This should show in handwriting specimens.

Today we are concerned more with organic forms of mercury than with the metal itself. Any mercury can be converted to organic mercury by living systems. Our awareness of the problems caused by mercury in the food supply and converted into the more highly toxic form of organic mercury compounds called methyl mercury started in the 1950s.

In 1953, a series of reports began appearing in the medical literature describing neurological disorders in the Minamata region of Japan. Eventually, the cause of the nervous system disease was traced to excessive amounts of methyl mercury in the local fish and shellfish due to contamination by factory effluents into Minamata Bay.[3-7] The disease was named Minamata disease, and it killed forty-six people and was known to affect 121 including infants born with serious defects. Seventy-two additional cases with six fatalities were uncovered in 1964 and 1965 in the Niigata area of Japan.

Since that time, the world has been more alert to methyl mercury poisoning. Other cases have appeared in Iraq, Guatemala and the Soviet Union.[8-10] However, the cause in these countries was not fish, but grains treated with organomercurial fungicides. These grains were intended for use as seeds, not food.

In 1970, several members of a U.S. family developed mercury poisoning after eating hogs that had consumed organomercurial-treated grains.[11,12]

Mercury in U.S. seafood

It was no wonder that a mercury-poisoning scare went out in 1970 when certain U.S. swordfish were said to have unacceptable amounts of mercury. Much debate also was initiated.

Large fish usually eat small fish which eat plants. The mercury level increases with each step up the food chain. Thus the larger fish have greater amounts of mercury.

In 1970, fish from Lake St. Clair, a fresh-water lake between Canada and the United States, were found to be high in mercury.[13] This touched off a hunt for other mercury contaminated fish, because it was believed that industrial dumping was the source of the contamination and it was feared to be widespread.[14-18]

In 1971, the Food and Drug Administration advised consumers not to eat swordfish because of their consistently high mercury levels.[19] The debate quickened and in 1972, Dr. Jack Kevorkian a pathologist at Detroit's Saratoga

General Hospital charged, "On very little data, the FDA has almost killed the swordfish industry, is injuring the tuna industry and has thrown thousands of people out of work."[20]

Dr. Kevorkian headed a team of researchers that measured mercury levels in a variety of human organs from fifty-nine autopsy cases collected by the University of Michigan from 1913 to 1970.[21,22] They concluded that mercury levels in the environment were probably lower in 1970 than they were in 1910. They suggested that mercury levels in humans were at their highest in 1913, dropped sharply between 1913 and 1938 and had remained fairly constant since then.

Note that the samples used were from individuals of various ages and dying from various causes. The number of samples in any one classification is thus limited and cannot be said to necessarily represent a trend in mercury exposure for an entire nation.

Also note that the tissues used had been stored for various times in preservative. No hair samples were used. When the reports of the Detroit research team was published in *Chemical and Engineering News*, Dr. K. Pillay of the Nuclear Research Center at the State University of New York in Buffalo commented:

In the light of these reports, I wish to bring to the attention of *Chemical and Engineering News* readers the results of a few simple experiments conducted at our laboratory. A gram of human brain tissue, kept in 30 ml of formaldehyde solution containing 3 micrograms of radioactive mercury (Hg + +) was found to accumulate about 12 percent of the mercury during the first eighteen hours. The absorption of mercury from the preservative continued and increased to 30 percent in twelve days and to 39 percent in nineteen days. Attempts made to leach out the mercury using fresh formaldehyde removed very little, if any, of the accumulated mercury from the tissues.

Several recent objective studies have pointed out that trace levels of mercury are present in almost all the chemicals and materials used around a laboratory. Also, some of the well-known fixatives like Zenker-Formal use large quantities of mercury in their formulation. I am also given to understand that an essential practice in the preservation of biological tissues is to periodically replace the preservatives. This practice in turn enables the preserved tissues to accumulate more mercury, the longer they are preserved and maintained properly. Therefore, it seems to me that it would be appropriate for those who ridicule mercury scare as based on "emotionalism and ignorance" to re-examine their sampling and analysis procedures before attempting flamboyant theories about mercury pollution. It would be a grave mistake to conclude that in spite of the nearly 100 million pounds of mercury consumed in the U.S. during the past twenty years alone, there has been a gratifying cleansing effect on the environmental mercury levels.[23]

Also in 1971, an analysis of tuna caught off both the East and West Coasts between 1878 and 1909 and preserved in formaldehyde at the Smithsonian Institution had the same mercury levels (0.3 to 0.6 ppm) as contemporary tuna.[24]

In 1972, high levels of mercury were found in the bones from twelve of seventeen samples of ancient fish (100 B.C. to A.D. 400).[25]

It is reasonable that the amount of mercury in solution in the oceans hasn't changed appreciably in hundreds of years. The amount of undissolved mercury on the ocean bottom may have increased. An estimate of the amount of mercury released into the environment annually by man is 10,000 tons compared to the 100,000,000 tons already in the ocean.[26] Thus, at the estimated levels, it would take one thousand years of pollution to increase the ocean's content by one-tenth.

Inland lakes and streams are another matter. The use of the Great Lakes as a waste basin and locating chemical dumps so that they can contaminate ground waters is of great concern.

Toxicity

Earlier we described the more severe forms of mercury poisoning as brain damage and other central nervous system disorders and birth defects. The toxic action of mercury is extensive ranging from effects due to binding on the cell membrane to inactivation of a number of enzymes.

Less severe symptoms of mercury toxicity include insomnia, dizziness, fatigue, drowsiness, weakness, depression, tremors, loss of appetite, loss of memory, nervousness, shyness, headache, uncoordination, dermatitis, numbness and tingling of the lips and feet, loss of vision and hearing, emotional instability and kidney damage.

Sources of contamination

There are many potential sources of mercury contamination. Tables 28.1 and 28.2 list common and occupational sources. However, the greatest mercury exposure to the public is from dental procedures, pesticides, cosmetics and medicines.

The American Dental Association News states, "Dentists should alert all personnel who handle mercury about the potential hazards of mercury vapor and the need for good mercury hygiene practices. . . . All amalgam scrap should be salvaged and stored in a tightly closed container. Handling amalgams requires extreme caution and that a *'no-touch'* technique should be employed."[27]

Dr. Bryan Hellewell, Advisor to Environmental Health Agencies on Toxic Metals warned Dr. David Owen, a Cabinet Minister of the Labor Government in Great Britain, in 1972: "In the face of mounting evidence of danger and an absence of evidence of safety, it is my duty to advise you that the use of mercury dental amalgam tooth fillings in the mouths of women who are pregnant should be discontinued."[28]

TABLE 28.1 MERCURY CONTAMINATION SOURCES

Mercury-silver amalgam (dental fillings)
Broken thermometers and barometers
Consumption of grain seeds treated with methymercury fungicide
Fish and marine mammals
Mercuric chloride (used in histology labs)
Calomel (body powders and talcs)
Mercury containing cosmetics
Latex and solvent-thinned paints
Organic mercurials (diuretics)
Air polluted by industrial mercury vapor
Mercury polluted industrial water
Clothing worn by mercury workers
Hemorrhoid suppositories using mercurials
Mercurochrome and thimerosal (Merthiolate)
Fabric softeners
Floor waxes and polishes
Air conditioner filters
Wood preservatives
Cinnabar (used in jewelry)
Batteries with mercury cells
Fungicides for use on lawns, trees, shrubs, etc.
Tanning leather
Felt
Adhesives
Laxatives (containing calomel)
Skin lightening creams
Psoriatic ointments
Photoengraving
Tatooing
Lab and industrial equipment using metallic mercury
Sewage sludge used as fertilizer contaminates soil.
Sewage disposal (may release 1000s of tons of Hg annually world wide)
Fungicides used in water-based, latex paint.

Source: MineraLab, Inc.

TABLE 28.2 MERCURY OCCUPATIONAL EXPOSURES

Amalgam makers	Chlorine makers
Bactericide makers	Dental amalgam makers
Barometer makers	Dentists
Battery makers, mercury	Direct current meter workers
Boiler makers	Disinfectant makers
Bronzers	Disinfectors
Calibration instrument makers	Drug makers
Cap loaders, percussion	Dye makers
Carbon brush makers	Electric apparatus makers
Caustic soda makers	Electroplaters
Ceramic workers	Embalmers

MERCURY OCCUPATIONAL EXPOSURES (*cont.*)

Explosives makers	Mirror makers
Farmers	Neon light makers
Fingerprint detectors	Paint makers
Fireworks makers	Paper makers
Fish cannery workers	Percussion cap makers
Fungicide makers	Pesticide workers
Fur preservers	Photographers
Fur processors	Pressure gage makers
Gold extractors	Refiners, mercury
Histology technicians	Seed handlers
Ink makers	Silver extractors
Insecticide makers	Switch makers, mercury
Investment casting workers	Tannery workers
Jewelers	Taxidermists
Laboratory workers, chemical	Textile printers
Lampmakers fluorescent	Thermometer makers
Manometer makers	Vinyl chloride manufacturing
Mercury workers	Wood preservative workers
Miners, mercury	

Source: MineraLab, Inc.

Dr. Jerry Mittelman of New York asks:

Where is the "health sense," much less the morality, of making these observations— and then permitting mercury amalgams to be placed in people's mouths?

The assumption is that the mercury is locked into the restoration. Not true. Mercury has been found in the urine and blood cells after an amalgam insertion. White cell differential counts change after amalgam removal from the mouth.[29]

Dentists and their assistants are particularly subject to mercury poisoning.[30,31] One in seven dental offices is so contaminated with mercury that the occupants are exposed to high mercury concentrations throughout the day.[31]

Cosmetics and medicines can be an unsuspected source of mercury. Learn to read the labels closely. Some skin bleach creams may contain ammoniated mercury or phenyl mercuric acetate, while others may contain no mercury.[32]

Protection from mercury

Organic mercury seems to be absorbed more readily and via a different mechanism than inorganic mercury. Pectin and alginate may offer some protection against inorganic mercury, but little against methyl mercury. A significant portion of mercury intoxication occurs via inhaled mercury vapor, absorbed mercury vapor, absorbed mercury from dental amalgams or skin absorption of cosmetics or pesticides. Fortunately, selenium binds both methyl mercury and inorganic mercury and protects against all of mercury's toxic effects.[33–36] Chelation therapy with EDTA is somewhat effective in increasing mercury excretion from the body.[37] Other chelating agents are also available for the treatment of mercury poisoning.

Hair analysis

Blood content of mercury reflects only recent exposure to mercury, whereas hair mercury content indicates an integrated history of long-term mercury exposure. Thus hair analysis is preferred because it can detect mercury exposure that might be missed by blood analysis.[38–42]

If your hair analysis indicates a significantly high level of mercury, then your next steps should be to obtain a confirmation as we have suggested.

Case histories

A.S. was a thirty-nine-year old lady who had worked for eleven years repairing, cleaning, calibrating and refilling medical instruments with mercury. During her years of work with mercury in a closed space with inadequate ventilation she developed many symptoms of recurrent depression, nightmares, weakness of her hand grip, arthritic pain in the joints of her fingers, a tendency to bruise easily, hemorrhagic menstrual flow, diminished lateral vision, increasing feelings of anxiety and numerous other psychiatric symptoms. Hair analysis revealed markedly elevated mercury concentration of 14.6 parts per million (upper acceptable 2.5 ppm).

She was subsequently seen by a specialist who confirmed elevated twenty-four hour urinary mercury excretions and treated her with dimercaprol (BAL), a mercury chelating agent. Her condition improved but only somewhat and very slowly. After four years of dimercaprol chelation therapy and intensive nutritional detoxification, her hair mercury returned to acceptable limits at 1.6 ppm. This is a well-documented, proven case of industrial mercury poisoning which was well diagnosed with hair analysis. Her improvement following treatment was also documented by a decrease in hair mercury. Clinically, this patient has never completely recovered from her poisoning. Mercury is difficult to remove from the body.

J.C. was a twenty-five-year-old male patient who presented symptoms of fatigue, lethargy, joint aches and excessive hair loss. Hair mercury was markedly elevated at 14 ppm (acceptable under 3 ppm). Twenty-four hour urinary mercury excretion was three times the upper limit of normal and increased to forty-four times the upper limit of normal on chelation with dimercaprol (BAL) injections. Following treatment hair mercury decreased from 14 ppm down to 5 ppm, much closer to an acceptable level. There was improvement of symptoms following treatment. The source of mercury toxicity for this patient was never identified.

F.G., a forty-eight-year-old dentist, was found on hair analysis to have a markedly elevated mercury of 14 ppm (upper acceptable 3 ppm). He was treated with dimercaprol (BAL) injections and nutritional detoxification. Six months later a repeat hair analysis was in the acceptable range of 2.2 ppm. This dentist had initially been extremely fatigued and depressed. He had given up his private dental practice because of his illness. After completion of his treatment for mercury toxicity he again resumed full employment and was enough improved clinically to teach and later to re-enter full-time private practice.

The exposure to mercury was his occupation as a dentist and his daily handling of mercury in the composition of amalgam (silver-mercury) fillings.

Prior to treatment his symptoms included unexplained recurrent leg pains, joint pains, fatigue, depression, lightheadedness, sleep disorder and increasingly severe headaches.

Without hair analysis this diagnosis might have been completely missed and this patient might have continued in his disabled state, depriving society of his services as a dentist with continued suffering, pain and disability.

REFERENCES

1 Broad, W. J. 1981. *Science* 213:1341–1344.

2 Spargo, P.E. and Pounds, C. A. 1979. *Notes and Records Royal Soc. London* 34:11.

3 Kurland, L. T., *et al.* 1960. *Wld. Neurol* 1:370–395.

4 Tokuomi, H., *et al.* 1961. *Wld. Neurol.* 2:536–545.

5 Irukayama, K. 1966. *Adv. Water Poll. Res.* 3:153–180.

6 Irukayama, K., *et al.* 1961. *Kumamoto Med. J.* 14:157–169.

7 McAlpine, D. and Araki, S. 1958. *Lancet* 2:629–631.

8 Abbasi, A. H. 1961. *Brit. J. Ind. Med.* 18:303–308.

9 Ordonez, J. V., *et al.* 1966. *Bol. Sanu Panam.* 60:510–519.

10 Mnatsakonov, T. S., *et al.* 1968. *Gig. Tr. Prof. Zabol* 12:39–42.

11 Storrs, B., *et al.* 1970. *Morbid. Mortal. Weekly Rep.* 19:25–26.

12 Curley, A., *et al.* 1971. *Science* 172:65–67.

13 Status Report on Mercury in the Food Chain, FDA , Wash., D.C. (Aug. 1, 1976).

14 Effects of Mercury on Man and the Environment, U.S. Senate Hearings, Committee on Commerce (May 8, 1970).

15 Study Group on Mercury Hazards. 1971. *Environ. Res.* 4:1–69.

16 Mercury Contamination in the National Environment, U.S. Dept. Inter. Wash., D.C. (1970).

17 Mercury in the Environment, U.S. Geological Survey, Prof. paper #713 (1970).

18 Symposium on Mercury in Man's Environment, Royal Soc. Canada, Ottawa (1971).

19 News Release, Food and Drug Administration (May 6, 1971).

20 Scripps-Howard Newspaper Syndicate (October 11, 1971).

21 Annual Meeting, Amer. Pub. Health Assoc., Minneapolis, Oct. 11, 1971.

22 *Chem. Eng. News*, 53, Oct. 18, 1971.

23 Pillay, K. K. S. Jan. 10, 1972. *Chem. Eng. News*, 48.

24 Kishore, R. and Guinn, V. Aug. 30, 1971. *Chem. Eng. News*, 14.

25 Wilmsen, E. Jan. 3, 1972. *Chem. Eng. News* 14.

26 *BioScience* 22 (1):24. 1972.

27 *Amer. Dent. Assoc. News* (Sept. 7, 1981).

28 Letter republished in "The Mittelman Letter" no. 133 (Oct. 1981).

29 Mittelman, J., Ibid.

30 Gutenmann, W. H., *et al.* 1973. *Bull Environ. Contam. Tox.* 9(5):318–320.

31 Gronka, P. A., *et al.* 1970. *J. Amer. Dental Assoc.* 81:923–926.

32 Marzulli, F. N. and Brown, W. C. 1972. *J. Soc. Cosmet. Chem.* 23:875–886.

33 Sugiura, Y., *et al.* 1976. *J. Amer. Chem. Soc.* (98(8):2339–2341.

34 Nordberg, G. F. In: *Effects and Dose Response Relationships of Toxic Metals*, 88–91.

35 Potter, S., *et al.* 1974. *J. Nutr.* 104(5):638–647.

36 Anon. 1975. *Nature:* 238–239.

37 Harvey, S. 1970. In: *Pharmacological Basis of Therapies*, Goodman, Chapter 36.

38 Phelps, R., *et al.* 1980. *Arch. Environ. Health* 35(3):161–166.

39 Nord, P. J., *et al.* 1973. *Arch. Environ. Health* 27(6):155–158.

40 Suzuki, T. and Miyama, T. 1975. *Tohuku J. Exp. Med.* 116:379–384.

41 Giovanoli-Jakubezak, T. 1974. *Arch. Environ. Health* 28(3): 139–143.

42 Hefferren, J. J. 1976. *J. Amer. Dent. Assoc.* 92(6):1213–1215.

29

ALUMINUM

Aluminum has not been shown to be essential to plants or animals. Yet aluminum is commonly ingested in food, medicine and cosmetics.

The toxicity of aluminum has only recently been recognized. Previously aluminum was considered to be virtually non-absorbable and was thus widely used in a variety of food additives and over-the-counter drugs such as antacids. Research now suggests that aluminum interferes with normal body processes causing neurological changes such as those recently incriminated in Alzheimer's disease (a form of senility often occurring at a young age), Parkinson's disease, and dialysis dementia.[1,2]

Recent research has shown that aluminum binds to DNA,[3] deposits in abnormal neurofibrillary tangles in the brain, may be a cause of these abnormal changes[4] and inhibits the enzyme, hexokinase.[5] Aluminum has also been linked to three different types of dementia diseases; senile dementia, parkinsonism dementia and dialysis dementia. (*Science News* 122, 292–293. Nov. 6, 1982).

Aluminum is absorbed in the intestine and is excreted via the kidney. In persons with abnormal kidney function, aluminum is deposited in the bones. Dr. R. Recker and colleagues studied aluminum absorption and excretion and report the following:

The gut barrier is permeable to aluminum under conditions of high oral aluminum intake, but accumulations in bone are uncommon since the element is cleared by the kidneys in individuals with normal renal function. Aluminum absorption in bone and tissue of long-term hemo-dialysis patients is a recognized phenomenon, but the possibility of absorption through the gut (important in peptic ulcer patients who ingest large quantities of aluminum in the form of antacids) has not previously been established because of a lack of precise analytic techniques.[6]

The increased level of aluminum in *bones* from the autopsied dialysis patients ranged from nine- to fifty-fold that of the normal nondialysis patients, which indicates that aluminum excretion occurs in those with normal renal function. The bone level of aluminum in peptic ulcer patients was midway between the nondialysis and dialysis autopsy specimens.

These researchers also conclude that the toxic action of aluminum is a direct action of aluminum rather than an indirect process such as phosphate depletion, as suggested by some researchers.

There was a striking decrease in urinary phosphorus levels during loading in all six subjects, while their serum phosphorus levels remained unchanged. Thus, it appears that renal conservation of phosphorus compensated for the decreased phosphorus absorption induced by the aluminum loading. Chronic hemodialysis patients, however, most often have elevated phosphorus levels in spite of aluminum ingestion—a fact that points to aluminum toxicity, not phosphate depletion, as the mechanism. Also, supporting this theory is the fact that the width of the osteoid seam was not increased in the osteoporosis patient in this series.

An earlier study had shown that increased levels of parathyroid hormone in the blood can increase aluminum absorption.[7]

There is suggestion that increased aluminum absorption further activates the parathyroid gland and exacerbates the whole process previously described in the calcium and phosphorus chapters, whereby the degenerative diseases are caused by the imbalanced calcium/phosphorus/magnesium/vitamin D in the diet.

There is even evidence that aluminum binds with phosphate in the diet. Dr. Karl Insogna believes that this direct action exists, whether other interactions exist or not. He comments, "Overuse of certain antacids to ease stomach trouble, especially in the elderly, can cause worse problems, such as weakened bones. Aluminum hydroxide, an ingredient of many popular brands of antacids, binds with phosphates in the diet, preventing them from being absorbed by the body's bones."[8] It may not be that simple, but the results are the same.

Senility

Aluminum was implicated as a cause of senility, sometimes at an early age, (presenile dementia or Alzheimer's disease) in 1977 by a team of researchers led by Dr. Donald Crapper of the University of Toronto.[9] They found four times as much aluminum in the neurons (nerve cells) of senile brains as in the neurons of normal brains. They noted that the aluminum was concentrated in areas of the senile brains that were abundant in neurofibrillary tangles. The tangles are characteristic of senility and presumably "tangle" the nerve transmissions causing confusion and loss of memory.

These findings were confirmed by Dr. Daniel Perl of the University of Vermont College of Medicine and Dr. Arnold Brody of the National Institute of Environmental Health Science in Research Triangle Park, North Carolina.[10] They concluded that aluminum accumulation is associated with Alzheimer's disease, which is the name given to the insidious senile deterioration of the mind that is becoming epidemic in the United States, often beginning in midlife rather than just in old age.

Dr. Lissy Jarvik of the University of California points out that at least 1.5 million to 2 million Americans suffer from Alzheimer's disease and 100,000 die of it each year. Dr. Jarvik warns, "It will be the worst public-health problem of the next century unless we do something about it."[11]

Dr. Leopold Liss of Ohio State University is studying the effects of removing the aluminum deposits with tetracycline.[12]

Aluminum has also been associated with hyperactivity in children.[13]

Dr. H. Richard Casdorph, Assistant Clinical Professor of Medicine at the University of California Medical School believes that aluminum is removed by intravenous EDTA (ethylene diamine tetra acetic acid) chelation therapy.[14] Dr. Casdorph reports cases of Alzheimer's disease improving following EDTA chelation therapy.

Research by one of the authors has revealed massive increases in urinary excretion of aluminum following EDTA chelation therapy.

Please see the Appendix to this chapter for additional information.

Aluminum pots and foil

There is debate over how much aluminum is added to foods by cooking in aluminum pots and pans or by wrapping in aluminum foil. Possible dangers from aluminum cookware appear occasionally in the medical journals[15] but are usually dismissed as being insignificant.[16,17] Aluminum cookware is definitely subject to destruction by acid and alkaline foods, but this source of aluminum in the diet is relatively small. The contribution from additives such as sodium aluminum sulfate in baking powder and cheese, potassium alum in white flour, and others, as well as antacids are the major dietary sources.

Hair analysis

Dr. Jeffrey Bland, Professor of Nutritional Biochemistry at the University of Puget Sound in Tacoma, Washington, and Director of the Bellevue-Redmond Medical Laboratory in Bellevue, Washington, has found in his clinical experience that hair aluminums above 60 ppm are highly significant in terms of elevated body burdens, but hair aluminums under 60 ppm are as yet uncertain. Laboratories are reporting a low toxic level under 10 ppm, borderline toxicity between 10 and 20 ppm, and toxicity above 20 ppm.

Dr. Bland has presented in his lectures a case history that concerned a physician's wife who had a routine hair analysis and found it contained a fairly high aluminum level. She was taking an aluminum-containing antacid. Upon discontinuing the aluminum-containing antacid, her hair aluminum gradually returned to normal. Recent animal research has been published to further confirm the significance of hair aluminum levels.

Dr. Robert Yokel has also reported that hair is a valid indicator of aluminum exposure.[18]

Case histories

Elizabeth Rees, M.D., reported[19] treating an eight-and-a-half-year-old hyperactive boy with elevated hair aluminum of 42 ppm (accepted limits are less than 10 ppm). This led Dr. Rees to investigate further the correlation between hair aluminum and hyperactivity. In 1977 the hair of ten severely delinquent and psychotic adolescent boys between the ages of twelve and eighteen was subjected to analysis. The hair of nine of the ten boys had elevated aluminum levels between 29 and 87 ppm with six of the ten above 52 ppm. The counselor who lived in the same institution with these boys also had elevated hair aluminum at 29 ppm. The tenth boy with low hair aluminum lived in a separate part of the institution and did not eat with the other boys. Some of these boys also had elevated levels of hair lead or hair copper and no definite conclusions could be made for scientific proof of clinical significance of the elevated hair aluminums and causal relationship with their disturbed behavior. There was certainly a strong circumstantial link.

Another case reported by Dr. Rees was F.J., a thirty-two-year-old male who worked for three years as an aluminum spray painter in a closed shop with no ventilation. He subsequently developed a diagnosis of paranoid schizophrenia. His hair aluminum was 130 ppm, three years after his exposure as an aluminum spray painter. Dr. Rees describes a series of patients with elevated hair aluminums and a variety of symptoms manifested as psychosis, depression, hyperactivity and behavior or learning disabilities. Loss of hair and brittle hair was frequently observed with high hair aluminums.[19]

Evidence is still inadequate to prove beyond any doubt that hair aluminum correlates well with brain or other organ aluminum concentrations. A certain amount of circumstantial evidence is developing however and it is quite possible that in the future we will be able to draw more definite conclusions concerning the clinical significance of hair aluminum.

Appendix to aluminum

Despite the similarity in aluminum between renal dialysis encepholopathy and Alzheimer's disease, there is no histopathology in renal dialysis dementia whereas there are neurofibrillatory tangles seen under the microscope with Alzheimer's disease and also with Parkinson's disease and elevated aluminum is concentrated in the nuclear DNA of these abnormal areas seen with the microscope.

Deferoxamine, an iron chelator, also chelates aluminum and increases aluminum excretion by two to three times. It increases iron excretion five times or more, so it is less efficient with aluminum. Nonetheless, it does increase aluminum excretion and it has been used. by Dr. D.R. Crapper-McLachan of the University of Toronto in patients with Alzheimer's disease. He has found that 30 to 40 percent of Alzheimer's patients improve or have slower progression of the disease by taking deferoxamine, 500 mg, every twelve hours, orally, for six months to two years. He gives the drug twice daily for three weeks and then a resting period of one week. He uses tetracycline as a chelating agent for aluminum during the seven days when they are not taking deferoxamine each month. In following these patients with electroencephalograms, he finds that in a controlled group 21 percent of EEGs remain unchanged if they are not treated, whereas 77 percent of the EEGs do not show progressive disease in the deferoxamine-treated group. He also reported that fluoride binds aluminum and he treats these patients with sodium fluoride. Fluoride apparently has an aluminum-lowering effect in the Alzheimer's regions of the brain. He gives the fluoride during the one week each month when deferoxamine is not being taken.

Dr. Crapper-McLachlan postulates, on the basis of his recent experience, that aluminum is only a part of the problem. He feels now that there is a defective metabolic breakdown in the aluminum blood-brain barrier which allows aluminum more readily into neurones of the brain. In addition, he feels that there is a metabolic defect by which the neurotransmitter enzymes, choline acetyl transferase and beta dopamine hydroxylase, are interfered with. Some improvement can be mediated in Alzheimer's disease by interfering with the aluminum aspect using chelation to remove the aluminum and using fluorides to bind the aluminum. Other reports have shown slight improvement in function using large doses of choline-containing substances, such as lecithin or others which increase production of acetyl choline within the brain or inhibit the enzyme cholinesterase which destroys acetyl choline.

Overall results have been slight, significant but not very dramatic and far from what would be desired in most of these patients.

REFERENCES

1 Crapper, D. R. *et al*. 1973. *Science* 180:511–513.

2 Alfrey, A. C. *et al*. 1976. *N. Engl. J. Med.* 294:184–188.

3 Karlik, S. J. *et al*. 1980. *Neurotoxicology* 1(4):83–88.

4 Perl. D. P. and Brody, A. P. 1980. *Science* 208:297–299.

5 Trapp, G.A. 1980. *Neurotoxicology* 1(4):89–100.

6 Recker, R. *et al*. 1978. *Modern Medicine* 130 (April 15).

7 Mayor, G. *et al*. 1977. *Science* 197:1187–1189.

8 Associated Press, *Phil. Inquirer*, p. 12A (February 1, 1981).

9 Crapper, D. R. *et al*. October 1, 1977. *Science News* 219.

10 Perl, D. P. and Brody, A. R. 1980. *Science* 208:297–299.

11 Clark, M. *Newsweek* 95 (November 5, 1979).

12 Liss, L. *Med. World News* 74 (November 12, 1979).

13 Rees, E. L. 1979. *Orthomolecular Psychiatry* 8(1):37–43.

14 Casdorph, H. R. 1981. *J. Holistic Med.* 3(2).

15 Levick, A. July 17, 1980. *N. Engl. J. Med.*

16 Trapp, G. A. and Cannon, J. B. January 15, 1981. *N. Engl. J. Med.* 172.

17 Koning, J. H. January 15, 1981. *N. Engl. J. Med.* 172.

18 Yokel, R.A. 1982. *Clin. Chem.* 28(4) 662–665.

19 Rees, E. 1979. *Orthomolecular Psychiatry* 8:37–43.

30

ARSENIC

Preliminary research indicates that arsenic may possibly be essential, but if so, very little seems to be required, whereas arsenic toxicity is a much greater problem than possible arsenic deficiency.

Dr. Forrest Nielsen of the U.S. Department of Agriculture's Human Nutrition Laboratory in Grand Fork, North Dakota, has found that laboratory rats deprived of arsenic evidenced slow growth rates, iron-ladened spleens and rough hair. The offspring of arsenic deprived rats had red blood cells which broke down more easily than normal.[1] By 1981, arsenic had been shown to be essential in three laboratories for at least four species.[2]

Healthy adults average about 20 milligrams of arsenic in their body with fairly even distribution throughout various body tissues. The exceptions are that hair and nails tend to accumulate more arsenic, perhaps as the body "dumps" or sequesters excess arsenic to these areas.

Responses to arsenic vary considerably from person to person, and from source to source. Arsenic occurs in both organic and inorganic forms and their effects on the body differ in several important respects. Organic arsenic, or arsenate, is rapidly excreted through the kidneys by a homeostatic mechanism so that accumulation doesn't occur.[3,4] It has a low toxicity,[4] is not inhibitory to most enzymes, and it can substitute for phosphate in some phosphorylases. It seems to be a normal constituent of some foods.[4] Inorganic arsenic, or arsenite, however, does accumulate in tissues and ranks second among the heavy metals as a cause of death.[5] Arsenite rapidly leaves the blood to be deposited in vital organs and tissues such as hair, skin, and nails.

Hair analysis

As arsenic intake increases, hair and urine levels also increase. However, the blood level of arsenic doesn't increase until chronic toxicity is reached.[6]

REFERENCES

1 Neilsen, F. H. Fed. Amer. Soc. Exp. Biol., Atlantic City, N.J. Meeting (April, 1975).

2 Frost, D. October 5, 1981. *Chem. Eng. News* 4.

3 Walkiw, O. *et al.* 1975. *Clin. Toxicol.* 8(3):325–331.

4 Schroeder, H. A. 1966. *J. Chronic Dis.* 19:85.

5 Harvey, S. 1970. In: *Pharmacological Basis of Therapies.* L. S. Goodman, ch. 46.

6 Valentine, J. L. *et al.* 1979. *Environ. Res.* 20:24–32.

Hair analysis interpretation and application: the techniques

31

STANDARDIZATION AND INTERPRETATION OF HUMAN HAIR FOR ELEMENTAL CONCENTRATION

Preface

In recent years numerous laboratories have offered their services to health care professionals in the measurement and interpretation of concentrations of various elements in human hair. Much confusion has resulted in the minds of health care professionals concerning the significance and interpretation of such measurements. A panel of five experts in this field has met and has resulted in a Hair Analysis Standardization Board, under the auspices of the American Holistic Medical Institute. The proceedings of that initial Board meeting are presented with specific recommendations concerning methods of specimen collection, analytical and reporting procedures and of the clinical significance of concentrations of specific elements in human hair.

In few areas of analytical chemistry as it is applied to medical problems is there so much doubt, confusion, uncertainty, indecision, skepticism and controversy as in the field of trace element analysis of human hair. As a first effort toward gathering meaningful information and stimulating scientific discussion of the present and potential problems and benefits of such analyses, a meeting was held in Burlingame, California, in August, 1981, under the temporary sponsorship of the International Foundation for Health Research.

This document results from the discussions of that meeting, and, while not always representing the unanimous views of the participants, is a majority consensus statement. The authors hope that the publication of this material will stimulate discussion and research in both analytical methodologies and clinical applications of the analysis of trace elements in human hair.

This committee functions independently of any commercial or proprietary affiliation and will be free of obligation to any segment of the hair analysis industry. Following the first meeting of the committee, it was accepted as a branch of the American Holistic Medical Institute, the educational and research institution of the American Holistic Medical Association, under the title of "Hair Analysis Standardization Board." Conclusions and recommendations expressed by Board members are their own and do not reflect the opinions of any segment of the hair analysis industry or of any organization or institution with which they are affiliated. The conclusions published in these proceedings of the first meeting of the Board are the result of prolonged and detailed discussions, including extensive review of both published and unpublished research by Board members in consultation with other experts in the field of hair analysis.

Board members fully recognize that these conclusions are preliminary in nature. Much research is in progress or remains to be done. All conclusions published in these proceedings are subject to modification and change with time as more scientific data become available. The Board also recognizes that advanced technology available to academic research laboratories may not be practical or economically feasible for use by commercial laboratories engaged in the screening of large populations, such as those laboratories available to most practicing health professionals. Therefore, some recommendations of this Board are of necessity a compromise between that which is possible and that which is practical and available to clinical practitioners. The Board also recognizes that the technology and the analytical techniques suitable for certain elements may not be suitable for other elements. More research is required before precise recommendations will be possible concerning the most appropriate technique for each element. Each technique that is employed, however, must be able to measure the concentration of the element(s) determined with acceptable accuracy, precision and reproducibility.

Recommendations

HAIR CUTTING PROCEDURES

This section contains recommendations as to the acceptable method(s) of gathering human hair specimens for trace element analysis.

1 A very strong recommendation is made that all hair specimens be collected under direct professional supervision, either in the office of a health professional or by a person trained in proper techniques for hair specimen collection. If a hair specimen has not been collected under professional supervision or by a thoroughly trained person, that fact should be so noted on the submittal form and on the final laboratory report *since contamination of the sample may invalidate the results.*

2 Because the preponderance of published data listing norms and reference ranges for elemental concentrations in hair deal specifically with nape-of-the-neck hair, the Board recommends that whenever possible collection of hair specimens should be from the nape of the neck. That portion of the scalp from which a hair specimen is collected should be stated on the hair analysis submittal form and on the final laboratory report. Hair from other portions of the scalp may be utilized, when so noted on the report, but only with the recognition that clinical interpretation may be somewhat less significant. The hair submitted should represent the first one to two inches of recent growth from the scalp and not include long hair ends.[1,2,3]

3 In the absence of scalp hair, other body hair such as beard hair, axillary hair or pubic hair may be analyzed. It must be fully recognized, however, that published data for such hair are inadequate for accurate interpretation. It has been suggested that hair from areas of the body other than the scalp may be useful to distinguish between exogeneous contamination of scalp hair as opposed to internal absorption of toxic elements.[4]

4 Sample size should range from 500 milligrams to one gram, depending upon the technology used, and should be obtained from at least five and preferably ten or more separate locations along the nape of the neck. Hair specimens should be cut as close to the scalp as possible and should be limited to the first five centimeters of recent growth.[3]

5 It is recommended that whenever possible instruments used to cut hair specimens be composed of plastic, quartz or some other suitable material which may not contaminate the hair specimen.[3] Further research is necessary to determine which types of cutting instruments will not contaminate the hair specimen. This information is especially needed by the hair analysis industry so that recommendations can be made to physicians utilizing hair analysis services in their practices. Until alternative instruments are available, it may be necessary to use cutting instruments composed of high quality, surgical grade, stainless steel.

6 Contamination from the hands or gloves of personnel collecting hair specimens should be avoided as much as possible. In practical terms, in a clinical setting, this is best obtained through washing and drying of the hands prior to collection of a hair specimen. Further research is necessary to determine whether gloves should be worn during the collection procedure, and if so, what type of glove would be suitable. Again, this information is particularly needed by the hair analysis industry so that recommendations can be made to practitioners about the best way to avoid the introduction of significant error in the analytical results due to contamination from the hands or gloves of personnel collecting the hair specimens.

7 As a final comment on collection procedures, the Board wishes to caution all personnel involved in hair analysis concerning the importance of meticulous general housekeeping, including the elimination of such sources of contamination as dust or other environmental contaminants, as well as the need for careful handling of hair specimens prior to and during packaging for shipment. A representative sample of each lot of containers used for shipping hair specimens should be tested prior to use to eliminate the possibility of introducing contamination from the shipping containers. As an example of potential contamination, it has been noted that some hair shipping envelopes with an adhesive flap have been licked with saliva and sealed with hair trapped beneath the adhesive material. This practice may introduce a number of potential elemental contaminants from saliva, from the adhesive and from exposure to the external environment prior to analysis of such a specimen.

LABORATORY HAIR WASHING PROCEDURES

This section contains tentative recommendations for appropriate hair washing procedures to be used by commercial hair element testing laboratories prior to sample digestion.

The Board urgently requests that research results and practical experience from various laboratories be provided to this Board to assist in further refining these recommendations. Board members distinctly recognize that much more scientific research must be accomplished to justify more definitive recommendations concerning hair specimen washing procedures prior to elemental analysis.

1 It is recommended that normal hair hygiene procedures, such as frequency of shampooing, be followed up to the time of specimen collection. Product names of hair treatment preparations, frequency of use, and last date of use should be recorded on the submittal form and on the final laboratory report. A delay of ten weeks should be required after cold wave (permanent wave) or bleaching treatments, after which only the first two and one-half centimeters of recent hair growth closest to the scalp should be gathered for analysis.[5]

2 Hair analysis laboratories should provide their clients with a complete list of hair preparations known to contain high concentrations of elements which could affect the final analytical result. The submittal form and the final laboratory report should list frequency of use and time lapse from last use of all such preparations.

3 Weighing hair samples *prior* to washing eliminates the possibility of contaminating the washed sample during the weighing procedure. This technique, however, requires

that weighing, washing, drying and digestion be performed in the same container to prevent the possible loss of hair during the wash procedure. Most laboratories, therefore, weigh the sample *after* washing the hair. This requires scrupulous attention to sample handling practices to avoid contaminating the washed sample during the weighing steps. Whether the specimen was weighed prior to or after washing should be stated in laboratory reports.

4 The Board recognizes that extensive and often conflicting literature exists on hair-washing techniques. The extremes are represented by (1) an organic solvent wash followed by a detergent wash and water rinse to (2) a detergent wash and water rinse. The Board agreed unanimously that further research was needed on this subject. The general (but not unanimous) consensus of the board was that tentative recommendations for hair specimen washing procedures should include:

a An organic solvent such as (but not limited to) acetone or ethanol, followed by
b An aqueous wash.

5 All aqueous solutions used for trace element analysis should be prepared from deionized or distilled water meeting NCCLS Type I Standards (National Committee for Clinical Laboratory Standards Approved Standard: ASC-3, "Specifications for Reagent Water Used in the Clinical Laboratory"; NCCLS, 771 E. Lancaster Avenue, Villanova, PA 19085). Water and all solutions used for preparing the hair sample for analysis should be tested and found free of trace element contamination at the time of preparation and use.

HAIR ELEMENT ANALYTICAL STANDARDS, DIGESTION TECHNIQUES AND ANALYTICAL PROCEDURES

This section contains standards for hair digestion and the analytical determination of element concentration in the digestant.

1 Any technique or equipment utilized, even a technique in which it is possible to analyze a very small specimen such as individual hairs or portions of individual hairs, must measure elemental concentrations of a homogeneous digestate of a 500 milligram sample or larger, obtained from at least five separate locations on the scalp, preferably the nape. Large variations in elemental concentrations from hair to hair and from segment to segment on individual hairs are felt to require a sample size of a total of at least 500 milligrams obtained from a minimum of five separate locations in order to allow significant clinical interpretations.

2 No measurement shall be reported by any laboratory when such a measurement falls below the level of that laboratory's detection limit, obtainable by the method used. The detection limit is defined by the American Chemical Society in "Guidelines for Data Acquisition and Data Quality Evaluation in Environmental Chemistry," *Analytical Chemistry* Vol. 52, No. 14, December, 1980, Pages 2242–2249. Because hair analysis is a screening test, this Board recommends that the detection limit be defined in terms of two times the standard deviation of the "noise" obtainable by the method used, rather than three times the standard deviation of the noise, which the

American Chemical Society requires for more precise analysis. Merely because a value is below or above its level of detectability, as defined above, does not necessarily mean that the subject from whom the hair specimen was obtained is deficient or in excess with respect to that element. Many other variables must be considered.

3 Each hair analysis laboratory should list its own detection limits in hair as defined above, for every element reported and on every report.

4 It is further recommended by this Board that every hair analysis laboratory report its results in the same standardized units of parts per million (ppm), or, synonymously, micrograms per gram (mg/g), of dry weight contained in the original sample.

5 Calibration Standards

a Before single-element standards are pooled to prepare a multi-element standard, they should be tested to ensure that the standard for a given element is not contaminated with other elements that are also to be added to the multi-element standard.

b Biological reference materials should also be utilized, in addition to non-biological standards, and should be formulated from a homogeneous human hair tissue sample prepared according to the published procedures of the International Atomic Energy Agency, Vienna, Austria.[6] A summary of the procedures utilized in preparation of such homogeneous biological standards are as follows:

i The hair should be thoroughly defatted and washed with acetone and water to remove contamination and ensure that it will freeze-fracture properly.

ii The hair should be powdered with a Braum Mikromembrator II according to IAEA instructions.

iii Sieving and mixing should be carried out essentially as the IAEA describes.

c Homogeneous human hair standards should be prepared by an independent group or agency such as the U.S. Public Health Service, Centers for Disease Control; by the National Bureau of Standards and/or by the International Atomic Energy Agency. Funding for this particular project may be requested from the commercial hair analysis industry.

Funds are needed to manufacture the sample, to accomplish the accurate elemental analysis of each lot of material, and to characterize each lot for homogeneity and stability. These materials will then be utilized for interlaboratory comparisons between those laboratories which voluntarily choose to adhere to the recommendations of this committee. Elemental concentrations in these homogeneous hair standards will be determined using best state of the art technology by several independent laboratories. Analytical methods employed must be described in great detail, including statistical estimates of error.

d Digestion procedures for destructive methods of analysis should produce a clear, homogeneous, particulate-free liquid medium. Procedures which might meet these criteria could include (but are not limited to) mixtures of nitric acid and perchloric acid or nitric acid and hydrogen peroxide.

e A number of pertinent statistics concerning the subject from whom each specimen was taken should be included on the submittal form and on the final report. These facts should include a minimum of the following: age, sex, geographical area of residence, type and frequency of shampoo, type and frequency of any other hair preparations such as conditioners and colorings, use of swimming pools, including frequency and most recent date, hair bleaching and cold-wave or "permanent wave" hair treatments, including most recent date, hair color, source of drinking water (well, spring, municipal supply), type of plumbing in the home (plastic, copper or galvanized pipe, etc.), occupation, medications and drugs consumed, vitamin and mineral supplements consumed, portions of the scalp from which the specimen was obtained, smoking habits and type, quantity and frequency of alcohol consumption. A number of other items may eventually prove to be important for accurate interpretation of results based on additional research and may require future revisions of this list.

UTILITY OF HAIR MINERAL ANALYSIS

This section contains a set of criteria by which the clinical utility of each hair tissue element can be evaluated in a screening sense.

1 Tightly bound e.ements in hair, not extractable in aqueous solutions, may be related to the metabolic control of these respective elements in the biologically active hair tissue. The hair concentrations of these elements may be influenced by many factors including dietary intake, overall nutritional status, endocrine and metabolic function, age, sex, general health status and other sociologic factors. Reduced or elevated concentrations of an element in human hair should not, therefore, be interpreted to necessarily indicate a respective nutritional deficiency or excess. Bound elements in hair are considered more likely to be endogenous and to have been deposited during protein synthesis. Water soluble elements in hair are considered more likely to have been exogenous in source and to be a result of environmental contamination or altered binding to hair protein. These factors relate to the ultimate strength and weakness of clinical interpretation and application of hair element analysis in human metabolic screening. It is essential, therefore, that a clinician develop expertise and interpretative skills in the application of hair element concentration profiles before applying this technique to patient management. *It is emphatically noted that hair element analysis is not a diagnostic, but a screening tool.* Hair analysis results require further confirmatory tests, taking into account other biomedical parameters before establishing a firm medical diagnosis.

2 The Board fully recognizes that scientific data concerning hair analysis are rapidly accumulating. As more scientific data are gathered and published, the interpretative characterization of the following elements will evolve and change. These conclusions, therefore, must be up-dated periodically as new data become available. The Board also recognizes that much information needs to be accumulated concerning elemental species, such as valence states and concerning synergism and interaction between various elements. In no way should aberrations in hair concentrations of any given element be considered to positively substantiate the firm diagnosis of a specific disease.

3 Characterization of Individual Elements:

    a *Elements of proven clinical significance based on hair concentrations*

CALCIUM: clinically significant.[7,8,9]

MAGNESIUM: clinically significant.[7,9,10]

ZINC: clinically significant. (Interpretation complicated by other factors such that both elevated or depressed hair zinc can be present in nutritional deficiency states.)[11,12,13,14,15,16,17,18,19]

COPPER: clinically significant in toxic states (literature conflicting in deficiency states).[20,21,22,23,24,25]

CADMIUM: clinically significant in toxic states.[24,40,45,57,61,66,67,68,69]

CHROMIUM: clinically significant for both toxic and deficiency states.[26,27,28,29,30,31,32,33]

NICKEL: clinically significant in toxic states only.[28,34,35,36,37]

LEAD: clinically significant in toxic states.[4,38,39,40,41,42,43,44,45]

MERCURY: clinically significant in toxic states.[46,47,48,49,50,51,52,53]

ARSENIC: clinically significant in toxic states.[54,55,56,57,58,59,60,61]

    b *Elements suggested to have possible clinical significance based on hair concentrations*

SODIUM: suggested clinical significance, may apply only to specific diseases.[7,8,62] (Sodium concentrations are variable depending on hair sample washing procedures.)

POTASSIUM: suggested clinical significance, may apply only to certain specific diseases.[7,8]

SELENIUM: suggested clinical significance. (The reason this element is not considered to have proven clinical significance is because of inherent difficulties with the methodology for measuring hair selenium and the small amount of published data.)[63,64,65]

ANTIMONY: suggested clinical significance for toxic states only.[66]

    c *Elements with unknown clinical significance because of absence of scientific data*

PHOSPHORUS: unknown clinical significance.

IRON: unknown clinical significance.

MANGANESE: unknown clinical significance.

MOLYBDENUM: unknown clinical significance.

BERYLLIUM: unknown clinical significance.

COBALT: unknown clinical significance.

LITHIUM: unknown clinical significance.

ALUMINUM: unknown clinical significance.

VANADIUM: unknown clinical significance.

TIN: unknown clinical significance.

STRONTIUM: unknown clinical significance.

IODINE: unknown clinical significance.

FLUORINE: unknown clinical significance.

SILICON: unknown clinical significance.

SILVER: unknown clinical significance.

The Hair Analysis Standardization Board considers it essential that clinicians utilizing hair trace element analysis in their practices consult the current and future literature to enhance their interpretation, recognizing that multiple variables may affect the results and that the interpretation of high and low measurements as being indicative of excess and deficiency states is overly simplistic. Because of the multiplicity of variables involved, in the case of certain elements high results may actually indicate deficiency states and in the case of certain other elements, low hair results may occur despite toxic body burdens.

REFERENCES

1 Strain, W. H.; Pories, W. J.; Flynn A.; Hill, D. A. 1971. Trace element nutriture and metabolism through head hair analysis. In: Hemphill D, ed. *Trace Substances in Environmental Health—V*. Missouri: University of Columbia, 383–397.

2 Gibson, R. S. 1980. Hair as a biopsy material for the assessment of trace element status in infancy. *J. Hum. Nutr.* 34:405–416.

3 International Atomic Energy Agency. October 1978. Activation analysis of hair an an indicator of contamination of man by environmental trace element pollutants. Vienna, Austria: IAEA/RL/50.

4 Marzulli, F. N., Watlington P. M., Maibach H. I., 1978. Exploratory skin penetration findings relating to the use of lead acetate hair dyes. *Curr. Probl. Dermatol* 7:196–204.

5 McKenzie, J. M. 1978. Alteration of the zinc and copper concentration of hair. *Am. J. Clin. Nutr.* 31:470–476.

6 M'Baku, S. B. and Parr, R. M. June 15–19, 1981. Interlaboratory study of trace and other elements in the IAEA powdered human hair reference material, HH-1. *Modern Trends in Activation Analysis*, 6th International Conference. Toronto, Canada 1–12.

7 Kopito, I., Elian, E. and Schwachman, H. 1972. Sodium, potassium, calcium, and magnesium in hair from neonates with cystic fibrosis and in amniotic fluid from mothers of such children. *Pediatrics* 49:620–624.

8 Kopito, L. and Schwachman, H. 1974. Alterations in the elemental composition of hair in some diseases. In: Brown A.C., ed. *First Human Hair Symposium*. New York: Medcom Press, 83–90.

9 Bland, J. 1979. Dietary calcium, phosphorus, and their relationship to bone formation and parathyroid activity. *J. John Bastyr College Naturopathic Med.* 1:3–6.

10 Cotton, D., Porters, J. and Spruit, D. 1976. Magnesium content of the hair in alopecia areata atopica. *Dermatologica* 152:60–62.

11 Strain, W. H.; Steadman, L. T.; Lankau, C. A.; Berliner, W. P.; Pories, W. J. 1966. Analysis of zinc levels in hair for the diagnosis of zinc deficiency in man. *J. Lab. Clin. Med.* 68:244–249.

12 Hambidge, K. M.; Hambidge, C.; Jacobs, H.; Baum J. D. 1972. Low levels of zinc in hair, anorexia, poor growth, and hypogeusia in children. *Pediatr. Res.* 6:868–874.

13 Hambidge, K.M. and Silverman. A. 1973. Pica with rapid improvement after dietary zinc supplementation. *Arch. Dis. Child.* 48:567.

14 Amador, M.; Hermelo, M.; Flores, P.; Gonzalez, A. 1975. Hair zinc concentrations in diabetic children. *Lancet* 2:1146.

15 Amador, M.; Pena, M.; Garcia-Miranda, A.; Gonzalez, A.; Hermelo, M. 1975. Low hair zinc concentrations in acrodermatitis enteropathica. *Lancet* 1:1379.

16 Prasad, A. S.; Ortega, J.; Brewer, G. J.; Oberleas, D.; Schoomaker, E. B. 1976. Trace elements in sickle cell disease. *JAMA* 235:2396–2398.

17 Jacob, R.; Sandstead, H.; Solomons, N.; Rieger, C.; Rothberg, R. 1978. Zinc status and vitamin A transport in cystic fibrosis. *Am. J. Clin. Nutr.* 31:638–644.

18 Atkin-Thor, E.; Goddard, B. W.; O'Nion, J.; Stephen, R. L.; Kolff, W. J. 1978. Hypogeusia and zinc depletion in chronic dialysis patients. *Am. J. Clin. Nutr.* 31:1948–1951.

19 Pekarek, R.; Sandstead, H.; Jacob, R.; Barcome, D. 1979. Abnormal cellular immune responses during acquired zinc deficiency. *Am. J. Clin. Nutr.* 32:1466–1471.

20 Rice, E. and Goldstein, N. 1961. Copper content of hair and nails in Wilson's disease. *Metabolism* 10:1085.

21 Harrison, W., Yurachek, J. and Benson, C. 1969. The determination of trace elements in human hair by atomic absorption spectroscopy. *Clin. Chim. Acta.* 23:83–91.

22 Epstein, O.; Boss, A. M. B.; Lyon T. D. B.; Sherlock, S. 1980. Hair copper in primary biliary cirrhosis. *Am. J. Clin. Nutr.* 33:965–967.

23 Pratt, W. and Phippen, W. 1980. Elevated hair copper levels in idiopathic scoliosis. *Spine* 5:230–233.

24 Capel, I. D.; Pinnock, M. H.; Dorrell, H. M.; Williams. D. C.; Grant, E. C. G. 1981. Comparison of concentrations of some trace, bulk and toxic metals in the hair of normal and dyslexic children. *Clin. Chem.* 27:879–881.

25 Porter, K.; McMaster, D.; Elmes, M.; Love, A. 1977. Anemia and low serum copper during zinc therapy. *Lancet* 2:774.

26 Hambidge, K. M.; Rodgerson, D. O. and O'Brien, D. 1968. Concentration of chromium in the hair of normal children and children with juvenile diabetes mellitus. *Diabetes* 17:517–519.

27 Benjanuvatra, N. and Bennion, M. 1975. Hair chromium concentration of Thai subjects with and without diabetes mellitus. *Nutr. Rep. Intl.* 12:40–45.

28 Creason, J. P.; Hinners, T. A.; Bumgarner, J. E.; Pinkerton, C. 1975. Trace elements in hair, as related to exposure in metropolitan New York. *Clin. Chem.* 21:603–612.

29 Jeejeebhoy, K. N.; Chu, R. C.; Marliss, E. B.; Greenberg, G. R.; Bruce-Robertson, A. 1977. Chromium deficiency, glucose intolerance, and neuropathy reversed by chromium supplementation, in a patient receiving long-term total parenteral nutrition. *Am. J. Clin. Nutr.* 30:531–538.

30 Tiefenbach, B., Jervis, R. and Tiefenbach, H. 1979. Chromium, zinc, mercury, and selenium levels of diabetic patients' hair determined by instrumental neutron activation analysis. In: Shapcott, D. and Hubert, J., eds. *Chromium in Nutrition and Metabolism.* New York: Elsevier/North-Holland Biomedical Press, 113–127.

31 Cote, M.; Munan L.; Gagne-Billon, M.; Kelly, A.; DiPietro, D.; Shapcott, D. 1979. Hair chromium concentration and arteriosclerotic heart disease. In: Shapcott, D. and Hubert, J., eds. *Chromium in Nutrition and Metabolism.* New York: Elsevier/North-Holland Biomedical Press, 223–228.

32 Vobecky, J.; Hontela, S.; Shapcott, D.; Vobecky, J. S. 1980. Hair and urine chromium content in 30 hospitalized female psychogeriatric patients and mentally healthy controls. *Nutr. Rep. Intl.* 22:49–55.

33 Al-Shahristani, H., Shihab, K. and Jalil, M. 1979. Distribution and significance of trace element pollutants in hair of the Iraqi population. *IAEA* SM—227/7, 515–525.

34 Nechay, M. and Sunderman, W. 1973. Measurements of nickel in hair by atomic absorption spectrometry. *Ann. Clin. Lab. Sci.* 3:30–35.

35 Hagedorn-Gotz, H. and Stoeppler, M. 1977. On nickel contents in urine and hair in a case of exposure to nickel carbonyl. *Arch. Toxicol.* 38:275–285.

36 Spruit, D. and Bongaarts, P. 1977. Nickel content of plasma, urine, and hair in contact dermatitis. In: Brown, S. S., ed. *Clinical Chemistry and Chemical Toxicology of Metals.* New York: Elsevier/North-Holland Biomedical Press, 261–264.

37 Chatt, A.; Secord, C. A.; Tieferbach, B.; Jervis, R. E. 1980. Scalp hair as a monitor of community exposure to environmental pollutants. In: Brown, A. C. and Crounse, R. G., eds. *Hair, Trace Elements, and Human Illness.* New York: Praeger, 46–71.

38 Kopito, L. Byers, R. K. and Schwachman, H. 1967. Lead in hair of children with chronic lead poisoning. *N. Engl. J. Med.* 276:949–953.

39 Kopito, L., Briley, A. and Schwachman, H. 1969. Chronic plumbism in children. *JAMA* 209:243–248.

40 Hammer, D.; Finklea, J. F.; Hendricks, R. H.; Hinners, T. A.; Riggan, W. B.; Shy, C. M. 1971. Trace metals in human hair as a simple epidemiologic monitor of environmental exposure. In: Hemphill, D., ed. *Trace Substances in Environmental Health—V.* Missouri: University of Columbia, 25–38.

41 Hasegawa, N.; Hirari, A.; Shibata, T.; Sugino, H.; Kashiwagi, T. 1971. Determination of Lead in hair by atomic absorption spectroscopy for simple screening of lead intoxication. In: Nagoya University, *Research Institute of Environmental Medicine—Annual Report* 18:1–5.

42 Speizer, F.; Ferris, B.; Burgess W.; Kopito, L. October 2–6, 1972. Health effects of exposure to automobile exhaust IV. Assessment of lead exposure in traffic policemen. In: Commission of European Communities. *Proc. Intl. Sympos. Environ. Health Aspects of Lead.* Amsterdam, 835–846.

43 Roberts, T.; Hutchinson, T.; Paciga, J.; Chattopadhyay, A.; Jervis, R.; VanLoon, J.; Parkinson, D. 1974. Lead contamination around secondary smelters: Estimation of dispersal and accumulation by humans. *Science* 186:1120–1123.

44 Johnson, D. E., Tillery, J. B. and Prevost, R. J. 1975. Trace metals in occupationally and nonoccupationally exposed individuals. *Environ. Health. Persp.* 10:151–158.

45 Pihl, R. and Parkes, M. 1977. Hair element content in learning disabled children. *Science* 198:204–206.

46 Yamaguchi, S.; Matsumoto, H.; Matsuo, S.; Kaku, S.; Hoshide, M. 1971. Relationship between mercury content of hair and amount of fish consumed.*HSMHA Health Rep.* 86:904–909.

47 Marzulli, F. and Brown. D. 1972. Potential systematic hazards of topically applied mercurials. *J. Soc. Cosmet. Chem.* 23:875–886.

48 Hibberd, J. and Smith, D. 1972. Systemic mercury levels in dental office personnel in Ontario: a pilot study. *J. Can. Dent. Assoc.* 38: 249–254.

49 Gutenmann, W. and Lisk, D. 1973. Elevated concentrations of mercury in dentist's hair. *Bull. Environ. Contam. Toxicol.* 9:318–320.

50 Cagnetti, P., Cigna-Rossi, L. and Clemente, G. June 24–28, 1974. Mercury pathways to man in "In Vivo" content of the population of the Mt. Amiata area. In: Commission of the European Communities. *Recent Advances in the Assessment of the Health Effects of Environmental Pollution.* Paris: EUR 5360, 1451–1460.

51 Yamaguchi, S.; Fujiki, M.; Shimojo, N.; Kaku, S.; Hirota, Y.; Mori, Y.; Sano, K. 1977. A background of geographical pathology on mercury in the East Pacific area. *J. Occup. Med.* 19:502.

52 Sexton, D. J.; Powell, K. E.; Liddle, J. Smrek, A.; Crispin-Smith, J.; Clarkson, T. W. 1978. A nonoccupational outbreak of inorganic mercury vapor poisoning. *Arch. Environ. Health* 33:186–191.

53 Phelps, R.; Clarkson, T.; Kershaw, T.; Wheatley B. 1980. Interrelationships of blood and hair mercury concentrations in a North American population exposed to methyl-mercury. *Arch. Environ. Health* 35:161–168.

54 Smith, H. 1962. Arsenic in biological tissue. *J. Forensic Med.* 9:143–149.

55 Lander, H., Hodge, P. R. and Crisp, C. S. 1965. Arsenic in hair and nails: Its significance in acute arsenical poisoning. *J. Forensic Med.* 12:52–67.

56 Boylen, G. and Hardy, H. 1967. Distribution of arsenic in nonexposed persons (hair, liver, and urine). *Am. Ind. Hyg. Assoc. J.* 28:148–150.

57 Hammer, D. I.; Finklea, J. F.; Hendricks, R. H.; Shy, C. M. 1971. Hair trace metal levels and environmental exposure. *Am. J. Epidemiol.* 93:84–92.

58 Jervis, R., Tiefenbach, B. and Chattopadhyay, A. 1977. Scalp hair as a monitor of population exposure to environmental pollutants. *J. Radioanal. Chem.* 37:751–760.

59 Bencko, V. and Symon K. 1977. Health aspects of burning coal with a high arsenic content: 1. Arsenic in hair, urine, and blood in children residing in a polluted area. *Environ. Res.* 13:378–385.

60 Valentine, J. L., Kang, H. K. and Spivey, G. 1979. Arsenic levels in human blood, urine, and hair in response to exposure via drinking water. *Environ. Res.* 20:24–32.

61 Baker, E. L., Hayes C. G., Landrigan, P. J., *et al.* 1977. A nationwide survey of heavy metal absorption in children living near primary copper, lead, and zinc smelters. *Am. J. Epidemiol.* 106:261–273.

62 Bowen, H. 1972. Determination of trace elements in hair samples from normal and protein-deficient children by activation analysis. *Sci. Total Environ.* 1:75–79.

63 Valentine, J., Kang, H. and Spivey, G. 1978. Selenium levels in human blood, urine, and hair in response to exposure via drinking water. *Environ. Res.* 17:347–355.

64 Keshan Disease Research Group of the Chinese Academy of Medical Sciences, Beijing. 1979. Epidemiologic studies on the etiologic relationships of selenium and Keshan disease. *Chinese Med. J.* 92:477–482.

65 Chatt, A.; Secord, C.; Tiefenbach, B.; Jervis R. 1980. Scalp hair as a monitor of community exposure to environmental pollutants. In: Brown A. C. and Crounse, R. G., eds. *Hair, Trace Elements, and Human Illness.* New York: Praeger, 46–73.

66 Chattopadhyay, A., and Jervis, R. 1974. Hair as an indicator of multi-element exposure of population groups. In: Hemphill, D., ed. *Trace Substances in Environmental Health—VIII.* Missouri: University of Columbia, 31–38.

67 Oleru, G. 1975. Epidemiological implications of environmental cadmium. 1: The probable utility of human hair for occupational trace metal (cadmium) screening. *Am. Indust. Hyg. Assoc. J.* 36:229–233.

68 McKenzie, J. and Neallie, J. 1974. Cadmium in urine and hair from New Zealand adults. In: *Trace Substances in Environmental Health—VIII.* Missouri: University of Columbia, 45–48.

69 Murray, T.; Walker, B.; Spratt, D.; Chappellea, R. 1981. Cadmium nephropathy: monitoring for early evidence of renal dysfunction. *Arch. Environ. Health* 36:165–171.

32

DOCUMENTATION OF THE UTILITY OF HAIR ELEMENT ANALYSIS
(as determined by the Hair Analysis Standardization Board)

Literature references addressing the utility of determining element levels in human hair have been compiled and summarized in this section. This review is intended to be comprehensive and representative of currently available literature, but should not be considered as providing exhaustive coverage. A number of additional available articles which deal primarily with analytical methodology or which were not directed towards the application aspects of the test have not been cited here.

Documentation for each element studied in hair has been summarized and, for the most part, arranged chronologically. The data, as available, has been tabulated in the following manner:

LOCALITY

DESCRIPTION OF SUBJECTS STUDIED

MEAN HAIR ELEMENT VALUES IN MG% (1 mg% = 10 ppm); ranges are also shown when available.

ANALYTICAL TECHNIQUES **1** Preparation of hair prior to analysis, i.e., washing and digestion methods, **2** Instrumentation used (Abbreviations used: AAS—Atomic Absorption Spectroscopy; INAA—Neutron Activation Analysis; IPAA—Photon Activation Analysis).

REMARKS A brief summary of findings is provided with most statements taken directly from the article.

CALCIUM

Ref.	Locality	No. and type of persons and special conditions	Analysis mg%		Technique — Preparation	Technique — Instrument	Remarks
			Water sol.	Water insol.			
1	United States	13 Newborns with cystic fibrosis	77.2	5.9	20–100 mg. hair washed in cold ion-free water. Wash water saved. Hair then boiled in water. Nitric and perchloric acid digestion.	AAS	Most of the Ca in hair of newborns with cystic fibrosis is water soluble whereas only a small fraction of the Ca from hair of healthy infants is water soluble. This may relate to a basic defect in this disease.
		34 Healthy newborns	24.1	61.2			
			Cold water sol.	Water insol.			
2	Iran	13 Pregnant women with geophagia	23	156	Cold water wash followed by boiling hair in water and comparing the two solutes. Hair acid digested to determine water-insoluble fraction	AAS	Women with geophagia had substantial portions of bound Ca in hair. Large amount of bound Ca in hair appears to relate to a metabolic need while the water-insoluble part represents Ca which may not be required or utilized.
		6 Non-pregnant women with geophagia	31	110			
		5 Controls-non-pregnant and no geophagia	70	35			

			Water insoluble	Method	Wash/Digestion	Comments
2	Japan	7 Male Japanese with PKU	11.4	AAS	(same)	Water insoluble Ca in hair of patients with PKU was significantly lower than controls.
		7 Female Japanese with PKU	17.6			
		100 Teenage controls:				
		males (Japanese)	31.5			
		females	70.8			
3	Venezuela	11 Amazonas Indians		INAA		An absence of detectable amounts of calcium in the hair reflects a condition of calcium deficiency in this area.
4	United States	40 Individuals on diets with different Ca:P ratios:				Significant differences in hair Ca were seen between the two groups. Elevated Ca (and Mg) are consistent with hyperparathyroidism of nutritional origin resulting from a low Ca/high P diet.
		Ca:P 0.58:1	95.2			
		Ca:P 1:1 (optimum)	30.3			
5	U.K.	73 Dyslexic children	22.0	AAS	Ethanol, diethyl ether, de-ionized water wash. Nitric/perchloric digestion	The differences in hair Ca observed were not considered significant.
		44 Controls	38.0			
6	Germany	2 Hyperthyroiditis patients	470.			Significant elevations in hair Ca seen in patients versus controls. Hair can be used for the examination of mineral status in different diseases.
		2 Nephrocalcinosis patients				
		male	1837			
		female	360			
		Controls	86			

CALCIUM, cont'd

1 Kopito, L., Elian, E. and Shwachman, H. 1972. Sodium, potassium, calcium, and magnesium in hair from neonates with cystic fibrosis and in amniotic fluid from mothers of such children. *Pediatrics* 49: 620–624.

2 Kopito, L. and Shwachman, H. 1974. Alterations in the elemental composition of hair in some diseases. *First Human Hair Symposium.* Algie C. Brown, ed. Medcom Press, pp. 83–90.

3 Perkons, A., Velandia, J. and Dienes, M. 1977. Forensic aspects of trace element variation in the hair of isolated Amazonas Indian tribes. *J. Forensic Science* 22(1): 95–105.

4 Bland, J. 1979. Dietary calcium, phosphorus and their relationships to bone formation and parathyroid activity. *J. John Bastyr College of Naturopathic Medicine.* 1(1): 3–6.

5 Capel, I. *et al.* 1981. Comparison of concentrations of some trace, bulk, and toxic metals in the hair of normal and dyslexic children. *Clin. Chem.* 27(6): 879–881.

6 Schneider, H. and Anke, M. 1966. Mineral content of human hair during various diseases. *Z. Gesamte. Inn. Med. Ihre. Grenzgeb.* 21(24): 802–806.

PHOSPHORUS

Ref.	Locality	No. and type of persons and special conditions	Analysis mg%	Technique Preparation	Instrument	Remarks
1	Egypt	30 Cases (M & F) with psoriasis of the scalp	24.9	Washed in ether, soap and water, distilled water.	Photoelectric Colorimeter	In cases of psoriasis of the scalp, there is a constant and significant increase in the amount of phosphorus in the hair.
		10 Cases (M & F) with psoriasis not affecting the scalp	15.0	0.5 g digested in sulphuric acid and hydrogen peroxide.		
		30 Controls	12.4			
2	United States	40 Individuals on two different diets: Ca:P 0.58:1 Ca:P 1:1	18.6 16.2			Slightly higher hair phosphorus levels seen in individuals on high P, lower Ca diet (dietary Ca/P - 0.58:1).

1 Abdel-Aal, H.; Soliman, A.; El Mahdy, H.; and El Saiee, L. 1976. Study of some minerals in scalp hair and blood sera of psoriatics. *Acta Dermatovener (Stockholm)* 56: 265–267.

2 Bland, J. 1979. Dietary calcium, phosphorus and their relationships to bone formation and parathyroid activity. *J. John Bastyr College of Naturopathic Medicine* 1(1): 3–6.

CALCIUM and PHOSPHORUS—ANIMALS

A number of references have indicated utility in measuring hair calcium and phosphorus in cattle. The Ca and P content of the hair has been shown to parallel that of the animals' feed. Ca and P levels in hair are suggested as indicators of the need and availability of these two elements for cattle. Hair is considered a more stable and objective indicator than blood in monitoring the Ca and P metabolism in calves. Ca and P in hair are low during bone formation and increase as the mineral process slows. In addition, high Ca in the hair of cattle indicates osteolysis.

1 Brochart, M. 1957. Phosphorus-calcium nutrition in dairy cows as determined by analysis of the hair. *Ann. Inst. Natl. Recherche Agron.* Ser. D, 6, 151–79, 185–235.

2 Vernichenko, A. *et al.* 1975. Hair as an indicator of the availability of calcium and phosphorus for animals. *S-kh. Bio.* 10(6): 938–940.

3 Vernichenko, A. 1975. Calcium and phosphorus content in the skin and hair cover of young bulls. *Dokl. TSKHA* 210: 203–206.

4 Neseni, R. 1970. Importance of the chemical hair analysis in animal production. *Arch. Tierzucht* 13(4): 297–313.

MAGNESIUM

Ref.	Locality	No. and type of persons and special conditions	Analysis mg%	Technique Preparation	Technique Instrument	Remarks
1	United States	13 Newborns with cystic fibrosis	Water soluble 10.8	(see Ca #1)	AAS	80% of the magnesium in hair of newborns with cystic fibrosis is water soluble, whereas only a small fraction of the Mg of hair of healthy infants is water soluble. This may relate to a basic defect with this disease.
		34 Healthy newborns	3.7			
2	Netherlands	14 Normal controls	3.7		AAS	A correlation between skin disease and low hair Mg was seen.
		21 Nonalopecia dermatological patients	~ 1.4			
		15 Alopecia areata atopica patients	~ 1.7			
3	United States	40 Individuals on two different diets: Ca:P 0.58:1 Ca:P 1:1	15.6 4.3			Significant differences in hair Mg (and Ca) were seen between the two groups. Elevated Mg (and Ca) are consistent with hyperparathyroidism of nutritional origin resulting from a low Ca/high P diet.

MAGNESIUM, cont'd

Ref.	Locality	No. and type of persons and special conditions	Analysis mg%	Technique Preparation	Instrument	Remarks
4	United States	Provisional ranges for hair Mg provided: Deficiency = <5.0 mg % Normal = 10–60 mg % Excess = >60 mg %		Ether wash. Tetramethyl-ammonium hydroxide digestion.	AAS	"Hair analysis provides a new way of measuring and investigating Mg deficiencies and excesses." **DISEASE ASSOCIATION WITH Mg LEVELS** (normal hair range: 10–60 mg %) **Deficiency** Learning difficulties, emotional problems, skin disorders, degenerative diseases, urolithiasis **Excess** Arthritis, psoriasis
5	U.K.	73 Dyslexic children 44 Controls	5.6 3.2	Ethanol, diethyl ether, deionized water wash. Nitric/perchloric digestion.	AAS	The significantly increased Mg content of the hair of dyslexic children could indicate increased excretion, and consequently, either a lower body-metal content or an increased body burden of this element.

6	Germany	2 Hyperthyroiditis patients
		2 Nephrocalcinosis patients
		   male
		   female
		Controls
			90
			
			534
			102
			22
						Significant elevations in hair Mg were seen in patients versus controls.

1 Kopito, L., Elian, E. and Shwachman, H. 1972. Sodium, potassium, calcium, and magnesium in hair from neonates with cystic fibrosis and in amniotic fluid from mothers of such children. *Pediatrics* 49: 620–624.

2 Cotton, D., Porters, J. and Spruit, D. 1976. Magnesium content of the hair in alopecia areata atopica. *Dermatologica* 152: 60–62.

3 Bland, J. 1979. Dietary calcium, phosphorus, and their relationships to bone formation and parathyroid activity. *J. John Bastyr College of Naturopathic Medicine* 1(1): 3–6.

4 Strain, W. *et al.* 1980. Hair analysis for the determination of magnesium deficiency or excess. *Magnesium in Health and Disease*. Englewood Cliffs: Spectrum Publ. pp. 25–29.

5 Capel, I. *et al.* 1981. Comparison of concentrations of some trace, bulk and toxic metals in the hair of normal and dyslexic children. *Clin. Chem.* 27(6): 879–881.

6 Schneider, H. and Anke, M. 1966. Mineral content of human hair during various diseases. *Z. Gesamte. Inn. Med. Ihre. Grenzgeb.* 21(24): 802–806.

POTASSIUM

Ref.	Locality	No. and type of persons and special conditions	Analysis mg%	Technique Preparation	Instrument	Remarks
1	United States	13 Newborns with cystic fibrosis	148	(see Ca)	AAS	Scalp hair of newborns with cystic fibrosis contains significantly elevated concentrations of sodium and potassium.
		34 Healthy newborns	66			
2	United States	22 Celviac disease patients	Na/K < 1.0	(See Ca)	AAS	Significantly elevated hair K in relation to sodium observed in celiac disease patients.
		150 Controls	Na/K ~ 3.4			
3	Germany	2 Hyperthyroiditis patients	52.6			Significant K elevations seen in patients versus controls.
		2 Nephrocalcinosis patients				
		male	143.3			
		female	60.3			
		Controls	16.7			

1 Kopito, L. 1972. Sodium, potassium, calcium, and magnesium in hair from neonates with cystic fibrosis and in amniotic fluid from mothers of such children. *Pediatrics* 49: 620–624.

2 Kopito, *et al.* 1974. Alterations in the elemental composition of hair in some diseases. *First Human Hair Symposium*, Algie C. Brown, ed. Medcom Press: 83–90.

3 Schneider, H. and Anke, M. 1966. Mineral content of human hair during various diseases. *Z Gesamte. Inn. Med. Ihre. Grenzgeb.* 21(24): 802–806.

SODIUM

Ref.	Locality	No. and type of persons and special conditions	Analysis mg%	Technique		Remarks
				Preparation	Instrument	
1	United States	13 Newborns with cystic fibrosis	552	Deionized water wash.	AAS	Concentrations of Na and K varied significantly in hair from cystic fibrosis patients versus controls.
		34 Healthy newborns	173	Nitric/perchloric acid digestion.		
2	United States	22 Celiac disease patients	Na/K < 1.0	(see Ca)	AAS	Significantly elevated hair K in relation to sodium observed in celiac disease patients.
		150 Controls	Na/K ~ 3.4			
3	Indonesia	41 Normal children	29.2	10–50 mg hair washed in ether.	INAA	Statistically significant differences in sodium found. Tissue retention of Na higher in protein-deficient children.
		40 Protein-deficient children	77.8			
4	Germany	2 Hyperthyroiditis patients	55.1			Sodium significantly elevated in hair of patients versus controls.
		2 Nephrocalcinosis patients				
		male	431.6			
		female	41.8			
		Controls	19.6			

1 Kopito, L. et al. 1972. Sodium, potassium, calcium, and magnesium in hair from neonates with cystic fibrosis and in amniotic fluid from mothers of such children. Pediatrics 49: 620–624.

2 Kopito, L. et al. 1974. Alterations in the elemental composition of hair in some diseases. First Human Hair Symposium, Algie C. Brown, ed. Medcom Press: 83–90.

3 Bowen, H. 1972. Determination of trace elements in hair samples from normal and protein-deficient children by activation analysis. Sci. Total Environment 1: 75–79.

4 Schneider, H. and Anke, M. 1966. Mineral content of human hair during various diseases. Z. Gesamte, Inn. Med. Ihre. Grenzgeb. 21(24): 802–806.

IRON

Ref.	Locality	No. and type of persons and special conditions	Analysis mg%	Technique Preparation	Instrument	Remarks
1	Canada	358 Normal individuals Males Females 14 Tuberculosis patients 12 Rheumatoid Arthritics 14 Diabetics Patients with Fe-deficiency anemia; pernicious anemia; hemochromatosis also tested.	2.5 (1.0–5.0) 4.0 (1.0–7.0) 3.5 3.9 5.1	Water wash. Sulphuric acid and hydrogen peroxide digestion.	Spectrophotometry	Iron content of scalp hair gives no indication as to the state of body Fe stores in individual patients. Iron in hair fell in some individuals when they were iron depleted and rose as Fe stores restored but findings not consistent. Some individuals with Fe depletion had high hair iron while those with excess iron storage had normal hair levels.
2	United States	15 Anemic, pregnant women before supplementation with ferric fructose Normal hair iron	2.3 (0.9–3.2) 1.9–3.9		AAS	Changes in hematocrit levels after supplementation correlated equally well with both percentage saturation levels and hair iron levels, suggesting that hair iron levels may be a good measure of body iron stores.
3	United States, Africa	African Bushmen, iron pots used for cooking: 12 Young women 11 Lactating women 15 Postmenopausal women 8 Men Bantu urban dwellers: 37 Lactating women	29.6 17.3 26.5 90.5 4.3	Acetone, detergent, deionized water wash. Nitric/perchloric and sulfuric acid digestion.	AAS	Hematological values confirmed high iron intake in Bushman women; no cases of anemia found. Significant differences in hair iron between groups. Cincinnati women had lowest hair iron levels and highest incidence of anemia (16%); all were receiving iron supplementation.

IRON, cont'd

Ref.	Locality	No. and type of persons and special conditions	Analysis mg%	Technique Preparation	Instrument	Remarks
		Inner city women, Cincinnati, Ohio: 50 Nonlactating	3.0			
4	Canada	76 Rural controls	3.1 (0.95–8.5)	Distilled water, ethanol, and diethyl ether wash.	INAA IPAA	Excessive ingestion of lead is most commonly associated with anemia, which is caused by the reduction of Fe level in the body. This was observed among the urban residents near smelters where the hair Fe content decreased with the increased Pb levels.
		81 Urban controls	4.2 (0.76–10.6)			
		153 Urban, near Pb smelters	2.5 (0.58–7.2)			
5	U.K.	86 Control subjects	2.1	Detergent, distilled water, acetone wash.	AAS	Hair Fe was significantly lower in mentally retarded patients.
		67 F Down's syndrome patients	1.5			Hair metal analysis can be useful as a diagnostic tool in the examination of trace metal exposure, including abnormal nutritional intake, and may possibly assist in the study of certain mental states.
		37 Schizophrenics	3.0	Sulfuric acid, H_2O_2 digestion.		
		25 Mentally retarded patients	0.63			
6	Germany	Patients w/ various diseases:				Iron higher in anemic patients receiving blood transfusions than controls. Also slightly higher in infectious hepatitis and high in hyperthyroiditis patients.
		11 Anemia	7.1			
		6 Infectious hepatitis	5.4			
		2 Hyperthyroiditis	7.1			
		Controls	4.0			

1 Green, P. and Duffield, J. 1956. The iron content of human hair. Canadian Services Med. J. 12: 980–996.

2 Eatough, D. et al. 1973. Ferric fructose and treatment of anemia in pregnant women. Trace Element Metabolism in Animals-2, Hoekstra et al., ed. Baltimore: University Park Press: pp. 659–663.

3 Baumslag, N. and Petering, H. Sept./Oct. 1976. Trace metal studies in bushman hair. *Arch. Environ. Health*, pp. 254–257.

4 Chatt, A. *et. al.* 1980. Scalp hair as a monitor of community exposure to environmental pollutants. *Hair, Trace Elements, and Human Illness*, Brown and Crounse, ed. New York: Praeger Publ., pp. 46–73.

5 Barlow, P. and Kapel, M. 1980. Metal and sulfur contents of hair in relation to certain mental states. *Hair, Trace Elements, and Human Illness*, Brown and Crounse, ed. New York: Praeger Publ., pp 105–127.

6 Schneider, H. and Anke, M. 1966. Mineral content of human hair during various diseases. *Z. Gesamte. Inn. Med. Ihre. Grenzgeb.* 21(24): 802–806.

ZINC

Ref.	Locality	No. and type of persons and special conditions	Analysis mg%	Technique Preparation	Instrument	Remarks
1	Egypt	10 Egyptian dwarfs	5.4	0.5 g hair washed with detergent.	Emission spectroscopy	"Hair analysis appears to be a reliable, simple, and atraumatic method of assessing body zinc stores."
		8 Egyptian dwarfs treated with Zn sulfate	12.1			
		12 Normal Egyptians	10.3			
		6 Normal males, New York	11.9			
2	Iran	49 Adult villagers with low zinc diets	12.6	Soap and water wash. Sulfuric, nitric, and perchloric acid digestion.	AAS	Zinc concentrations in hair of villagers were depleted presumably as a result of limited intake and possibly increased losses of zinc.
		36 Control subjects	22.0			

ZINC, cont'd

Ref.	Locality	No. and type of persons and special conditions	Analysis mg%	Technique Preparation	Instrument	Remarks
3	Panama	52 Males, 0–5 yr.	14.7	0.1 g hair extracted with acetone and ether, washed with sodium lauryl sulfate and water.	AAS	If hair is to be used as a biopsy material for comparing the zinc nutriture of individuals or groups, only age-matched individuals or groups may be compared.
		64 Females, 0–5 yr.	14.8			
		31 Males, 6–10 yr.	12.7			
		52 Females, 6–10 yr.	11.3			
		29 Males, 11–15 yr.	12.6			
		38 Females, 11–15 yr.	14.8			
		14 Males, 16–20 yr.	16.3			
		19 Females, 16–20 yr.	21.0			
		64 Males, > 20 yr.	14.2			
		70 Females, > 20 yr.	16.7			
4	Iran	75 Iranian village children	19.9 (15.1–25.4)	Detergent, water wash. Perchloric acid and H_2O_2 digest.	AAS	No significant correlation was found between hair and plasma zinc levels.
5	United States (Denver)	25 Newborns	17.4	Hair washed in hexane, ethanol, deionized water.	Emission spectroscopy	After zinc supplementation, taste acuity normalized in children with hypogeusia and hair zinc levels increased. Low levels of zinc in hair indicate that low stores of zinc in the body are common in infants and young children.
		93 Infants and preschool children (3 mo.–4 yr.)	8.8			
		132 Children & adolescents (4–17 yrs.)	15.3	Digested in HC1.		
		88 Young adults (17–40 yrs.)	18.0			

#	Country	Sample	Value	Method	Comments
		10 Children > 4 yr. with poor appetite, poor growth, and hypogeusia	< 7.0		
6	United States	18 Mo. female with pica After 2 mo. Zn therapy	7.0 12.7		Diagnosis of zinc deficiency suggested by history of poor appetite, declining growth centiles, and low hair zinc level.
7	Cuba	201 Normal children 31 Children with protein-energy malnutrition 23 Children with celiac disease 4 Children with acrodermatitis enteropathica	21.9 16.2 17.4 5.3	AAS	Highly significant differences in hair zinc found between patients with A.E. and patients with other diseases. Hair zinc considered to be a reliable method to measure body-zinc stores.
8	Cuba	17 Diabetic children, before insulin 25 Diabetic children, after insulin 25 Healthy children	11.5 26.1 21.5	AAS	Very low zinc in hair of diabetic children. Normal levels in treated children correlated with insulin requirements.
9	United States (Denver)	74 Head Start children aged 3–5 yrs. 42 Controls, middle-income children aged 3–5 yrs.	8.7 13.1	Hexane, ethanol, deionized water wash. HC1 digestion. Emission spectroscopy	Hair and plasma zinc levels used as biochemical indices in evaluating zinc nutritional status. Inadequate zinc nutrition observed in over two-thirds of children from low income families.

ZINC, cont'd

Ref.	Locality	No. and type of persons and special conditions	Analysis mg%	Technique Preparation	Instrument	Remarks
10	United States (Detroit)	43 Sickle cell disease patients 24 Controls	12.1 19.0	Hexane and ethanol wash. Digested with HNO_3.	AAS	Zinc in plasma, hair, and red blood cells was decreased in sickle cell disease patients. Low hair zinc suggested chronic zinc depletion.
11	China	16 Normal subjects 19 Patients with esophageal cancer 4 Patients with other types of cancer 8 Patients with other disorders	19.5 16.2 16.9 21.2	50 mg. hair washed with hexane, ethanol, and water. Digested with HNO_3.	AAS	Zinc in hair of patients with esophageal cancer was lower than in normal subjects. Hair appears to reflect previous zinc intake; thus, this may be a sign of possible zinc deficiency. Zinc in serum and esophageal tissue was also low in these patients.
12	United States (Indiana)	183 Adolescent females, in fall 184 Adolescent females, in spring	21.6 19.1		AAS	Hair zinc levels represent zinc nutritional status of a subject at an earlier time when the hair was formed. Serum zinc affected by many factors, including diet, when sample was collected, only 3–4% of subjects in this study classified as marginal zinc status.
13	New Zealand	32 Polynesian men 34 Polynesian women	25.0 15.5		AAS	Zinc levels in hair, serum, urine, and toenails appeared adequate despite the low dietary zinc intake. Copper intakes were also low.
14	United States (Indiana)	25 Elderly subjects with marginally impaired taste acuity before supplementation	15.9	Hair washed.	AAS	Zinc supplementation significantly increased hair Zn levels but did not affect taste acuity. The decline in taste acuity among the aged may be due to a variety of factors besides poor nutritional status.

319

No.	Location	Subjects	Value	Method	Preparation	Comments
		24 Elderly control subjects before supplementation	17.0			
		25 Subjects after 15 mg. zinc for 95 days	21.0			
		24 Control subjects after placebo	17.0			
15	United States (Chicago)	17 Adolescents with cystic fibrosis	11.7	AAS	15–20 mg. samples washed with acetone, ether, detergent. Nitric and sulfuric acid digestion.	Zinc status of cystic fibrosis group judged to be low-normal as determined by low hair zinc. Plasma zinc was not significantly lower than controls. Zinc may be a contributing factor to low plasma vitamin A/retinol binding protein levels of CF patients with marginal or deficient Zn status.
		39 Adolescent controls	16.2			
16	Turkey	Healthy subjects:		AAS	Hair washed in distilled water and carbon tetrachloride. Digested with HC1.	Hair zinc in healthy subjects increased with age. Serum zinc of protein-calorie malnourished children lower than healthy subjects while hair zinc was higher than healthy subjects. The authors feel that hair zinc may be useful if it is low, but that high or normal hair zinc may not be a good index of body zinc status.
		9 F age 0–5	13.3			
		21 F age 6–10	14.3			
		20 F age 11–15	16.7			
		19 M age 0–5	11.9			
		21 M age 6–10	16.8			
		25 M age 11–15	19.2			
		Protein-calorie malnourished:				
		11 F age 0–3	17.1			
		6 M age 0–3	15.7			

ZINC, cont'd

Ref.	Locality	No. and type of persons and special conditions	Analysis mg%	Technique Preparation	Instrument	Remarks
		Normal children:				
		8 F age 0–3	10.9			
		9 M age 0–3	10.2			
17	United States (Utah)	20 Dialysis patients with hypogeusia: before Zn supplementation after supplementation	11.5 (6.2–23.4) 18.4 (9.8–32.1)	Hexane, ethyl alcohol, deionized water wash.	AAS	Improvement in taste acuity of dialysis patients after Zn supplementation was significant. Zinc concentrations in hair increased in 85% of patients. Dialysis patients appear to be depleted of body Zn stores.
		9 Normal control subjects: before supplementation after supplementation	18.3 22.7	Tetramethyl ammonium hydroxide digestion.		
18	Turkey	20 Patients with homozygous B-thalassemia	10.5		AAS	Plasma, erythrocyte, and hair zinc levels were significantly lower in thalassemic children. Zinc content of hair reflects total body zinc more accurately because of its slower turnover.
		20 Controls	19.7			
19	United States (New York)	38 Normal adults	18.6	60–80 mg. hair digested in nitric: perchloric acid.	AAS	Normal parents of children with achondroplasia have significantly reduced zinc and increased copper in their hair, suggesting that Zn deficiency may be a contributing factor in the pathogenesis of this mutation.
		27 Parents of achondroplasia children	16.2			
		11 Achondroplasia children	13.0			
		109 Children with constitutional growth delay	16.3			
		43 Children with familial short stature	18.0			

20	England (Southampton)	Normal children: 92 Males, age 10–11 127 Females, age 10–11	11.8 14.6	Acetone, detergent, distilled water wash. Nitric acid digestion.	AAS	There was no evidence of serious Zn deficiency in these children. Lower hair zinc for boys may indicate smaller body zinc reserves than girls.
21	Ireland	Subjects free of acute illness aged 65–95 yr. 28 M, no supplements 76 F, no supplements 7 M, with supplements 35 F, with supplements	20.3 21.4 24.6 24.7	Detergent wash.	AAS	No correlation between hair and plasma zinc values found. Females receiving multivitamin supplementation had significantly higher mean zinc concentration.
22	New Zealand	13 Oyster openers 9 Industrial workers nongalvanizers galvanizers 11 Leg ulcer patients 19 Dermatosis patients	16.9 18.2 421.0 17.8 17.6	8 cm. lengths of hair were washed with nonionic detergent, 0.1 EDTA $HNO_3/HC10_4$ digestion.	AAS	Only external exposure to zinc from an industrial source or from use of zinc-based creams increased the zinc level in hair and toenails. Concluded that zinc in serum, urine, hair, and toenails is not a sensitive indicator of zinc status.
23	Greece	34 Control subjects 20 Nondialyzed uremics 18 Hemodialyzed uremics Predialysis Postdialysis	20.3 (13.4–28.5) 16.6 (8.5–23.5) 19.3 (15.1–25.0)	Hexane, ethanol, distilled water wash. Nitric and perchloric digest.	AAS	Hair zinc levels were low in nondialyzed uremics but partially restored to normal in patients on hemodialysis. Tissue zinc depletion was evidenced by low hair zinc levels.

ZINC, cont'd

Ref.	Locality	No. and type of persons and special conditions	Analysis mg%	Technique Preparation	Instrument	Remarks
24	United States	17 Yr. old male, decerebrate from head injury with facial seborrhea and decubitus ulcer		Acetone, ether, sodium lauryl sulfate, water.	AAS	Slightly elevated zinc in hair pre-therapy increased shortly after initiation of zinc supplementation and subsequently decreased to normal levels. Hair growth was impaired by severe zinc deficiency and zinc accumulated in the slow growing hair. This is in contrast to the decrease in hair zinc which occurs in less severe zinc deficiency.
		$^5/_{25}$ pre-therapy	~ 30.0			
		$^8/_2$ zinc supplementation	~ 39.0			
		$^8/_2$ zinc supplementation	~ 24.0			
		$^8/_{22}$ zinc supplementation	~ 16.0			
		$^8/_{29}$ zinc supplementation	~ 15.5			
25	United States	90 Hispanic-American 4 yr. old children in California	13.1 (6.9–21.9)	Hexane, ethanol, deionized water wash. HCl digestion.	Emission spectroscopy	These data confirm the finding that normally growing Hispanic-American children have normal hair zinc values and suggest that the low hair zinc values reported for children in the lower height percentiles are more likely to be related to poor growth than to genetic factors.
26	United States	79 Vegetarians	23.6		AAS	The decreased levels of hair zinc in vegetarians are presumably the result of a decreased ingestion or absorption of dietary zinc over an extended period of time.
		41 Non-vegetarians	27.6			
27	Germany	4 Cases hyperthyroiditis	17.2			Zinc in hair significantly decreased in patients with hyperthyroiditis. Cu was increased in hair.
		Controls	23.9			

28	United States	Maternal scalp hair obtained at delivery:		Hexane, ethanol, deionized water wash. Nitric acid digestion.	AAS	Hair zinc of women with chronic vaginitis or borderline diabetes was significantly elevated compared with controls. No differences in hair zinc were observed for women taking antinausea pills, antibiotics, sleeping pills, B vitamins or folic acid.
		Kidney infection				
		with	20.7			
		without	19.8			
		Chronic vaginitis				
		with	31.7			
		without	19.5			
		Diabetes (borderline)				
		with	37.4			
		without	19.7			
29	U.K.	73 Dyslexic children	31.3 (12.6–111)	Detergent wash. Nitric and perchloric acid digestion.	AAS	Zinc in hair of dyslexics higher than in control children. No comments made by authors.
		44 Control children	22.0 (8.6–52)			

1 Strain, W. *et al.* 1966. Analysis of zinc levels in hair for the diagnosis of zinc deficiency in man. *J. Lab. Clin. Med.* 68(2): 244–249.

2 Reinhold, J. *et al.* 1966. Zinc and copper concentrations in hair of Iranian villagers. *Am. J. Clin. Nutr.* 18: 294–300.

3 Klevay, L. 1970. Hair as a Biopsy Material: I. Assessment of zinc nutriture. *Am. J. Clin. Nutr.* 23: 284–289.

4 McBean, L. *et al.* 1971. Correlation of zinc concentrations in human hair and plasma. *Am. J. Clin. Nutr.* 24: 506–509.

5 Hambidge, K. *et al.* 1972. Low levels of zinc in hair, anorexia, poor growth and hypogeusia in children. *Pediat. Res.* 6: 868–874.

6 Hambidge, K. M. and Silverman, A. 1973. Pica with rapid improvement after dietary zinc supplementation. *Arch. Dis. Child.* 48, 567.

7 Amador, M. *et al.* June 21, 1975. Low hair zinc concentrations in acrodermatitis enteropathica. *Lancet*, p. 1379.

8 Amador, M. Hermelo, M. *et al.* December 6, 1975. Hair zinc concentrations in diabetic children. *Lancet*, p. 1146.

9 Hambidge, K. M. *et al.* 1976. Zinc nutrition of pre-school children in the Denver Head Start Program. *Am. J. Clin. Nutr.* 29: 734–738.

10 Prasad, A. *et al.* 1976. Trace elements in sickle cell disease. *JAMA* 235-22, 2396–2398.

11 Lin, H., Chan, W., Fong, Y. and Newberne, P. 1977. Zinc levels in serum, hair and tumors from patients with esophageal cancer. *Nutr. Reports Intl.* 15(6): 635–643.

12 Greger, J. 1978. Nutritional status of adolescent girls in regard to zinc, copper, and iron. *Am. J. Clin. Nutr.* 31: 269–275.

ZINC, cont'd

13 McKenzie, J. et al. 1978. Zinc and copper status of Polynesian residents in the Tokelau Islands. Am. J. Clin. Nutr. 31: 422–428.

14 Greger, J. and Geissler, A. 1978. Effect of zinc supplementation on taste acuity of the aged. Am. J. Clin. Nutr. 31: 633–637.

15 Jacob, R.; Sandstead, H.; Solomons, N.; Kieger, C.; and Rothberg, R. 1978. Zinc status and vitamin A transport in cystic fibrosis. Am. J. Clin. Nutr. 31: 638–644.

16 Erten, J. et al. 1978. Hair zinc levels in healthy and malnourished children. Am. J. Clin. Nutr. 31: 1172–1174.

17 Atkin-Thor, E. et al. 1978. Hypogeusia and zinc depletion in chronic dialysis patients. Am. J. Clin. Nutr. 31: 1948–1951.

18 Dogru, U. 1979. Zinc levels of plasma, erythocyte, hair, and urine in homozygote Beta-Thalassemia. Acta. Haemat. 62: 41–44.

19 Collipp, P. et al. 1979. Zinc deficiency in achondroplastic children and their parents. J. Pediatrics 94(4): 609.

20 Heinersdorff, A. and Taylor, G. 1979. Concentration of zinc in the hair of school-children. Arch. Dis. Child 54: 958–960.

21 Vir, S. and Love, A. 1979. Zinc and copper status of the elderly. Am. J. Clin. Nutr. 32: 1472–1476.

22 McKenzie, J. 1979. Content of zinc in serum, urine, hair, and toenails of New Zealand adults. Am. J. Clin. Nutr. 32: 570–579.

23 Mountokalakis, Th. et al. 1979. Hair zinc compared with plasma zinc in uremic patients before and during regular hemodialysis. Clinical Nephrology 12(5): 206–209.

24 Pekarek, R. et al. 1979. Abnormal cellular immune responses during acquired zinc deficiency. Am. J. Clin. Nutr. 32: 1466–1471.

25 Bradfield, R. and Hambidge, K. February 16, 1980. Problems with hair zinc as an indicator of body zinc status. Lancet, 363.

26 Freeland-Graves, J. et al. 1980. Zinc Status of Vegetarians. J. Am. Dietet. Assoc. 77: 655–661.

27 Schneider, H. and Anke, M. 1966. Mineral content of human hair during various diseases. Z. Gesamte. Inn. Med. Ihre Grenzgeb. 21(24): 802–806.

28 Kohrs, M. et al. 1978. The relationship of tissue levels of zinc, copper, and magnesium to disease and drug usage in pregnant women. Trace Substances in Environmental Health-XII. Columbia: Univ. Missouri, pp. 258–263.

29 Capel, I. et al. 1981. Comparisons of concentrations of some trace, bulk, and toxic metals in the hair of normal and dyslexic children. Clin. Chem. 27(6): 879:881.

COPPER

Ref.	Locality	No. and type of persons and special conditions	Analysis mg%	Technique Preparation	Instrument	Remarks
1	United States (Minnesota)	18 Male control subjects	1.5	Cleaned with iso-propanol.	Spectro-photometry	There is no abnormal deposition of copper in hair of Wilson's disease patients, in contrast to most other organs and tissues.
		18 Female control subjects	3.9	HC1 and tri-chloroacetic acid extraction.		
		10 Wilson's disease patients	1.1			

				Hair washed.	Spectro-photometry	
2	Uganda	10 Children with Kwashiorkor	1.6			Kwashiorkor is not necessarily accompanied by a reduction of Cu in hair (normal approx. 1.8).
		3 Control children	0.89			
3	United States	17 Adult males	1.4	0.5 g hair washed with detergent. Nitric and perchloric acid digestion.	AAS	High Cu level in drinking water resulted in high hair Cu.
		1 Adult male with high Cu in drinking water (from well)	34.8			
4	Panama	121 Male children and adults	2.2	Acetone, ether, sodium lauryl sulfate.	AAS	If hair is to be used as a biopsy material for the purpose of comparing the copper nutriture of individuals or groups, only age and sex-matched individuals may be compared.
		159 Female children and adults	1.6			
5	United States (Boston)	11 Mo. male with Menkes Kinky Hair Syndrome	0.61		AAS	Very low Cu levels in blood, urine, and hair found.
6	India	18 Pellagrins	1.6	Alcohol, ether wash. HC1 digestion.		Hair and urinary Cu levels were significantly higher in subjects with pellagra.
		6 Controls	0.87			
7	United States	Schizophrenic patients:			AAS	High copper levels in hair may indicate schizophrenia.
		F age 1–12	7.7			
		13–30	6.4			
		31–60	5.3			
		M age 1–12	2.8			
		13–30	5.6			
		31–60	3.5			

COPPER, cont'd

Ref.	Locality	No. and type of persons and special conditions	Analysis mg%	Technique Preparation	Instrument	Remarks
		Normal individuals:				
		F age 1–12	2.0			
		13–30	2.8			
		31–60	2.2			
		M age 1–12	3.4			
		13–30	3.3			
		31–60	1.8			
8	Egypt	30 Patients with psoriasis of scalp	11.6	Ether rinse. Soap and water wash. Sulphuric and hydrogen peroxide.	Colorimetric	A significant increase in copper in hair of psoriatics is observed.
		10 Psoriasis not affecting scalp	10.7			
		30 Normals	7.9			
9	United States	175 Adolescent females	3.1	Hair washed. Acid digested.	AAS	Copper levels in serum and hair were not correlated to age or dietary intake. Only 3–4% of subjects classified as in marginal nutritional status for Zn & Cu.
10	New Zealand	32 Polynesian men	1.1	Hair washed.	AAS	Hair Cu was at the low end of the normal range. Serum Cu was high; dietary Cu low; urinary Cu excretion relatively low.
		34 Polynesian women	1.0			
11	Canada	42 Controls	2.9	Distilled water with ultrasonic.	INAA	Highly significant differences in hair levels of Cu, I. Mn, S, Se, and V were noted.
		40 Multiple sclerosis patients	0.9			

12	England	11 F patients with primary biliary cirrhosis	1.2–2.6	AAS	Acetone, deionized water wash. Nitric and perchloric acid digestion.	Hair Cu did not reflect liver Cu and is considered of no value as a biopsy material for Cu analysis.
		Normal	0.7–2.3			
13	United States (Pennsylvania)	68 Patients with idiopathic scoliosis	6.5	AAS	Washed in 1,1,1-trichlorothane. Digested in nitric & perchloric acids.	The significantly elevated Cu in hair of scoliosis patients suggests that scoliosis is in some way related to a disorder of Cu metabolism.
		25 Controls	3.6			
14	United States	10 Mo. old Cu-deficient male		AAS	Non-ionic detergent, deionized water, ether, and ethanol. HC1 digestion.	Hair Cu appeared normal even in gross Cu deficiency (low serum Cu). Cu supplementation brought serum Cu to normal levels but did not raise hair Cu above normal levels.
		on admission	3.6			
		recovery	5.6			
		11 Mo. old Cu-deficient male				
		on admission	1.3			
		recovery	2.2			
		11 Control children	1.9			
		25 Kwashiorkor, admission	2.9			
		9 Kwashiorkor, recovery	2.1			
		14 Marasmus, admission	2.5			
		9 Marasmus, recovery	2.1			

COPPER, cont'd

Ref.	Locality	No. and type of persons and special conditions	Analysis mg%	Technique Preparation	Instrument	Remarks
15	England	73 Dyslexic children	5.7 (2.1–10.7)	Detergent wash. Nitric and perchloric acid digestion.	AAS	Hair from dyslexic children had significantly higher hair copper levels than controls.
		44 Controls	3.1 (0.8–7.8)			
16	Germany	Patients w/ various diseases:				Cu increased in hair of patients with infectious hepatitis and hyperthyroiditis.
		11 Anemia	2.8			
		6 Infectious hepatitis	4.6			
		2 Hyperthyroiditis	4.3			
		Controls	1.4			

1 Rice, E. and Goldstein, N. 1961. Copper content of hair and nails in Wilson's disease. *Metabolism* 10: 1085.

2 Lea, C. and Luttrell, V. 1965. Copper content of hair in kwashiorkor. *Nature* 206: 4982, 413.

3 Harrison, W., Yurachek, J. and Benson, C. 1969. The determination of trade elements in human hair by atomic absorption spectroscopy. *Clin. Chim. Acta* 23(1): 83–91.

4 Klevay, L. 1970. Hair as a biopsy material—assessment of copper nutriture. *Am. J. Clin. Nutr.* 23(8): 1194–1202.

5 Singh, S. and Bresnan, M. 1973. Menkes kinky-hair syndrome (trichopoliodystrophy). *Am. J. Dis. Child* 125: 572–578.

6 Krishnamachari, K. 1974. Some aspects of copper metabolism in pellagra. *Am. J. Clin. Nutr.* 27: 108–111.

7 Pfeiffer, C. 1974. Observations on trace and toxic elements in hair and serum. *Orthomol. Psycho.* 3(4): 259–264.

8 Abdel-Aal, H. *et al.* 1976. Study of some minerals in scalp hair and blood sera of psoriatics. *Acta Dermatovenor (Stockholm)* 56: 265–267.

9 Greger, J. *et al.* 1978. Nutritional status of adolescent girls in regard to zinc, copper, and iron. *Am. J. Clin. Nutr.* 31: 269–275.

10 McKenzie, J. 1978 (see zinc reference #13).

11 Ryan, D. *et al.* 1978. Trace elements in scalp-hair of persons with multiple sclerosis and of normal individuals. *Clin. Chem.* 24: 11.

12 Epstein, O. *et al.* 1980. Hair copper in primary biliary cirrhosis. *Am. J. Clin. Nutr.* 33: 965–967.

13 Pratt, W. and Phippen, W. 1980. Elevated hair copper levels in idiopathic scoliosis. *Spine* 5(3): 230–233.

14 Bradfield, R. *et al.* August 16, 1980. Hair copper in copper deficiency. *Lancet*, pp. 343–344.

15 Capel, I. *et al.* 1981. Comparison of concentrations of some trace, bulk, and toxic metals in the hair of normal and dyslexic children. *Clin. Chem.* 27(6): 879–881.

16 Schneider, H. and Anke, M. 1966. Mineral content of human hair during various diseases. *Z. Gesamte. Inn. Med. Ihre. Grenzgeb.* 21(24): 802–806.

MANGANESE

Ref.	Locality	No. and type of persons and special conditions	Analysis mg%	Technique Preparation	Instrument	Remarks
1	Morocco	Manganese miners: apparently healthy miners	36.5			Elimination of Mn by affected individuals thought to be extremely slow or deficient as compared to apparently healthy subjects. Hair considered excretory route.
		subjects suspected of Mn poisoning	23.2			
		subjects who had been away from work for several years	10.5			
		patient, 17 yrs. after stopping work	7.2			
		patient, 11 yrs. after stopping work	25.4			
		patient, 2 yrs. after	17.4			
2	India	Non-occupationally exposed: 12 Male residents, Bombay	0.46 (0.11–0.76)	Washed with distilled ether, soap, ethanol, distilled water. 100–200 mg. samples.	Benzidine colorimetric method	Higher manganese levels in Indians appears to be due to differences in dietary habits.
		12 Female residents, Bombay	1.0 (0.32–1.9)			

MANGANESE, cont'd

Ref.	Locality	No. and type of persons and special conditions	Analysis mg%	Technique Preparation	Instrument	Remarks
	France	4 Male residents, Paris	0.32 (0.18–0.53)			
		18 Female residents, Paris	0.44 (0.07–1.09)			
3	United States	11 Control individuals	0.15	Water and ethyl alcohol wash.	INAA	Hair Mn in uremics appears lower than either control or dialysis groups, although not considered statistically significant.
		18 Dialysis patients	0.11			
		8 Uremic patients	0.05			
4	United States	Male patient with chronic manganism from working in a steel foundry.			AAS	Threefold level of Mn in chest hair compared to scalp hair was considered to be of diagnostic significance.
		scalp hair	2.9			
		chest hair	10.7			
		Scalp hair levels of people living around industrial complexes	0.47			
5	Poland	58 Normal controls	0.16 (0.03–0.46)		Colorimetric	Mn level of hair reflected exposure but did not correlate with length of service.
		31 Factory workers (dry electric cells)				
		<5 years at job	1.57			
		5–10 years at job	1.37			
6	Indonesia	40 Normal controls	0.29	10–50 mg hair washed in ether.	NAA	Some, but not all, protein-deficient children had markedly elevated manganese in hair. The increases were significant but not consistent enough for diagnosis of protein deficiency in individuals.
		40 Protein-deficient children	1.47			

7	India United States Thailand	11 Adults, Chandigarh 18 Adults, Denver 25 Adults, Bangkok	0.029 0.019 0.38	Washed in hexane, ethanol, deionized water. HC1 digest.	Emission spectroscopy (silver-argon dc-arc)	Significantly higher Mn levels were observed for adults in Bangkok. Differences in nutritional intake may account for this variation.
8	Germany	Welders Non-welders	0.7 0.14		NAA	Hair Mn values correlated well with daily welding time, working place conditions, and welding procedure.
9	United States	Tardive dyskinesia patients All other patients	0.046 0.08		AAS	Significant difference in mean hair Mn level observed. Dietary supplementation with Mn usually followed by increase in hair Mn level.
10	U.K.	86 Control subjects 67 F Down's syndrome patients 37 Schizophrenics 25 Mentally retarded patients	0.23 0.021 0.12 0.086	Detergent, distilled water, acetone wash. Soluene-350 digestion.	AAS	Significantly lower hair Mn levels were seen in patients with Down's syndrome, schizophrenia, and mental retardation. Hair metal analysis can be useful as a diagnostic tool in the examination of trace metal exposure, including abnormal nutritional intake, and may possibly assist in the study of certain mental states.

1 Rodier, J. 1955. Manganese poisoning in Moroccan miners. *Brit. J. Industr. Med.* 12: 21–35.

2 Umarji, G. and Bellare, R. 1966. Hair manganese levels in normal subjects. *Indian J. Exp. Biol.* 4: 212–214.

3 Mahler, D. *et al.* 1970. A study of trace metals in fingernails and hair using neutron activation analysis. *J. of Nuclear Medicine* 11(12): 739–742.

4 Rosenstock, H., Simons, D. and Meyer, J.S. 1971. Chronic manganism. *JAMA* 217(10): 1354–1358.

5 Byczkowski, S. *et al.* 1971. Manganese level of hair as a factor of exposure. *Chem. Abstr.* 75: 132689q.

6 Bowen, H. 1972. Determination of trace elements in hair samples from normal and protein-deficient children by activation analysis. *Sci. Total Environ.* 1:75–79.

7 Hambidge, K. M. and Walravens, P. 1974. Chromium, zinc, manganese, copper, Iron and cadmium concentrations in the hair of residents of Chandigarh, India and Bangkok, Thailand. *Trace Substances in Environmental Health*—VIII. Columbia: Univ. Missouri, pp. 39–44.

8 Grund, W., Schneider, W., and Wiesener, W. 1980. Manganese content of the hair, a criterion for evaluating exposure risks for electric welders. *J. Radioanal. Chem.* 58(1), 319–326 (German); *Chem. Abstr.* 93: 172952y.

9 Kunin, R. 1976. Manganese and niacin in the treatment of drug-induced dyskinesias. *J. Orthomol. Psych.* 5(1): 4–27.

10 Barlow, P. and Kapel, M. 1980. Metal and sulfur contents of hair in relation to certain mental states. *Hair, Trace Elements, and Human Illness.* Brown and Crounse, eds. New York: Praeger Publ., pp. 105–127.

IODINE

Ref.	Locality	No. and type of persons and special conditions	Analysis mg%	Technique — Preparation	Technique — Instrument	Remarks
1	Jerusalem	Children drinking water with high or low I levels				Both groups had similar contents of Iodine in their hair; urine levels reflected high or low intake of I.

1 Ganor, S., Gedalia, I. and Brand, N. 1964. Iodine in children's hair: its relation to urinary iodine levels. *J. Invest. Dermatol.* 43, 5–6.

CHROMIUM

Ref.	Locality	No. and type of persons and special conditions	Analysis mg%	Technique — Preparation	Technique — Instrument	Remarks
1	United States	19 Juvenile diabetic children	0.056 (0.026–0.119)	1 g hair washed in hexane, ethyl, alcohol deionized H_2O; digested w/ nitric, perchloric, & sulfuric acid.	AAS	Highly significant difference in Cr between the two groups was noted.
		33 Normal children	0.085 (0.036–0.187)			
2	United States	25 Newborn (0–7 days)	0.091	Hexane, ethanol, deionized water wash.	Emission spectroscopy	Results strongly suggest that hair analyses can provide a useful index of chromium nutrition.
		14 Infants (3–8 mo.)	0.11	1.5 N HC1 digestion.		
		23 Infants (1–2 yrs.)	0.052			
		20 Infants (2–3 yrs).	0.041			

#	Country	Study	Values	Preparation	Analysis	Comments
3	United States	Comparison of washing procedures, shampoos, environment		Hexane, ethanol, detergent wash. 1.5 N HCl digestion.	Emission spectroscopy	Chromium content of hair after washing is endogenous in origin and is likely to reflect the Cr nutritional status of the individual.
4	United States	Variation in Cr along hair shaft measured		Hexane, ethanol, deionized water. HCl digestion.	Emission spectroscopy	Chromium in hair not related to Cr from external environment. Changes reflect past fluctuations in Cr nutritional status of individual.
5	Thailand	28 Adult-onset diabetics 28 Nondiabetic controls	0.009 (.004–.030) 0.024 (.008–.047)	0.1 g washed in hexane, ethanol, deionized H_2O.	AAS w/ Graphite Furnace	Significantly lower hair Cr of diabetics suggests possible relationship between glucose tolerance and Cr nutrition.
6	Turkey	50 Newborns 50 Mothers	0.012 0.02	100 mg washed in hexane, ethanol, deionized H_2O.	AAS w/ Graphite Furnace	Interrelationship between hair Cr of mother and newborn probably depends on Cr nutrition state of mother.
7	New York	261 Children Riverhead (low exposure) Queens (intermediate) Bronx (high exposure)	0.052 0.045 0.080	Detergent wash sulfuric acid digestion.	Emission spectroscopy	Cr environmental exposure gradients reflected in children's hair only.

CHROMIUM, cont'd

Ref.	Locality	No. and type of persons and special conditions	Analysis mg%	Technique Preparation	Instrument	Remarks
8	Canada	Woman on TPN developed glucose intolerance & neuropathy Normal hair Cr	0.015–0.018 > 0.05	Washed in hexane, ethanol, water. Nitric acid digestion.	AAS w/ Graphite Furnace	Evidence of Chromium deficiency observed through low levels of blood and hair.
9	Canada	67 Diabetics age 27–89 yrs. 109 Healthy controls	0.09 0.053	Washed twice with diethyl/ether 20–150 mg.	INAA	INAA of scalp hair is a sensitive and accurate analytical method for the assessment of Cr in man and for the detection of low Cr states. Diabetes is associated with lower hair Cr concentration.
10	Canada	Literature review				Hair analysis is the method of choice to identify populations at greater risk for chromium deficiency.
11	Canada	64 Males with arteriosclerotic heart disease 44 Normal males	0.045 0.082	Washed with hexane and triton x 100; nitric acid digest.	AAS	Correlation between low hair chromium levels and arteriosclerotic heart disease was significant.
12	Canada	30 Psychogeriatric females: 16 Senile dementia 6 Schizophrenia 2 Affective disorder 5 Others 26 Mentally healthy females	 0.024 0.029 0.032 0.035 0.0499		AAS	Significant differences in hair chromium found. 92.6% of patients values < 0.05 mg % 57.7% of controls < 0.05 mg %.

No.	Country	Subjects	Value	Wash/Digestion	Method	Comments
13	Iraq	Workers in a leather factory where Cr compounds used	0.95	Ether, acetone, water wash.	INAA	Occupationally exposed individuals had higher average Cr levels in hair than unexposed persons.
		General population	0.41			
14	U.K.	11 F insulin-treated diabetics	0.015	Acetone, detergent, distilled water wash. Nitric acid digestion.	AAS w/ Graphite Furnace	Age and sex-matched groups were measured. Hair Cr was lower in female diabetics than controls but male diabetics and controls were not significantly different.
		11 F controls	0.027			
		12 M diabetics	0.019			
		12 M controls	0.026			
15	Turkey	17 Nulliparous women	0.022	50–100 mg hair washed in hexane, ethanol, deionized water. 1 N HC1 digestion.	AAS w/ Graphite Furnace	Results show that 1) hair Cr in multiparous women is lower than in nulliparous women, 2) depending on Cr nutrition, hair Cr of pregnant women shows a decrease with advancing pregnancy, 3) if adequate amounts of Cr are not taken during pregnancy, deficiency may result with increasing frequency.
		73 Multiparous women	0.016			

1 Hambidge, K. M. et al. August 1968. Concentration of chromium in the hair of normal children and children with juvenile diabetes mellitus. Diabetes 17: 8, 517–519.

2 Hambidge, K. M. and David Baum. April 1972. Hair chromium concentrations of human newborn and changes during infancy. Am. J. Clin. Nutr. 25: 4, 376–379.

3 Hambidge, K. M., M. Franklin and M. Jacobs. April 1972. Hair chromium concentration: effects of sample washing and external environment. Am. J. Clin. Nutr. 25: 4, 384–389.

4 Hambidge, K. M., M. Franklin and M. Jacobs. April 1972. Changes in hair chromium concentrations with increasing distances from hair roots. Am. J. Clin. Nutr. 25:4, 380–383.

5 Benjanuvatra, N. and H. Bennion. November 1975. Hair chromium concentration of Thai subjects with and without diabetes mellitus. Nutr. Reports Intl. 12: 5, 40–45.

6 Saner, G. and Gürson, T. August 1976. Hair chromium concentration in newborns and their mothers. Nutr. Rep. Intl. 14: 2, 155–164.

7 Creason, J. et al. 1975. Trace elements in hair, as related to exposure in metropolitan New York. Clin. Chem. 21: 4, 603–612.

8 Jeejeebhoy, K. et al. April 1977. Chromium deficiency, glucose intolerance, and neuropathy reversed by chromium supplementation, in a patient receiving long-term total parenteral nutrition. Am. J. Clin. Nutr. 30: 531–538.

9 Tiefenbach, B., Jervis, R., and Tiefenbach, H. 1979. Chromium, zinc, mercury, and selenium levels of diabetic patients' hair determined by instrumental neutron activation analysis. Chromium in Nutrition and Metabolism. D. Shapcott and J. Hubert, eds. New York: Elsevier/North-Holland Biomedical Press, pp. 69–78.

CHROMIUM, cont'd

10 Shapcott, D. 1979. The detection of chromium deficiency. *Chromium in Nutrition and Metabolism.* D. Shapcott and J. Hubert, eds. New York: Elsevier/North-Holland Biomedical Press, pp. 113–127.

11 Cote, Michael *et al.* 1979. Hair chromium concentration and arteriosclerotic heart disease. *Chromium in Nutrition and Metabolism.* D. Shapcott and J. Hubert, eds. New York: Elsevier/North-Holland Biomedical Press, pp. 223–228.

12 Vobecky, J. *et al.* July 1980. Hair and urine chromium content in 30 hospitalized female psychogeriatric patients and mentally healthy controls. *Nutrition Reports International* v. 22:1, 49–55.

13 Al-Shahristani, H., Shihab, K. and Jalil, M. 1979. Distribution and significance of trace element pollutants in hair of the Iraqi population. IAEA-SM-227/7, 515–525.

14 Rosson, J. *et al.* 1979. Hair chromium concentrations in adult insulin-treated diabetics. *Clinica Chimico Acta* 93: 299–304.

15 Saner, G. 1981. The effect of parity on maternal hair chromium concentration and the changes during pregnancy. *Am. J. Clin. Nutr.* 34: 853–855.

SELENIUM

Ref.	Locality	No. and type of persons and special conditions	Analysis mg%	Technique Preparation	Instrument	Remarks
1	Italy (Amiata Mt.)	7 Males, Hg smelter workers	0.045 (0.21–0.066)	A few mg. of hair washed in acetone and ether.	INAA	Se content in blood was higher with higher Hg exposure, but Se in hair was not correlated with higher Hg exposure.
		13 Males, Hg miners	0.043 (0.41–0.045)			
		12 Males, unexposed controls	0.033 (0.022–0.051)			

	Location	Description	Value	Preparation	Method	Comments
2	United States (New Mexico)	39 Residents drinking well water high in Se.	0.046 (0.002–0.2)	Washed with non-ionic detergent, ethyl alcohol, and deionized water. Nitric and perchloric acid digest.	AAS with hydride generation	Se in urine and hair significantly correlated with well water Se. Data suggests hair would serve as useful monitor of Se exposure. Blood Se alone is not adequate monitor of body burden at levels below chronic toxicity and hair or urine should be monitored simultaneously.
3	United States (So. Dakota)	6 Individuals living in area where chronic selenosis in some livestock observed	0.077 (0.025–0.11)	Acetone wash (some).	Fluorometry	Use of Se-containing shampoos reduces reliability of determining Se status for those individuals.
4	China	Inhabitants in areas affected by Keshan disease	< 0.012			Significant correlations observed between Se in hair and in blood. Endemic distribution of Keshan disease closely related to variation in hair Se levels. Se content of hair considered an important criterion of body Se status. Se content of hair and activity of glutathione peroxidase in blood increased after sodium selenite supplementation.
		Inhabitants in unaffected areas located both within and away from affected zone	> 0.02			
		Nonaffected areas located close to affected zone	0.012–0.02			
		Nonaffected areas located far from affected zone	0.03–0.06			

SELENIUM, cont'd

Ref.	Locality	No. and type of persons and special conditions	Analysis mg%	Technique Preparation	Technique Instrument	Remarks
5	Canada	153 Urban residents near lead smelters	0.26 (0.022–0.77)	Distilled water, ethanol, ether wash.	INAA IPAA	Se higher in exposed urban residents compared to controls. Se present as co-contaminant of smelter emissions and was also elevated in local dust fall and soil samples.
		81 Urban controls	0.18 (0.026–0.64)			
		76 Rural controls	0.18 (0.032–0.48)			
6	United States	22 "Well-nourished" individuals (age 24–45)	0.02–0.06			Serum tocopherols, blood Se, erythrocyte hemolysis, glutathione peroxidase activity in erythrocytes, dietary Se, and hair Se determined. No good correlation found between diet and hair Se. Good clinical correlation found between hair Se and glutathione peroxidase levels: the higher the hair Se levels within the normal range, the more active the glutathione peroxidase. Hair Se levels considered a good screening tool. Values < 0.012 mg % suggest compromised antioxidant defense.

1 Cigna Rossi, L., Clemente, G. and Santaroni, G. 1976. Mercury and selenium distribution in a defined area and in its population. *Arch. Env. Health* 31(3): 160–165.

2 Valentine, J. Kang, H. and Spivey, G. 1978. Selenium levels in human blood, urine, and hair in response to exposure via drinking water. *Environ. Research* 17: 347–355.

3 Howe, M. 1979. Selenium in the blood of South Dakotans. *Arch. Environ. Health* 34(6): 444–448.

4 Keshan Disease Research Group. 1979. Epidemiologic studies on the etiologic relationship of selenium and Keshan disease. *Chinese Medical Journal* 92(7): 477–482.

5 Chatt, A. *et al.* 1980. Scalp hair as a monitor of community exposure to environmental pollutants. *Hair, Trace Elements, and Human Illness.* Brown and Crounse, eds. New York: Praeger Publishers, pp. 46–73.

6 Bland, J. October 1980. Trace elements in human health: selenium and aluminum. *Am. Acad. Medical Preventics Symposium* (Uni-Mar, Sacramento, CA.—taped program).

SILICON

Ref.	Locality	No. and type of persons and special conditions	Analysis mg%	Technique Preparation	Instrument	Remarks
1	Poland	Welders in shipyard:			Colorimetric	Parallel X-ray examinations of lungs of the welders were made which showed increasing incidence of silicosis with increasing length of service.
		0 years working	4.4			
		0–5 years working	5.99			
		5–10 years working	7.94			
		> 10 years working	8.68			
2	Poland	247 Males, aged 3–75 yrs.			Colorimetric	Hair Si levels did not differ in non-occupationally exposed individuals.
		Fair haired	4.2			
		Dark haired	4.1			
		Auburn haired	3.98			

1 Byczkowski, S. and Wrzesniowska, K. 1975. Silicon level of welders hair. *Gdansk. Tow. Nauk. Rozpr. Wydz.* 3(8): 43–47, 1971. *Chem. Abstracts* 132691j.

2 Byczkowski, S. and Wrzesniowska, K. 1975. Physiological hair silicon content in men. *Toxicology* 5(1): 123–124.

VANADIUM

Ref.	Locality	No. and type of persons and special conditions	Analysis mg%	Technique Preparation	Instrument	Remarks
1	United States	Environmental exposure: 265 Children (0–15) low exposure moderate exposure high exposure 193 Adults low exposure moderate high	 0.020 0.024 0.040 0.012 0.020 0.035	Detergent wash.	Emission spectroscopy	Vanadium in scalp hair in adults and children was significantly correlated with environmental exposure gradients.
2	Canada	42 Controls 40 Multiple sclerosis patients	0.006 0.0036	Distilled water wash with ultra-sonic sound.	INAA	Higher values are observed for hair V in controls versus multiple sclerosis patients.

1 Creason, J. et al. 1975. Trace elements in hair as related to exposure in metropolitan New York. *Clin. chem.* 21(4): 603–612.

2 Ryan, D., Holzbecher, J. and Stuart, D. 1978. Trace elements in scalp-hair of persons with multiple sclerosis and of normal individuals. *Clin. Chem.* 24(11): 1996–2000.

NICKEL

Ref.	Locality	No. and type of persons and special conditions	Analysis mg%	Technique Preparation	Instrument	Remarks
1	United States	20 Healthy subjects, ages 21–80 yr.	0.022 (0.013–0.051)	Detergent wash.	AAS	A slight decrease in Ni concentrations in hair was seen with advancing age. Measurements of Ni in hair may supplement Ni analyses of serum and urine as indices of the body burden of Ni.
		Woman with dyed hair	0.22	Nitric and perchloric acid digestion.		
		Permanent-waved hair	0.095			
2	United States	Environmental exposure 265 children (0–15)		Detergent wash.	Emission spectroscopy	Ni in scalp hair of children was correlated with environmental exposure gradients.
		Riverhead (low)	0.05			
		Queens (moderate)	0.04			
		Bronx (high)	0.07			
3	Germany	5 Persons accidentally exposed to nickel carbonyl	0.7–4.8	Hair washed in methanol/acetone.	AAS	An exponential decrease in the amount of Ni in hair was observed which was considered to be probably the result of the Ni $(Co)_4$ inhalation during the accidental exposure.
		Ni in hair 169 days after exposure	< 0.04–1.7	Digested in nitric acid.		
4	Netherlands	8 Occupationally exposed subjects	1.45		AAS	Ni concentrations in blood plasma, urine, and scalp hair do not differ between hypersensitive subjects with Ni-eczema and non-hypersensitive subjects. Occupationally exposed individuals have about ten times the Ni in plasma, urine, and hair of control subjects.
		Non-occupationally exposed:				
		10 Men	0.06			
		14 Women	0.10			

NICKEL, cont'd

Ref.	Locality	No. and type of persons and special conditions	Analysis mg%	Technique Preparation	Instrument	Remarks
5	Canada	76 Rural controls 81 Urban controls 153 Urban, near lead smelters	0.21 (0.16–1.7) 0.24 (0.12–2.1) 0.40 (0.10–3.8)	Washed with distilled water, ethanol, diethyl ether.	IPAA	Ni levels in hair were progressively higher from rural to exposed urban residents. Ni present as cocontaminant with Pb of smelter omissions.

1 Nechay, M. and Sunderman, W. 1973. Measurements of nickel in hair by atomic absorption spectrometry. *Annals of clinical Laboratory Science* 3(1): 30–35.

2 Creason, J. *et al.* 1975. Trace Elements in hair as related to exposure in metropolitan New York. *Clin. Chem.* 21(4): 603–612.

3 Hagedom-Götz, H. and Stoeppler, M. 1977. On nickel contents in urine and hair in a case of exposure to nickel carbonyl. *Arch. Toxicology* 38, 275–285.

4 Spruit, D. and Bongaarts, P. 1977. Nickel content of plasma, urine, and hair in contact dermatitis. *Clinical Chemistry and Chemical Toxicology of Metals.* New York: Elsevier/North-Holland Biomedical Press, pp. 261–264.

5 Chatt, A. *et al.* 1980. Scalp hair as a monitor of community exposure to environmental pollutants. *Hair, Trace Elements, and Human Illness.* New York: Praeger Publ., pp. 46–71.

TIN

Ref.	Locality	No. and type of persons and special conditions	Analysis mg%	Technique Preparation	Instrument	Remarks
1	United States (New York)	265 Children with varying environmental exposure levels: Riverhead (low) Queens (intermediate) Bronx (high)	0.054 0.044 0.083	Detergent wash.	Emission spectroscopy	Tin in scalp hair of children correlated with environmental mental exposure gradients.

1 Creason, John *et al.* 1975. Trace elements in hair as related to exposure in metropolitan New York. *Clinical Chemistry* 21(4): 603–612.

LITHIUM

Ref.	Locality	No. and type of persons and special conditions	Analysis mg% 1975/76	Analysis mg% 1977	Technique Preparation	Instrument	Remarks
1	Canada	31 Learning-disabled children	0.022	0.068		AAS	Discriminant function analysis using Cd, Co, Mn, Cr, and Li allowed subjects to be classified as learning disabled or not with 98% accuracy. Significant differences in Li were seen both initially and in follow-up study, but in opposite directions. Also, as Pb and Cd levels decreased, Li increased.
		22 Normal children	0.040	0.049			

1 Pihl, R., Drake, H. and Vrana, F. 1980. Hair analysis in learning and behavior problems. *Hair, Trace Elements, and Human Illness*. Brown and Crounse, eds. New York: Praeger Publ., pp. 128–143.

STRONTIUM

Ref.	Locality	No. and type of persons and special conditions	Analysis mg%	Technique Preparation	Instrument	Remarks
1	United States	Strontium 90 and stable strontium were measured in hair, plasma, and diets of children and in hair and plasma of adults.		Detergent wash.	INAA (stable Sr)	No correlation could be made between the quantity of 90Sr in hair and dietary intake. Lack of correlation between the specific activities of 90Sr in adult hair and plasma indicated that additional evaluation was required.
2	United States	794 Outpatients		Nonionic detergent and de-ionized water.	Emission spectroscopy ICAP	Mean Sr values increase until age 25; females were higher by a factor of two or more. A strong positive correlation was found between Sr and Ca. Further investigation of Sr and Ca in hair is necessary.

1 Magno, P., Baratta, E. and Leonard, I. 1966. Strontium-90 in human hair and blood. *Health Physics* 12(10): 1493–1496.

2 Lord, R. and Trawick, W. 1980. Trace element patterns in hair from outpatient clinical laboratory data. *Hair, Trace Elements, and Human Illness.* Brown and Crounse, eds. New York: Praeger Publ., pp. 102–104.

COBALT

Ref.	Locality	No. and type of persons and special conditions	Analysis mg%	Technique Preparation	Instrument	Remarks
1	United States	19 Male subjects 11 Female subjects	0.017 0.028	Carbon tetrachloride wash. D.1 N HC1 digestion.	AAS	Cobalt levels remained relatively constant at all ages. Significant differences in hair Co for males and females observed.

2	England	16 Patients with metallic total hip replacements	0.042 (.006–0.23)	INAA	Although mean Co levels not statistically significant, three patients had Co levels outside range of control values suggesting that in certain subjects the implant does give rise to a raised cobalt level in the body. Blood and urine Co levels increased after implant insertion showing wear of components of metallic implants.
		20 Control subjects	0.022 (.007–0.049)		
3	Canada	76 Rural controls	0.041 (0.012–0.18)	Distilled water, ethanol, and diethyl ether wash. INAA IPAA	Co levels were progressively higher from rural to exposed urban residents. Co was present as a co-contaminant of smelter emissions.
		81 Urban controls	0.047 (0.01–0.27)		
		153 Urban, near lead smelters	0.053 (0.01–0.36)		
4a,b	Canada	31 Learning disabled children	0.016	AAS	Discriminant function analysis using Cd, Co, Mn, Cr, and Li allowed subjects to be classified as learning disabled or not with 98% accuracy. (1977)
		22 Normal children	0.023		Follow-up study employing discriminant analysis yielded only 66% accuracy. (1980)

COBALT, cont'd

Ref.	Locality	No. and type of persons and special conditions	Analysis mg%	Technique		
				Preparation	Instrument	Remarks
5	United States	794 M and F outpatients	0.02	Nonionic detergent and de-ionized H_2O wash.	Emission Spectroscopy ICAP	Significant correlations between Co and Fe in hair found.

1 Schroeder, H. and Nason, A. 1969. Trace metals in human hair. *J. Investigative Dermatology* 53(1): 71–78.

2 Coleman, R., Herrington, J. and Scales, J. 1973. Concentration of wear products in hair, blood, and urine after total hip replacement. *British Medical Journal* 1: 527–529.

3 Chatt, A. *et al.* 1980. Scalp hair as a monitor of community exposure to environmental pollutants. *Hair, Trace Elements, and Human Illness.* Brown and Crounse, eds. New York: Praeger Publ., pp. 46–73.

4a Pihl, R. and Parkes, M. 1977. Hair element content in learning disabled children. *Science*, 198: 204–206.

b Pihl, R., Drake, H. and Vrana, F. 1980. Hair analysis in learning and behavior problems. *Hair, Trace Elements, and Human Illness.* Brown and Crounse, eds. New York: Praeger Publ., pp. 128–143.

5 Lord, R. and Trawick, W. 1980. Trace element patterns in hair from outpatient clinical laboratory data. *Hair, Trace Elements, and Human Illness,* Brown and Crounse, ed. New York: Praeger Publ., pp. 102–104.

MERCURY

Ref.	Locality	No. and type of persons and special conditions	Analysis mg%	Technique Preparation	Technique Instrument	Remarks
1	Japan	178 Japanese, no abnormal Hg exposure; ate average of 84 g fish/day			AAS Cold vapor	Amount of Hg in scalp hair correlated with fish consumption. "The amount of Hg in a hair sample can be used as a diagnostic criterion in Hg poisoning." The amount of methylmercury in the samples was 57% of total Hg content.
		111 males	0.44			
		67 females	0.39			
		89 Japanese fishermen; 270 g fish/day	0.48			
		14 American men living in Japan; ate fish 3–4 times/week	0.19			
		7 Americans, Cleveland	0.24			
		31 Nepalese men; ate no fish during survey	0.02			
2	United States	5 Women with symptoms of mercurialism who used mercurial skin bleach creams			INAA	Hair offers certain advantages over blood as an index of Hg absorption as it contains a long-term depot of fixed Hg. Urinary Hg values were also elevated in three subjects.
		1% Hg cream used	0.03–0.52			
		3% Hg cream used	0.74, 12.8			
		50 Adult controls	0.19			

MERCURY, cont'd

Ref.	Locality	No. and type of persons and special conditions	Analysis mg%	Technique Preparation	Instrument	Remarks
3	Canada	60 Dentists 49 Dental assistants	0.68 0.86	Ether wash.	INAA	10% of subjects tested had twice normal Hg levels (70.7 mg %) in hair indicating that a significantly large group of dental personnel are exposed to Hg. Blood analyses confirmed elevated values but urinalyses did not correlate well. A need for routine monitoring of dental personnel is suggested.
4	United States	115 Dentists	0.95		AAS	A major portion (89%) of the hair samples in this study were above the normal range of 0.001–0.25 mg%.
5	Scotland	87 Dentists 80 Dental surgery assistants 16 Other staff	0.95 0.76 0.24		INAA	Bodily contamination as reflected in hair and nail Hg levels was significantly higher in staff handling Hg. Dental personnel should be monitored to assess Hg contamination using hair and nail analyses.
6	United States	99 Pasadena women 147 Los Alamos women	2.96 2.08	Washed.	AAS Cold vapor	The results suggest a difference in environmental exposure to Hg between the two groups.
7	Scotland	35 African adults with nephrotic syndrome used Hg skin cream in last 6 months discontinued Hg skin cream 6 mo. prior no skin cream used	2.1–922.0 0.27–76.8 0.05–2.3		INAA	Estimation of Hg in hair and nails is reliable and safe and offers a direct means of detecting previous exposure to the metal. Levels of Hg in scalp hair, pubic hair, and fingernails reflected use of Hg-containing skin creams, the causal agents of many cases of adult nephrotic syndrome in Kenya.

349

No.	Country	Subject	Sample prep / Values	Method	Remarks
8	Canada	Residents of Cree Indian communities		INAA	Good correlation between blood and hair Hg levels seen. Some relationship between fish consumption and blood Hg observed. Recommend that blood and/or hair should be screened for Hg periodically in areas where high environmental Hg found.
9	Iraq	48 Patients who had ingested treated grains	Detergent, distilled water, alcohol wash.	INAA	The biological half-life which was calculated from the distribution of Hg along the head hair indicated that some persons may face a much higher risk than others with the same body burden. Hair is an excellent indicator of Hg poisoning.
10	Italy	7 Males with highest occupational Hg exposure — 2.5; 13 Male miners, inhalation and ingestion of Hg ore — 0.40; 8 Controls, relatives — 0.18	Washed.	INAA	Hg levels in blood, hair, urine, and feces correlated with degree of exposure.
11	Iraq	3 Females, ate bread made with methyl-mercury treated wheat for 2–2½ months	53.5–64.9	AAS	Measurements of total and inorganic mercury in hair were used to trace the history and extent of methyl mercury exposures.
12	Japan	14 Japanese females exposed to elemental mercury vapor — Inorganic Hg / Organic Hg: 0 months exposure 0.032/0.20, 4 months exposure 0.047/0.20, 8 months exposure 0.050/0.18		AAS Cold vapor.	Level of organic Hg in hair remained constant but inorganic Hg increased, possibly due to external contamination with mercury vapor. Urine value did not change significantly; Hg in plasma increased.

MERCURY, cont'd

Ref.	Locality	No. and type of persons and special conditions	Analysis mg%	Technique Preparation	Instrument	Remarks
13	Japan	Maternal hair Newborn hair	0.33 0.43	Detergent, distilled water, acetone wash.	AAS	A significant correlation between Hg in newborn hair and maternal blood, and newborn hair and newborn blood.
14	Japan	19 Nonvegetarian Indians, Bombay 23 Vegetarians, Bombay	0.21 0.08			The amount of Hg in urine samples is not a good index of body burden of methylmercury intake via food. However, human scalp hair and blood will reflect the dose response relationship.
15	United States	11 Individuals exposed to inorganic mercury vapor 15 Controls	0.07–11.4 < 0.5		AAS	Endogenous excretion of Hg in hair is supported by the observed shifts in peak Hg concentration with increasing time from last exposure.
16	Canada	945 Residents of Indian reserve exposed to methylmercury contaminated fish.		Not washed.	AA	Hair should be the indicator medium of choice in clinical and epidemiological studies of individuals suspected of methylmercury exposure. The relationship between total Hg in hair and organic Hg in hair is consistent thus, measurement of total Hg in hair is just as satisfactory in populations consuming methylmercury from fish.
17	England	Dental students & faculty: 9 unexposed to amalgam 8 worked 4 mo. with amalgam	1.3 0.4	Not washed.	INAA	Significant results were found for head hair and fingernail Hg despite considerable dispersion. There is a need to monitor Hg levels and fully implement Hg hygiene procedures.

8 students, 1½ yr. w/ amalgam	12.8
13 students, 2½ yrs. exposure	20.8
7 hospital interns	1.0
9 practitioners, < 5 yrs. exp.	1.2
7 practitioners, > 15 yrs.	5.0

1 Yamaguchi, S. *et al.* 1971. Relationship between mercury content of hair and amount of fish consumed. *HSMHA Health Reports* 86: 904–909.

2 Marzulli, F. and Brown, D. 1972. Potential systemic hazards of topically applied mercurials. *J. Soc. Cosmet. Chem.* 23: 875–886.

3 Hibberd, J. and Smith, D. 1972. Systemic mercury levels in dental office personnel in Ontario: a pilot study. *J. Canad. Dent. Assoc.* 38: 249–254.

4 Gutenmann, W. and Lisk, D. 1973. Elevated concentrations of mercury in dentists' hair. *Bull. Environ. Contam. Toxic.* 9(5): 318–320..

5 Lenihan, J., Smith, H. and Harvey, W. 1973. Mercury hazards in dental practice. *British Dental Journal* 135: 363–367.

6 Nord, P., Kadaba, M. and Sorenson, J. 1973. Mercury in human hair. *Arch. Environ. Health* 27: 40–44.

7 Barr, R. *et al.* 1973. Tissue mercury levels in the mercury-induced nephrotic syndrome. *Am. J. Clin. Pathol.* 59: 515–517.

8 Bernstein, A. D. 1974. Clinical investigation in northwest Quebec Canada of environmental organic mercury effects. *Intl. Symp. Proc. Recent Adv. Assess. Health Effects Environ. Pollution I*, pp. 105–117.

9 Al-Shahristani and Shibab, K. 1974. Variation of biological half-life of methylmercury in man. *Arch. Environ. Health* 28: 342–344.

10 Cagnetti, P., Cigna-Rossi, L. and Clemente, G. 1974. Mercury pathways to man and "in vivo" content of the population of the Mt. Amiata area. *Intl. Symp. Proc. Recent Advances Assess. Health Effects of Environ. Pollution III*, pp. 1451–1460.

11 Giovanoli-Jakubczak, T. and Berg, G. 1974. Measurement of mercury in human hair. *Arch. Envir. Health* 28: 139–144.

12 Ishihara, N., Urushiyama, K. and Suzuki, T. 1977. Inorganic and organic mercury in blood, urine, and hair in low level mercury vapour exposure. *Int. Arch. Occup. Environ. Health* 40: 249–253.

13 Fujita, M. and Takabatake, E. 1977. Mercury levels in human maternal and neonatal blood, hair and milk. *Bull. Environ. Contam. Toxicol.* 18(2): 205–209.

14 Yamaguchi, S. *et al.* 1977. A background of geographical pathology on mercury in the east Pacific area. *J. Occup. Med.* 19(7).

15 Sexton, D. *et al.* July/August 1978. A nonoccupational outbreak of inorganic mercury vapor poisoning. *Arch. Environ. Health*, pp. 186–191.

16 Phelps, R., Clarkson, T., Kershaw, T. and Wheatley, B. 1980. Interrelationships of blood and hair mercury concentrations in a North American population exposed to methylmercury. *Arch. Environ. Health* 35(3): 161–168.

17 Sharry, J. 1980. Mercury levels in dental students and faculty measured by neutron activation analysis. *J. Prosthetic Dentistry* 43(5): 581–585.

CADMIUM

Ref.	Locality	No. and type of persons and special conditions	Analysis mg%	Technique Preparation	Instrument	Remarks
1	United States	4th Grade boys with varying exposures: I. high exposure II. high exposure III. low exposure IV. low exposure V. low exposure	0.21 0.15 0.10 0.10 0.07	Detergent, distilled water, alcohol, hot EDTA.	AAS	Mean hair levels for Cd accurately reflected community exposure.
2	United States	Follow-up study one year after study cited in reference 1.		(same)	AAS	Results were virtually identical to those of original study. Hair Cd again reflected environmental exposure.
3	United States	Cincinnati residents: 83 Females (14–84 yr.) 95 Males (2–88 yr.)	0.24 0.22	Organic solvents, detergent, deionized H_2O, acetone wash. Nitric/perchloric acid digestion.	AAS	Cd and Pb were highly correlated in both sexes. A possible unknown factor in Pb poisoning of children may be associated Cd exposure. Blood Cd is inadequate to demonstrate associated exposure, while analysis of hair might lead to important findings.
4	Canada	76 Rural controls 45 Urban controls 121 Urban residents, near refineries	0.12 0.20 0.41	Ether, alcohol, distilled water wash.	INAA	Hair Cd levels reflected environmental exposure gradients.

343

#	Country	Subjects	Value	Preparation	Method	Comments
5	United States	Houston residents: I. policemen on foot patrol	0.11	Hair washed. Nitric/perchloric acid digestion.	AAS	Levels of Cd considered low in all specimens. These low levels pushed the analytical methods to the limit of effectiveness.
		IA. office workers (controls)	0.11			
		II. garage attendants	0.10			
		IIA. orderlies/custodians (control)	0.22			
		III. females living 2 blocks from freeway	0.06			
		III. females living away from the freeway	0.07			
6	United States (New Jersey)	17 Men occupationally exposed to Cd	0.25	Deionized water, detergent, acetone wash. HNO$_3$ digestion.	AAS	Hair Cd levels correlated significantly with Cd in kidney and liver. Hair sampling can distinguish between occupational and non-occupational exposure.
		Non-occupationally exposed	0.20			
		Hair, kidney, liver, and lung specimens also obtained from 50 autopsies.				
7	United States (New York)	23 Subjects (age to 12 yrs.)	0.17			Hair Cd levels were highest in adults living closest to Cd usage areas (golf course). High Cd levels in hair correlated with elevated diastolic blood pressure.
		16 Subjects (age 13–21)	0.17			
		7 Subjects (age 22–35)	0.45			
		86 Subjects (over 36 yrs.)	0.38			

354

CADMIUM, cont'd

Ref.	Locality	No. and type of persons and special conditions	Analysis mg%	Technique Preparation	Instrument	Remarks
8	Canada	31 Learning disabled children	0.17		AAS	Discriminant function analysis using Cd, Co, Mn, Cr, and Li enabled subjects to be classified as learning disabled or not with 98% accuracy. Elevated Pb and Cd in the learning disabled group is viewed as being of particular importance.
		22 Normal children	0.11			
9	United States	Children in smelter and comparison towns:		Detergent, water wash.	AAS	Hair Cd significantly elevated in children living near Zn smelters and Pb smelters. Blood Cd levels also high near several smelters. Cd levels in hair provided evidence of external Cd exposure.
		126—Pb smelter towns	0.53			
		872—Cu smelter towns	0.19			
		295—Zn smelter towns	0.56			
		160—Comparison towns	0.09			
10	England	73 Dyslexic children	0.26	Detergent wash. Nitric/perchloric acid digestion.	AAS	Significantly higher levels of Cd were observed in hair of dyslexic children. Excessive Cd burden could be implicated in this form of learning disorder.
		44 Controls	0.01			
11	New Zealand	13 Oyster openers (consume 2.5–12.5 dozen oysters/week)	0.07	NOH_3 $HCCO_4$ digestion.	AAS	Cd low in both urine and hair of oyster openers. Urinary excretions and hair concentrations of Cd might not be suitable media for detecting exposure to Cd except when the exposure is high.
		9 Factory workers	0.13			
		1 Electroplater (for 25 yrs.)	0.34			
		11 Leg ulcer patients	0.06			
		19 Dermatosis patients	0.10			

1 Hammer, D. et al. 1971. Hair trace metal levels and environmental exposure. Am. J. Epidemiology 93(2): 84–92.

2 Hammer, D. et al. 1971. Trace metals in human hair as a simple epidemiologic monitor of environmental exposure. Trace Substances in Environmental Health—V. Columbia: Univ. Missouri, pp. 25–38.

3 Petering, H., Yeager, D. and Witherup, S. 1973. Trace metal content of hair, II: cadmium and lead of human hair in relation to age and sex. Arch. Environ. Health 27: 327–330.

4 Chattopadhyay, A. and Jervis, R. 1974. Hair as an indicator of multi-element exposure of population groups. Trace Substances in Environmental Health—VIII, Columbia: Univ. Missouri, pp. 31–38.

5 Johnson, D., Tillery, J. and Prevost, R. 1975. Trace metals in occupationally and nonoccupationally exposed individuals. Environmental Health Perspectives 10: 151–158.

6 Olevu, George. 1975. Epidemiological implications of environmental cadmium. 1.

The probable utility of human hair for occupational trace metal (cadmium) screening. Am. Indust. Hyg. Assoc. J. 36: 229–233.

7 Keil, J. et al. 1975. Biologic observations of a population adjustment to cadmium usage. Intern. Conf. on Heavy Metals in the Environ. Toronto. Abstracts B-38-40.

8 Pihl, R. and Parkes, M. 1977. Hair element content in learning disabled children. Science 198: 204–206.

9 Baker, E. et al. 1977. A Nationwide survey of heavy metal absorption in children living near primary copper, lead, and zinc smelters. Am. J. Epidemiology 106(4): 261–273.

10 Capel, I. et al. 1981. Comparison of concentrations of some trace, bulk, and toxic metals in the hair of normal and dyslexic children. Clin. Chem. 27(6): 879–881.

11 McKenzie, J. and Neallie, J. 1974. Cadmium in urine and hair from New Zealand adults. Trace Substances in Environmental Health—VIII. Columbia: Univ. Missouri, pp. 45–48.

LEAD

Ref.	Locality	No. and type of persons and special conditions	Analysis mg%	Technique Preparation	Technique Instrument	Remarks
1	Japan	Lead workers:				Symptoms of Pb poisoning were found in workers with elevated hair Pb. Correlations between Pb in blood, urine and hair were seen. Lead in hair of men is classified:
		9 men, electric storage battery plant	21.7 (3.7–55.0)			< 3.0 mg% .non-occupational and normal Pb exposure
		9 men, rayon manu-facturing plant	16.8 (4.7–61.7)			3.0–11.0 ....occupational normal Pb exposure
		55 men, printing workers	5.5 (0.4–19.6)			> 11.0 ....warning or dangerous Pb exposure
		22 women, printing	10.0 (1.3–21.5)			
		5 workers making scales	1.1			

LEAD, cont'd

Ref.	Locality	No. and type of persons and special conditions	Analysis mg%	Technique Preparation	Instrument	Remarks
		6 auto-painting workers	0.6			
		6 bobbin-painting workers	2.3			
		Healthy controls: 13 men	0.99			
		9 women	1.5			
2	United States (Boston)	41 Control children	2.4 (0.2–9.5)	Hair washed. Digested with nitric/ perchloric acids.	AAS	Measurement of Pb in hair may provide a simple means for screening children exposed to possible lead intoxication. Good correlation was found between the major clinical and laboratory findings, including Pb in bones.
		16 Children with lead intoxication	28.2 (4.2–97.5)			
3	United States (Boston)	5 Children with Pb intoxication confirmed with Pb chelation test	Before Treatment / After Treatment: 16.5 / 2.4; 5.3 / 1.7; 7.6 / 1.6; 21.3 / 4.2; 16.6 / 5.9		AAS	Determination of Pb in scalp hair is a valuable diagnostic aid in chronic or mild Pb intoxication, particularly when other clinical or laboratory evidence is of questionable diagnostic quality.
4	United States	Non-occupationally exposed boys:	Median / Arith. Mean: highest 4.6 / 8.0; high 1.9 / 3.2; low 1.1 / 1.4; low 0.73 / 1.3; lowest 0.68 / 0.81	Detergent, alcohol, EDTA wash. Nitric acid digest.	AAS	Hair metal levels reflect non-occupational exposure to Pb. Hair and blood Pb levels correlated well indicating that hair Pb reflects endogenous Pb absorption in addition to any exogenous deposition.

	Country	Group	Concentration	Wash/Digestion	Method	Comments
5	Japan	11 Healthy persons 12 Lead workers	1.7 (0.4–3.2) 5.7–25.0	1% EDTA, acetone, ether wash. Nitric/perchloric digestion.	AAS	Hair analysis for Pb may provide a simple screening method for lead workers who are exposed to possible lead poisoning.
6	United States	265 Boston policemen Hair 0–1.5 cm from scalp Hair 1.5–3.5 cm from scalp	 1.8 2.9	Hair washed. Digested with perchloric acid.	AAS	Hair levels of Pb correlated well with exposure to traffic and suggest that these men have increased burden of lead. Hair can be used as an indicator of chronic automobile exhaust exposures.
7	Canada	Residents living close to secondary Pb smelter Urban controls	4.1 (1.4–16.6) 1.3 (0.3–3.9)		IPAA	A relationship between hair and blood lead levels was established. In children with excessive Pb absorption, 10–15% showed subtle neurological dysfunctions and minor psychomotor abnormalities.
8	Egypt	27 Controls Pb-exposed workers 46 workers 12 workers 8 workers	0.94 < 2.0 2.0–3.0 > 3.0	Detergent, distilled water, hot nitric acid (1%) wash.	USPHS dithizone Method	Levels of Pb in hair correlate with the degree of Pb absorption and toxicity based on biochemical and medical tests (blood, urine coproporphyrin). Lead in hair > 3.0 mg% could be taken as a sign of excessive lead exposure.
9	United States	83 Females 95 Males	2.4 1.8	Acetone, ether, detergent wash. Nitric/perchloric acid digestion.	AAS	Pb and Cd in hair were highly correlated. Studies of Pb and Cd in blood would be inadequate to demonstrate associated exposure while hair might lead to important findings. Comparisons should be limited to age and sex matched groups.

LEAD, cont'd

Ref.	Locality	No. and type of persons and special conditions	Analysis mg%	Technique Preparation	Instrument	Remarks
10	United States	Boston, Mass. 56 Children 68 Adults	2.8 1.9	Hair washed. Nitric and perchloric acid digestion.	AAS	The most significant variables which influenced the level of Pb in hair were ingestion of lead-containing substances, exposure to Pb of environmental origin, place of residence, site from which hair specimen sampled (distance from scalp), and age.
		Tokyo, Japan 57 Children 17 Adults	2.1 1.4			
		Yugoslavia, near Pb smelter 15 Children 15 Adults	0.3 2.3 3.7			
		Yugoslavia, controls (10) Iran villagers 6 Children 27 Adults	 0.9 0.9			
11	United States (Houston, TX)	Policemen on foot patrol Office workers (control)	2.35 1.31	Hair washed. Digested in nitric/perchloric acid.	AAS	Policemen and garage attendants had significantly higher blood and hair Pb levels due to airborne exposures.
		Garage attendants	4.8			
		Orderlies & custodians (control)	3.0			
		Females living 2 blks from freeway	0.74			
		Females living away from freeway (controls)	0.60			

	Country	Subjects	Value	Method	Comments
12	New Zealand	28 M occupations with probable Pb exposures	3.3	AAS	Detergent wash. HCl digestion.	No specific age- or sex-related hair Pb levels were found. Highly significant elevations were found only in a group of occupations which would be expected to have above-normal exposure to Pb.
		44 M students, clerical, teachers, etc.	1.0			
		61 M other occupations, farmers, salesmen	1.1			
13	United States	3 Adult men fed ^{204}Pb for 100 days		Mass spectrometry	Soap and water wash. Nitric acid digestion.	Blood showed immediate response to intake of Pb, facial hair showed more gradual response and a delay of about 35 days. Hair Pb values are the integral of blood Pb values in this study.
14	Nigeria	8 Sickle cell anemia patients	11.8	AAS	Ultrasonic water bath with acetone, alcohol, water. HNO$_3$ and H$_2$O$_2$ digestion.	Hair Pb levels were significantly higher in sickle cell anemia subjects.
		25 Control subjects	1.3			
15	Canada	76 Rural controls	1.0	IPAA	Distilled water, ethanol, diethyl ether wash.	Hair can be used to assess the body burden of Pb and other toxic metals and to investigate the interrelationships among them in an effort to evaluate the overall health effects arising from environmental metal exposure.
		45 Urban controls	1.7			
		121 Urban residents near smelter	4.5			
16	United States	Children in smelter & comparison towns:		AAS	Non-ionic detergent wash.	Increased external exposure to Pb, as evidenced by increased amounts in hair was occurring in smelter areas. Blood or urine Pb levels were not elevated.
		126 Pb smelter towns	7.7			
		872 Cu smelter towns	2.2			

LEAD, cont'd

Ref.	Locality	No. and type of persons and special conditions	Analysis mg%	Technique Preparation	Instrument	Remarks
		294 Zn smelter towns	4.4			
		160 Comparison towns	1.3			
17	United States	9 Adult males using 2% lead acetate hair dye			X-ray spectroscopy	Scalp hair Pb analysis confirmed use of Pb and pubic and axillary hair indicated systemic absorption of Pb occurs with use of Pb-acetate hair dyes.
18	United States	31 Learning disabled children	2.3		AAS	Elevations of Pb and Cd in hair of learning disabled children were viewed as being of particular importance. Significant group differences and a discriminant function separated the groups with 98% accuracy.
		22 Normal children	0.4			

1 Suzuki, Y., Nishiyama, K. and Matsuka, Y. 1958. Studies on lead content and physical properties of the hair of lead poisoning. *Tokushima J. Exp. Med.* 5: 111–119.

2 Kopito, L. *et al.* 1967. Lead in hair of children with chronic lead poisoning. *N. Eng. J. Med.* 276: 949–953.

3 Kopito, L., Briley, A. and Shwachman, H. 1969. Chronic Plumbism in Children. *JAMA* 209(2): 243–248.

4 Hammer, D. *et al.* 1971. Trace metals in human hair as a simple epidemiological monitor of environmental exposure. *Trace Substances in Environmental Health—V.* Columbia: Univ. Missouri, pp. 25–38.

5 Hasegawa, N. *et al.* 1971. Determination of lead in hair by atomic absorption spectroscopy for simple screening of lead intoxication. *Annual Report of the Research Institute of Environ. Med., Nagoya Univ.* 18: 1–5.

6 Speizer, F. *et al.* October 2–6, 1972. Health effects of exposure to automobile exhaust IV. Assessment of lead exposure in traffic policemen. *Proc. Intl. Symp. Environ. Health Aspects of Lead.* Amsterdam, pp. 835–846.

7 Roberts, T. *et al.* 1974. Lead contamination around secondary smelters: estimation of dispersal and accumulation by humans. *Science* 186: 1120–1123.

8 El-Dakhakhny, A. and El-Sadik, Y. January 1972. Lead in hair among exposed workers. *Am. Ind. Hyg. Assoc. J.* 33.

9 Petering, H. *et al.* 1973. Trace metal content of hair. II. Cadmium and head of human hair in relation to age and sex. *Arch. Environ. Health* 27: 327–330.

10 Kopito, L. and Shwachman, H. 1975. Lead in human scalp hair: some factors affecting its variability. *J. Investigative Dermatology* 64: 342–348.

11 Johnson, D.E. *et al.* 1975. Trace metals in occupationally and non-occupationally exposed individuals. *Environmental Health Perspectives* 10: 151–158.

12 Reeves, R., Jolley, K, and Buckley, P. 1975. Lead in human hair: relation to age, sex and environmental factors. *Bull. of Environ. Contam. Toxicol.* 14(5): 579–587.

13 Rabinowitz, M., Wetherill, G. and Kopple, J. July/August 1976. Delayed appearance of tracer lead in facial hair. *Arch. Environ. Health*, pp. 220–223.

14. Olatunbosun, O. *et al.* 1976. Trace element content of hair from Nigerians with sickle cell anemia. *Trace Substances in Environ. Health—X*, Columbia: Univ. Missouri, pp. 383–388.

15. Chattopadhyay, A., Jervis, T. H. and Jervis, R. E. September–October 1977. Scalp hair as a monitor of community exposure to lead. *Arch. Environ. Health*, pp. 226–235.

16. Baker, *et al.* 1977. A nationwide survey of heavy metal absorption in children living near primary copper, lead, and zinc smelters. *Am. J. Epidemiology* 106(4): 261–273.

17. Marzulli, F., Watlington, P. and Maibach, H. 1978. Exploratory skin penetration findings relating to the use of lead acetate hair dyes. *Current Problems in Dermatology.* 7: 196–204.

18. Pihl, R. and Parkes, M. Hair element content in learning disabled children. *Science*, pp. 204–206.

ALUMINUM

Ref.	Locality	No. and type of persons and special conditions	Analysis mg%	Technique Preparation	Instrument	Remarks
1	U.S.S.R.	Workers in contact with aluminum	3.5–22.1			The content of Al in the hair depended on the intensity of occupational contact with Al.
		Workers not in contact	2.9			
2	Canada	Dialysis patients				Elevated Al levels noted for patients on dialysis with encephalopathy syndrome.
3	United States	10 Delinquent, psychotic, or prepsychotic boys, age 12–18			Emission spectroscopy	Ten delinquent, psychotic, or prepsychotic boys had 90% incidence of elevated hair aluminum whereas only 12.4% of 595 patients had elevated levels.
		9 boys	2.9–8.7			
		1 boy (lived in separate building)	1.6			
		595 Patients: 74 patients or 12.4%	> 2.0			

ALUMINUM, cont'd

Ref.	Locality	No. and type of persons and special conditions	Analysis mg%	Technique Preparation	Instrument	Remarks
4						Excess aluminum concentrations in hair ($>$ 5 mg%) may be associated with excess body burden of Al. Cases of amyotrophic lateral sclerosis in Guam may be result of Al-induced toxicity. Hair analysis may be a general screening tool for Al excess.
5	United States	794 Cases, age:		Nonionic detergent and deionized water wash. HNO_3 and H_2O digestion.	Emission spectroscopy	Al levels highest in youngest age group. Hair Al may be reflecting excretion rates. Al and Cd in hair were positively correlated.
		2–8	1.2			
		9–14	0.8			
		15–25	0.4			
		26–35	0.2			
		36–50	0.2			
		51–60	0.3			
		61–75	0.3			
		76–98	0.13			
6	England	73 Dyslexic children	0.23 (0.04–0.59)	Detergent wash. Nitric/perchloric acid digestion.	AAS	Statistical differences noted.
		44 Controls	0.13 (0.03–0.35)			

1 Bryukhanov, V. 1968, 1972. Accumulation of aluminum in the hair of persons in contact with aluminum compounds during their production. *Uch. Tr. Gor'k. Gos. Med. Inst.* 27: 226–9; *Chem. Abstr.* 58828d.

2 Pankhurst, C. and Pate, B. 1978. *Trace Elements in Hair*, University of British Columbia, Vancouver, B.C.—referred to Horsky, S.J., Private Communication, Dept. Pathology, U.B.C.

3 Rees, E. L. 1979. Aluminum toxicity as indicated by hair analysis. *Orthomol. Psych.* 8(1): 37–43.

4 Bland, J. July/August 1980. Diagnostic usefulness of trace elements in human hair—Part II. *Am. Chiropractor* p. 98.

5 Lord, R. and Trawick, W. 1980. Trace element patterns in hair from outpatient clinical laboratory data. *Hair, Trace Elements, and Human Illness.* New York: Praeger Publ., pp. 102–104.

6 Capel, I. *et al.* 1981. Comparison of concentrations of some trace, bulk, and toxic metals in the hair of normal and dyslexic children. *Clin. Chem.* 27(6): 879–881.

ARSENIC

Ref.	Locality	No. and type of persons and special conditions	Analysis mg%	Technique Preparation	Instrument	Remarks
1	Canada	2 Cases as poisoning: I. Chronic poisoning II. Acute poisoning proximal hair after 30 hr. fatal illness	0.44 0.32 0.77		Marsh-Berzelius test	As detected in hair in both acute and chronic poisoning cases.
2	United States	12 Cases peripheral neuropathy	2–8			Diagnosis of arsenic intoxication based on high As levels in hair or urine.
3	Scotland	1200 Subjects	0.081		Radio-activation analysis and chemical separation	Those with hair As > 0.3 mg% (3 ppm) have been exposed to As to some extent. Those between 0.2–0.3 mg (2–3 ppm) should be further examined. Hair As content is important in the investigation of homicidal and industrial poisoning cases.
4	Australia	18 Cases acute arsenical poisoning 6 Cases 12 Cases	< 0.4 0.5–70.0	Nitric and sulfuric acid digestion.	Colorimetric	Results demonstrate unequivocally that excessive quantities of As may be found in the hair and nails within a few hours of poisoning.

ARSENIC, cont'd

Ref.	Locality	No. and type of persons and special conditions	Analysis mg%	Preparation	Instrument	Remarks
5	United States	Normal subjects	.03 (0.006–0.10)	Nitric-sulfuric-perchloric digestion.	Colorimetric	Hair analysis for As is considered to be useful in demonstrating whether long-term absorption to small doses occurred, thus, "normal" levels in hair determined in this study.
6	United States	4th Grade boys environmentally exposed to As:		Detergent, alcohol, EDTA wash.	AAS	Mean hair levels for As accurately reflected community exposure: highest = Cu smelting high = Pb and Zn smelting intermediate = Pb and Zn mining and smelting intermediate = government and commercial low = education and farm trading
		31 highest	0.91			
		16 high	0.30			
		32 intermediate	0.12			
		13 intermediate	0.07			
		28 low	0.03			
7	Czechoslovakia	10 Yr. old boys; distance from source of As emission:		Washed in saporate, water, alcohol, benzene, 10% HCl, alcohol.	Colorimetric	Determination of As in hair in non-occupational exposure conditions can be applied as an exposure test of the population to As.
		1.5 km	0.32			
		3.0 km	0.33			
		4.0 km	0.26			
		7.5 km	0.36	Sulphuric, nitric, perchloric acids.		
		7.5 km	0.18			
		10 km	0.12			
		10 km	0.20			
		14 km	0.18			
		Control	0.10			

	Country	Subjects	As level	Wash/Ref	Method	Comments
8	United States	Individuals drinking high As well-water			Colorimetric	A statistically significant association of water As and hair As levels demonstrated.
9	Canada	76 Rural subjects	0.068 (0.045–0.17)	Distilled water, ethanol, and diethyl ether wash.	INAA RNAA IPAA	Hair can be reliably used as a monitor of environmental exposure to toxic elements.
		45 Urban subjects	0.075 (0.04–0.21)			
		121 Urban subjects near refineries	0.19 (0.063–0.49)			
		Residents of Detah, Yellowknife with minimum amount of As in drinking water	0.34 (0.09–0.6)			
		Letham Island, Yellowknife with large quantities As in water from gold refinery.	0.74 (0.29–2.25)			
10	Czechoslovakia	10 Yr. old boys residing in polluted communities: most heavily polluted	0.33	(see ref. 7)	Colorimetric	As levels in blood, urine, and hair measured; the most advantageous for estimation of non-occupational exposure to As was hair.
		36 km from As source	0.29			
		control group outside polluted area	0.15			

ARSENIC, cont'd

Ref.	Locality	No. and type of persons and special conditions	Analysis mg%	Technique Preparation	Instrument	Remarks
11	United States	Communities with varying As levels in drinking water:		Washed with non-ionic detergent, ethyl alcohol, water.	AAS Hydride generation	Results show that hair and urine mirror As intake. Blood does not seem to be useful in assessing As exposure.
		6 mcg/liter	0.015			
		51 mcg/liter	0.048			
		98 mcg/liter	8.0	Nitric and perchloric acid digestion.		
		123 mcg/liter	0.05			
		393 mcg/liter	22.9			
12	United States	872 Children in Cu smelter towns	0.26	Detergent, deionized water wash.	AAS Hydride Generation	Hair As levels were significantly higher than comparison values in every Cu smelter town. Urine As levels were higher in 10 of 11 copper smelter towns than comparison towns. Hair As tended to reflect urine As concentrations.
		160 Children in comparison towns	0.009			

1 Young, E. G. and Smith, R. P. February 21, 1942. The arsenic content of hair and bone in acute and chronic arsenical poisoning. *Brit. Med. J.*, pp. 251–253.

2 Heyman, A. *et al.* 1956. Peripheral neuropathy caused by arsenical intoxication. *N. Eng. J. Med.* 254(9): 402–409.

3 Smith, H. 1962. Arsenic in biological tissue. *J. Forensic Med.* 9(4): 143–149.

4 Lander, H. *et al.* 1965. Arsenic in the hair and nails: Its significance in acute arsenical poisoning. *J. Forensic Med.* 12(2): 52–67.

5 Boylen, G. and Hardy, H. 1967. Distribution of arsenic in nonexposed persons (hair, liver, and urine). *Am. Ind. Hyg. Assoc. J.* 28: 148–150.

6 Hammer, D. *et al.* 1971. Hair trace metal levels and environmental exposure. *Am. J. Epidemiology* 93(2): 84–92.

7 Bencko, V. *et al.* 1971. Arsenic in the hair of a non-occupationally exposed population. *Atmospheric Environment* 5: 275–279.

8 Goldsmith, J. *et al.* 1972. Evaluation of health implications of elevated arsenic in well water. *Water Research* 6: 1133–1136.

9 Jervis, R., Tiefenbach, B. and Chattopadhyay, A. 1977. Scalp hair as a monitor of population exposure to environmental pollutants. *J. Radioanalytical Chem.* 37: 751–760.

10 Bencko, V. and Symon, K. 1977. Health aspects of burning coal with a high arsenic content: 1. Arsenic in hair, urine, and blood in children residing in a polluted area. *Environ. Res.* 13: 378–385.

11 Valentine, J. *et al.* 1979. Arsenic levels in human blood, urine, and hair in response to exposure via drinking water. *Environ. Res.* 20: 24–32.

12 Baker, E. *et al.* 1977. A nationwide survey of heavy metal absorption in children living near primary copper, lead, and zinc smelters. *Am. J. Epidemiology* 106(4): 261–273.

FLUORINE

Ref.	Locality	No. and type of persons and special conditions	Analysis mg%	Technique Preparation	Technique Instrument	Remarks
1	England					In cases of fluoride poisoning, appreciable amounts of F are found in nails and hair.
2	Czechoslovakia	6–14 Yr. old children living near Al factory				Amount of F in teeth, nails, hair, and urine of children living near Al factory was 2–3 times as high as in control groups.
3	Poland	Welders exposed to fluorides for < 5 yrs. and > 10 yrs.				F levels in hair and skin were directly related to duration of fluoride exposure and to concentrations of fluoride in air and drinking water.

1 Spira, L. 1948. Some sources of intake and methods of elimination of fluorine. *Acta. Med. Scand.* 130: 78–96.

2 Balazova, G., Macuch, P. and Rippel, A. 1969. Effects of fluorine emissions on the living organism. *Fluoride Quart. Rep.* 2(1): 33–6.

3 Byczkowski, S. *et al.* 1971. Attempt to evaluate exposure to fluorides based upon fluoride levels in hair. *Fluoride* 4(2): 98–100.

ANTIMONY

Ref.	Locality	No. and type of persons and special conditions	Analysis mg%	Technique Preparation	Technique Instrument	Remarks
1	Canada	76 Rural residents	0.79	Ether, alcohol, distilled water wash.	IPAA	Environmental location significantly influenced the antimony content of hair.
		45 Urban residents	0.97			
		121 Urban residents, near smelters	1.46			

1 Chattopadhyay, A. and Jervis, R. 1974. Hair as an indicator of multi-element exposure of population groups. *Trace Substances in Environmental Health—VIII.* Columbia: Univ. Missouri, pp. 31–38.

INDEX

Aamodt, R., 137
Abraham, Abraham, 184
Acetoacetyl-CoA deacyclase, and
    vanadium, 223
Acne, and zinc, 134, 135
Acrodermatitis enteropathica, and
    zinc, 125–126
Adenosine triphosphate (ATP), 61
Adult Market Basket(s)
    lead content of, 250
    potassium content of, 84
    sodium content of, 84, 95
Age, and chromium decrease,
    179–180, 189–190
Aging, and copper, 152
Albanese, A., 36, 47
Alcohol, and zinc excretion, 125, 128
Alcohol dehydrogenase, 125
Alcoholism, lithium for, 232
Aldehyde oxidase, 209
Aldosterone
    and magnesium, 70
    and sodium intake, 93

Alfalfa tea, 164
Algin, for lead poisoning, 256
Alginate, in protection from
    mercury, 277
Alkaline phosphatase, and zinc,
    123, 130
Allergies. *See also* Food allergies
    and hair calcium, 52, 54–55
Altura, Burton, 65
Aluminum, 11, 281–286
    absorption, 281–282
    and Alzheimer's disease, 281, 283
    cookware, 283–284
    and dialysis dementia, 281, 285
    dietary intake of, 253, 254–255
    excretion, 281–282
    and food additives, 284
    and hair analysis, 53, 284
    and hair analysis documentation,
        361–363
    and hyperactivity in children, 283
    and parathyroid activity, 74, 282
    and Parkinson's disease, 281, 285–286

368

Aluminum *(continued)*
lead content of in cans, 257
and phosphate, 282
Alzheimer's disease, 74
and aluminum, 281, 283,
285–286
American Society of Elemental
Testing Laboratories, 27
Amino acids, 2
sulfur-containing, 240
Anderson, M. P., 43
Anderson, T. W., 65
Anemia. *See specific type*
Animal foods, iron absorption from,
108, 114
Animals, and hair analysis
documentation of calcium and
phosphorus, 309
Antacids, 61, 282
Anti-inflammatory drugs, 150
Anxiety, calcium for, 47
Arsenic, 3, 6, 287–288
in body, amount of, 287
deficiency, 287
hair analysis interpretation of, 24
and hair analysis documentation,
363–366
toxicity, 287–288
Arthritis
and calcium, 35
and copper, 149–150
and copper bracelets, 149–150
gouty, and molybdenum, 210
rheumatoid
and manganese, 164
and silicon, 218
and zinc, 136
Ashmead, Harvey, 228
Aspartate, as medium-strength chelate,
15
Atherosclerosis
and chromium, 184
and diabetes, 188–189
and lead and cadmium, 266
and silicon, 216, 217, 218
Atomic absorption spectrophotometer,
122
Atoms, in body, 2

Barnes, Broda, 152
Bassler, Tom, 218

Battarbee, Harold, 82, 84
B-complex vitamins
for lead poisoning, 254
and phosphate, 60
Behavior, and zinc, 126
Behavioral and learning disorders, and
aluminum, 283
Benign prostatic hypertrophy,
133–134, 143
Berenshtein, T. F., 203
Berry, Charles, 81
Billick, Irwin, 248
Biorck, Gunnar, 38
Birth defects, and zinc, 125
Bjorksten, Johann, 201
Bland, Jeffrey, 26, 51
Blood
calcium content of, 32, 33, 40
and lead, 245
magnesium in, 70
Blood pressure
and cadmium, 262, 264–265
and calcium, 39
and magnesium, 67
and potassium, 81–82
and sodium, 82, 94–95
and sodium-potassium ratio, 80,
82, 95
and zinc-cadmium ratio, 132
Blood studies
of calcium, as unreliable, 53
of chromium, 182, 183
deficiencies of, 18, 19
of magnesium, 72
need for, 19
of phosphorus, as unreliable, 53
Blood sugar, and potassium, 82–83
Bois, P., 66
Bond decalcification, 35–37, 51
Bone fractures, and silicon, 219
Bonemeal, 50
lead in, 252, 257–258
phosphorus in, 252
Bones
calcium in, 31, 33
finger, radiological examination of,
to determine calcium balance,
40
lead in, 246
magnesium in, 64, 65
mineral content of, 33

Bones *(continued)*
phosphorus in, 60
silicon in, 216
sodium in, 93
strontium in, 239
zinc in, 123
Boynton, Herbert H., 217
Brain, lead in, 246
Bran, and iron absorption, 108
Bratton, Gerald, 254
Breast cancer, and iodine, 172, 173
Breast dysplasia, and iodine, 172–173
Brewer, George E., 137
Brewer's yeast
and cholesterol, 185, 187
and chromium, 181, 185, 187, 192
for diabetes, 189, 190
and GTF activity, 181, 189
Bricklin, Mark, 35
Brody, Arnold, 283
Buettner, Garry, 164
Bunney, William, 231
Burch, G. E., 66
Burnet, F. M., 137
Bush, I. M., 134

Cadmium, 11, 262–271
in cigarette smoke, 264
deficiency, 262
dietary intake of, 253, 254–255,
263, 264, 266–267
in food, 266–267
and hair analysis, 263, 267
and hair analysis documentation,
352–355
hair analysis interpretation of, 24
and kidney damage, 262–265
and lead, 266
relationship of, to other nutrients,
267, 268
selenium in detoxification of, 202
and sludge-fertilized soil, 264, 266
and soil, 266
in water, and blood pressure, 39
women at risk for toxicity of,
263
and zinc, 132
Cadmium poisoning, 262, 263
protection against, 262–263
symptoms of, 262, 263
Cadmium-zinc ratio, 264–265

Calabresi, Paul, 232
Calcitonin, and blood level of
calcium, 32
Calcitriol, and calcium absorption,
41
Calcium, 31–59
absorption, 40, 41–42, 43, 44, 45,
52, 54–55
and age, 51
in American diet, 1
amount of, 31, 50
amount of, in body, 3, 31–32, 33
amount needed, 46–47
and anxiety, 47
and arthritis, 35
and blood pressure, 39, 262,
264–265
blood studies of, as unreliable,
53
daily intake of, 44
in environment, 265–267
excretion, 40–41, 42, 45
and exercise, 32, 35, 46
food sources of, 47–48, 49
forms of, in body, 32
functions of, 31–32, 53
and hair analysis, 40, 51–54
hair analysis documentation of,
306–308
in animals, 309
hair analysis interpretations of,
21–22
and heart disease, 38–40
and iron absorption, 107
and lactose, 45
for lead poisoning, 254
and muscle spasms, 34, 35
and osteoporosis, 35–37, 46–47,
51, 75
and oxalic acid, 45
and periodontal disease, 37–38, 51,
55–56, 75
as protection against cadmium
absorption, 262, 265
release of, from bone, 32, 33
and salt, 45
in teeth, 33–34
Calcium antagonists, 165
Calcium balance, 40–41
and exercise, 36
and osteoporosis, 35, 36, 37

Calcium deposits, in heart, and magnesium, 65
Calcium excretion studies, 52
Calcium fluoride, 45
Calcium-magnesium ratio, 34, 70, 72–75
Calcium phosphate, 33
Calcium-phosphorous ratio, 32, 42–44, 50, 55–56, 61, 75
    and periodontal disease, 37
    of selected foods, 49
Calcium supplements, 50
Calmodulin, 32
Calorie intake, decreased, effects of, 8
Cancer
    breast, and iodine, 172, 173
    esophageal, and molybdenum, 209, 210
    and lithium, 232
    and manganese, 164
    prostate, and zinc, 133
    and rubidium, 234–236
    and selenium, 172, 201
    thyroid, and radioactive fallout, 173
    and zinc, 128
Canfield, Wesley, 183, 190
Cans, lead-soldered, 250, 251–252
Carbohydrates, 2
Carbon, 215
Carbonic anhydrase, 130
Carboxypeptidase, and zinc, 123
Carlisle, Edith, 216
Casdorph, H. Richard, 283
Celiac disease, 97
Cell membranes, maintenance of electrical potential across
    and calcium, 53
    and magnesium, 53, 64, 66–67
    and potassium, 53
    and sodium, 53
Ceruloplasmin, 148, 151, 156
Charnot, A., 218
Chatt, A., 26
Chelates, mineral, 14–16
    stabilities of, 15
Chelation, 10, 14–16
Chelation therapy, 16
    in aluminum toxicity, 285–286
    for mercury poisoning, 278
Cheraskin, Emanuel, 69, 246
Chloride, 92

Chobanian, Aram, 94
Cholesterol
    and chromium, 183, 184–185
    and copper, 130, 131, 132
    and Glucose Tolerance Factor, 185, 187
    and silicon, 218
    and vanadium, 222–223
    and zinc, 130, 131, 132
Choline acetyl transferase, 286
Christopher, Carole, 8
Chromium, 6, 179–199
    absorption, 182
    and age, 179–180, 189–190
    in American diet, 192
    amount needed, 194
    in body, amount of, 179–180, 186
    and brewer's yeast, 181, 185, 187, 192
    and cholesterol, 183, 184–185
    and culture, 180
    and diabetes, 181–182, 188–192
    excretion, 179, 182–183
    food sources of, 192, 193
    forms of, 182, 195
    functions of, 180
    and glucose tolerance, 180
    and Glucose Tolerance Factor, 180, 181–182, 194
    and hair analysis, 182, 191, 195–197
    and hair analysis documentation, 332–336
    hair analysis interpretation of, 23
    and heart disease, 183–187
    hexavalent, toxicity of, 182, 195
    for lead poisoning, 254
    and longevity, 183
    in mammals, 186
    nature of, 180–181
    and processed foods, 179, 183, 194
    storage, 182
    toxicity, 195
    transport, 182
Cigarette smoke. See also Tobacco
    cadmium in, 264
Cobalt, 241
    and hair analysis documentation, 344–346
Collagen, and silicon, 216, 217
Cook, Irving, 133

Cook, James, 108
Copper, 147–160. *See also*
　Zinc-copper ratio
　absorption, features affecting, 148,
　　157
　and aging, 152
　in American diet, 153
　and arthritis, 149–150
　in body, amount of, 147
　chelated, 15
　and cholesterol, 130, 131, 132
　depletion of, from stomach lining,
　　150, 151
　and enzymes, 147, 148, 150, 172
　excretion, 148, 149
　food sources of, 153, 154
　functions of, 137, 147, 148
　and gastric ulcers, 151
　and hair analysis, 155–157
　and hair analysis documentation,
　　324–329
　hair analysis interpretation of, 22
　and heart disease, 149
　and hypothyroidism, 152
　and iron, 148
　and laboratory studies, 156
　for lead poisoning, 254
　and liver, 155, 156
　and molybdenum, 210
　and oral contraceptives, 151, 156
　and pregnancy, 151
　in protection from cadmium, 263
　and schizophrenia, 151
　and soil, 153, 154
　storage, 148–149
　from swimming pools, and hair
　　analysis, 25
　and thyroid gland, 173
　toxicity, 154–155
　transport, 148
　and water, 155–156, 158–159
Copper bracelets, for arthritis,
　149–150
Copper transport diseases, 152–153
Coronary artery spasms and
　magnesium, 65–66, 75–76
Cortisol, and calcium metabolism,
　32
Cosmetics, mercury in, 277
Cranton, Elmer M., 26
Crapper-McLaughlin, D. R., 283, 285

Crawford, Margaret D., 38, 39
Cystic fibrosis, 97

Dailey, John, 82
Dairy products, and iodine, 174
David, Oliver J., 259
Davis, George, 148
Davis, W., 67
Deferoxamine, in aluminum
　chelation, 285
Deoxythymidine kinase, and zinc,
　123
Depression, lithium for, 231–232
Diabetics
　and atherosclerosis, 188–189
　brewer's yeast for, 189, 190
　and chromium, 181–182,
　　188–192
　complications of, 188
　and food allergy, 191–192
　Glucose Tolerance Factor for,
　　188, 189, 190–191
　and manganese, 164
　and zinc, 142
Dialysis dementia, and aluminum,
　281, 285
2-Diaminocyclohexane disodium
　zinc tetraacetate, for cadmium-
　caused high blood pressure,
　265
Diet, balanced, 9
Dietary fiber
　description of, 219
　for lead poisoning, 254
　and silicon, 218, 219, 220
　and zinc absorption, 124, 138, 139
Diet diary, 54
Diets, reducing, and calcium, 36
Dimercapto-l-propanol, with
　EDTA, for lead poisoning, 256
Diseases, hair analysis in early
　detection of, 20, 51–52
DNA dependent RNA polymerase,
　123
DNA synthesis, and zinc, 122–123,
　137
Doisy, Richard, 185, 187, 190,
　191, 192
Dolomite, 50, 252
Drachman, Daniel, 232
Duffield, Joyce, 119

EDTA
   in aluminum toxicity, 283
   with dimercapto-l-propanol, 256
   for mercury poisoning, 278
   as strong chelating agent, 15
   for vanadium poisoning, 224
Egg shell calcium supplements, 50
Elderly, and chromium, 189
Electrolyte minerals. *See* Chloride;
   Potassium; Sodium
Elements, essential, 3, 4. *See also*
   specific element
   definition of, 4
   ranges of, in intake, 5
Elements, toxic. *See* Toxic
   elements
Energy
   and magnesium, 67, 83
   and manganese, 162
   and potassium, 82–83
Enzymes. *See also specific enzyme*
   and copper, 147, 148, 150, 172
   and magnesium, 64, 67, 68
   and manganese, 161, 162, 163, 164
   and minerals, 7
   and molybdenum, 209, 210
   and potassium, 83
   and zinc, 122, 123, 130, 137, 150,
   172
Epstein, O., 155
Eskin, Bernard A., 172, 173
Esophageal cancer, and molybdenum,
   209, 210
Estrogen, and breast dysplasia, 173
Ethylenediamine dihydroiodide
   (EDDI), 174
Exercise
   and calcium, 32, 35, 46
   and phosphorous excretion, 61
   and silicon, 268
   and sodium, 93, 96

Fatty acids, 2
Ferritin, 105, 107, 110
Ferrous fumerate, 10
Ferrous gluconate, 10
Ferrous sulfate, 16
Fertility, and zinc, 133
Fertilizers, and decreased absorption
   of trace elements, 138
Fetal alcohol syndrome, and zinc, 125

Fiber. *See* Dietary fiber; Plant fiber
Fluoride, 3
   and aluminum toxicity, 286
   and calcium, 45
Fluorine, 3
   and hair analysis documentation,
   367
Flour
   enriched, 116–118
   refined. *See also* Refined flour
Food additives
   and aluminum, 284
   and iodine, 171
   phosphates in, 37, 61, 108
   and diabetes, 191–192
   and malabsorption of minerals,
   157–158
Food coloring, and iodine, 175, 176
Food preparation
   and potassium, 84
   and zinc, 140
Food "substitutes," 8
Food supplements
   lead in, 252
   for lead poisoning, 254
Foods
   animal. *See also* Animal foods
   fortification of, with iron, 108,
   115–118
   plant. *See also* Plant foods
   processed. *See also* Processed foods
Food utensils
   aluminum in, 283–284
   lead in, 252
Frazer, A., 232
Freeland-Graves, Jeanne, 131
Free radicals, and copper, 152
Frommer, Donald, 136
Fumerates, 15–16

Gasoline, lead from, 249, 250
Genetic defects, and copper,
   152–153, 156–157
Gershoff, Stanley, 68
Giles, T. D., 66
Gluconate, 15
Glucose intolerance, and manganese,
   163–164
Glucose Tolerance Factor (GTF)
   and chromium, 180, 181–182,
   194

(GTF) *(continued)*
  and cholesterol, 185, 187
  for diabetes, 188, 189, 190–191
  food sources of, 192, 193
Glutathione peroxidase, 200
Glycerol kinase, 180
Glycogen, and potassium, 83
Glycosyltransferase enzymes, and
  manganese, 161
Goddard, James L., 150
Goiter
  and breast cancer, 172
  and iodine, 170–171, 176
Goitrogens, 171
Goodwin, Frederick, 232
Gordon, Gary, 246
Gordus, Adon, 127
Gouty arthritis, and molybdenum,
  210
Gram, 2
Green, Paul, 119
Growth
  and nickel, 227
  and silicon, 216
  and zinc, 125, 142–143, 216

Haeger, Knut, 135
Hair analysis, 18–27
  advantages of, 19–24
  and aluminum, 53, 284
  argon plasma emission, method of,
    195, 205
  atomic absorption technique, 205
  and cadmium, 263, 267
  and calcium, 51–54
  and chromium, 182, 191,
    195–197
  and copper, 155–157
  and digestion techniques, 295–297
  factors leading to
    misinterpretation of, 25, 51, 52,
    73, 142, 205
  flameless, graphite furnace atomic
    absorption method of, 196
  hair cutting procedures in, 293–294
  and iron, 119, 120, 121
  laboratory hair washing procedures
    in, 294–295
  and lead, 247, 248, 256, 257
  and lithium, 233
  and magnesium, 52, 54, 71–72

  and manganese, 167–168
  and mercury, 278
  need for skilled professional in,
    19–20
  and nickel, 228
  and phosphorus, 61, 75
  and potassium, 85–86, 96–97
  as screening test, 53
  and selenium, 205
  and silicon, 220
  and sodium, 96–97
  utility of, 297–299. *See also*
    specific element
  and vanadium, 224
  and zinc, 141–142
Hair analysis documentation, 304–367
  and aluminum, 361–363
  and animals, 309
  and arsenic, 363–366
  and cadmium, 352–355
  and calcium, 306–308
    in animals, 309
  and chromium, 332–336
  and cobalt, 344–346
  and copper, 324–329
  and flourine, 367
  and iodine, 332
  and iron, 313–315
  and lead, 355–361
  and lithium, 343
  and magnesium, 309–311
  and manganese, 329–331
  and mercury, 347–351
  and nickel, 341–342
  and phosphorus, 308
    in animals, 309
  and potassium, 311
  and selenium, 336–338
  and silicon, 339
  and sodium, 312
  and strontium, 344
  and tin, 343
  and vanadium, 340
  and zinc, 315–324
Hair analysis interpretation, 20, 21–24
  and correction of abnormalities,
    20, 21–24
Hair analysis standardization,
  25–27, 291–297
Hair Analysis Standardization
  Board, 26–27, 291, 292

Hair color, and hair analysis, 25, 51, 54, 73, 142
Hair dyes, lead in, 253
Hair growth, 18–19, 25
Hair preparations and treatments and misinterpretation of hair analysis, 25, 51, 52, 73, 142, 205
Hanes survey, 1
Hansen, Gaurth, 96
Hass, George, 66
Healing, and zinc, 127–128, 132, 135, 136
Heart beat, calcium controlling, 32, 38
Heart disease
    and calcium, 38–40
    and chromium, 183–187
    and copper, 149
    and magnesium, 65–66, 75–76
    and manganese, 164–165
    and selenium, 201–203, 205
    and soft water, 38–40
    and vanadium, 222, 223
    and zinc, 129–132
    and zinc-copper ratio, 130–132
Heart rhythm, and potassium, 81
Heath, Hunter, 44
Hegsted, Mark, 44
Hellewell, Bryan, 275
Hemochromatosis, 111, 116, 119–120
Hemoglobin, iron in, 105
Hemosiderin, 107, 110
Hemosiderosis, 111
Henkin, Robert, 137
Henzel, John, 127, 129
High density lipoprotein-to-low density lipoprotein ratios, and chromium, 185
Histapenia. See Schizophrenia
Huntington's chorea, lithium for, 232
Husain, Latafat, 135
Hyperparathyroidism, 42, 44, 96–97
    subclinical, and calcium, 51, 73, 74
    subclinical, and magnesium, 73, 74
Hypothyroidism
    and copper, 152
    and zinc, 152

Immune system
    and selenium, 203–204
    and vitamin E, 203, 204
Immunity, and zinc, 128
Inorganic salts, 10
Insogna, Karl, 282
Insomnia, and magnesium, 67
Insulin, and calcium metabolism, 32
Insulin injections, 189
Intelligence, and zinc, 126–127
Intestinal mucosa, electrical barrier of, 15
Iodine, 170–176
    absorption, 171–172
    in American diet, 174, 175–176
    amount needed, 174
    in body, amount of, 171
    and breast cancer, 172, 173
    and breast dysplasia, 172–173
    in dairy products, 174
    excretion, 172
    in food coloring, 175, 176
    food sources of, 174, 175
    and goiter, 170–171, 176
    and hair analysis documentation, 332
    and radioactive fallout, 173
    and soil, 173
    storage, 172
    symptoms of deficiency of, 171
    and thyroid gland, 171, 172
    toxicity, 175–176
Iodophors, 174
Ionization, 10
Ionized serum calcium, 52
Iron, 105–121
    absorption, 10, 106–108, 114
    active, 105
    in American diet, 1, 109, 113
    in body, amount of, 105
    chelated, 15, 17
    and copper, 148
    deficiency, 106, 109–110
    elemental, 108
    female's intake of, 1
    food sources of, 112–113
    forms of, 10
    fortification of food with, 108, 115–118
    functions of, 105
    and growth, 109

Iron *(continued)*
  in hair, and poor correlation with
    body stores of, 19
  and hair analysis, 119, 120, 121
  and hair analysis documentation,
    313–315
  heme, 108, 114
  in infancy, 109
  for lead poisoning, 254
  loss, by cell loss, 105–106
  non-heme, 108
  in pregnancy, 109
  in protection from cadmium, 263
  storage, 107
  stored, 105, 106, 107, 109, 111
  toxicity, 106, 110–111, 114–115
  transport, 107
Iron deficiency anemia, 106, 110,
  120–121
Iron supplements, 106, 109, 110–111,
  114–115, 118–119
  in pregnancy, 109
  and toxicity, 106, 110–111,
    114–115
Iseri, Lloyd, 66

Jarvik, Lissy, 283
Jick, Hershel, 264

Kark, Robert, 94
Keshan disease, and selenium,
  202–203, 205
Kevorkian, Jack, 273, 274
Kidney damage, and cadmium, 262,
  265
Kidney stones, and magnesium, 68
Klevay, Leslie, 130, 132, 153, 155
Kobayashi, J., 38
Krakoff, Lawrence, 94
Krakovitz, Rob, 26
Krook, Lennart, 37
Kuller, Lewis, 82

Laboratory studies
  in calcium disorder, 52, 53
  and copper, 156
  and iron deficiency, 110
  and magnesium, 72
  and vanadium, 224
Lactation
  and cadmium accumulation, 263

  and iron, 109
Lactic acid dehydrogenase, 130
Lactose, and calcium, 45
Langford, Herbert, 82
Laragh, John, 94
Lead, 11, 245–261
  airborne, 245, 246, 247, 248, 249,
    250
  in blood, amount of, 245
  in bone, amount of, 246
  in brain, 246
  and cadmium, 266
  daily excretion of, 248
  daily intake of, 248
  dietary, 250–253, 254–255
  and environmental contamination,
    245, 246, 247, 248–249
  in food supplements, 252
  from gasoline, 249, 250
  and hair analysis, 247, 248,
    256–257
  and hair analysis documentation,
    355–361
  hair analysis interpretation of, 23
  in hair dyes, 253
  in improperly glazed food
    utensils, 252
  increase in, through time,
    245–246
  occupational sources of, 253,
    255–256
  in paint, 245, 247, 248–249
  in soldered cans, 250, 251–252
  in water, 266
  from water pipes, 253
  and zinc protoporphyrin in
    screening for, 248, 256
Lead acetate, in hair preparations,
  and hair analysis, 25
Lead poisoning, 245
  and behavioral and learning
    impairments, 247, 259
  early symptoms of, 246–247
  in market basket survey, 250
  prevalence of, 245, 247
  treating, 254, 256
Lecithin, for Alzheimer's disease,
  286
Lee, C. J., 36
Lee, Kenneth, 108
Lewis, George P., 264

Libido, and zinc, 133
Lindsay, Allen, 42
Linkswiler, Hellen, 42, 43
Liss, Leopold, 283
Lithium, 3, 231–232
  for alcoholism, 232
  amount needed, 231
  and cancer, 232
  for depression, 231–232
  and hair analysis, 233
  and hair analysis documentation,
    343
  for Huntington's chorea, 232
  and lymphocytes, 232
  for mania, 231
  for Ménière's disease, 232
  for tardive dyskinesia, 232
  toxicity, 233
Liu, Victoria, 183, 187
Liver, and copper, 155, 156
Ljunghall, Sverker, 68
Longevity, and chromium, 183
Lund-Olesen, Knud, 150
Lutwak, Leo, 37, 38, 43, 44, 46
Lymphocytes, and lithium, 232

McCarron, David, 39
McCay, C. M., 190
Macro-minerals, 3. See Calcium;
  Magnesium; Phosphorus
Magnesium, 64–76. See also
  Calcium-magnesium ratio
  absorption, 69–70
  in American diet, 69
  amount needed, 65, 69
  and blood pressure, 67
  in body, amount of, 64
  and cancer, 66–67
  chelated, 15
  and electrical potential across cell
    membranes, 53, 64
  and energy, 67, 83
  and epilepsy, 68
  excretion, 70
  food sources of, 70–71
  functions of, 64
  and hair analysis, 52, 54, 71–72
  and hair analysis documentation,
    309–311
  hair analysis interpretation of, 22
  and heart disease, 65–66, 75–76

  and kidney stones, 68
  and menstrual cramps, 68
  and osteoporosis, 72, 73, 75
  and periodontal disease, 72, 73, 75
  and potassium, cellular, 80
  and sleep, 65
  supplements, 71
  symptoms of deficiency of, 68
  and tension, 67–68
Mammals, amount of chromium in,
  186
Man
  ancient, trace elements in,
    186–187
  modern, trace elements in,
    186–187
Mandell, Marshall, 191
Manganese, 161–169
  absorption, 162, 164, 165
  in American diet, 167
  amount needed, 166–167
  in body, amount of, 161
  and cancer, 164
  and diabetes, 164
  and enzymes, 161
  and epilepsy, 163
  excretion, 162, 165
  food sources of, 165–166
  functions of, 161–162
  and glucose intolerance, 163–164
  and hair analysis, 167–168
  and hair analysis documentation,
    329–331
  and heart disease, 164–165
  and phenothiazines, 163
  and processed foods, 166
  and rheumatoid arthritis, 164
  and schizophrenia, 151, 163
  signs of deficiency of, 161
  and soil, 166
  supplements, when to take, 165
  and tardive dyskinesia, 163
  toxicity, 166
  transport, 162
Mania, lithium for, 231
Manic-depression
  lithium for, 232
  and vanadium toxicity, 224
Martin, John, 204
Maseri, Attilio, 66
Medicine, mercury in, 277

Menander-Huber, Kerstin B., 150
Mendels, J., 231, 232
Ménière's disease, lithium for, 232
Menkes' disease, 152–153
Menstrual cramps
  and calcium, 34
  and magnesium, 34, 68
Menstrual iron loss, 109
Mercury, 11, 272–280
  in cosmetics, 277
  and dental fillings, 275–276, 277
  dietary intake of, 253, 254–255
  and hair analysis, 278
  and hair analysis documentation,
    347–351
  hair analysis interpretation of, 23
  inhaled, 277, 278
  in medicines, 277
  occupational sources of, 275,
    277–278
  protection from, 277–278
  in seafood, 273–275
  sources of contamination of, 276.
    See also specific source
  symptoms of toxicity of, 275
Mercury poisoning, 272–273
Mertz, Walter, 4, 8, 181, 189, 192,
    194
Microgram, 2
Miller, George, 82
Milligram, 2
Minamata disease, 273
Mineral balance, complete, 44
Mineral supplements, when to take,
    20
Minerals
  in bones, 33
  and enzymes, 7
  forms of, 10
  importance of, 7
  interference of, with other minerals,
    5, 6
  in teeth, 33–34
  today's problems with, 7–10
  and topsoil loss, 9
  use of word, 3
Mittelman, Jerry, 277
Molecules, 2
Molybdenum, 209–211
  amount needed, 210
  in body, amount of, 209

and copper, 210
diseases associated with deficiency
  of, 209–210
and enzymes, 209, 210
food sources of, 209, 210, 211
functions of, 210
Morris, Steven, 183
Muscle spasms, and calcium
  deficiency, 34, 35
Myers, John, 173

Nandi, Manis, 264
Nanogram, 2
Needleman, Herbert L., 247
Nerve(s)
  calcium's effect on, 32–33
  resting potential of, 32–33, 34
Newton, Isaac, 272–273
Nickel, 3, 227–229
  amount needed, 228
  deficiency, 227
  dust and gases, toxicity of, 228
  food sources of, 228–229
  functions of, 228
  and growth, 227
  and hair analysis, 228
  and hair analysis documentation,
    341–342
  hair analysis interpretation of, 23
  and taste, 137
  in tobacco, 228
Nickel carbonyl, toxicity of, 228
Nielsen, F. H., 227, 287
Nucleoproteins, 61

Oberly, Larry, 164
Occupational sources
  of lead, 253, 255–256
  of mercury, 275, 277–278
Offenbacher, Ester, 187
Oral contraceptives, and copper, 151,
    156
Organic complexes, absorption of, 10,
    15–16
Osteomalacia, 35
Osteoporosis
  and calcium, 35–37, 46–47, 51, 75
  and magnesium, 72, 73, 75
  and phosphorus, 43
Oxalic acid
  and calcium, 45

Oxalic acid *(continued)*
  food sources of, 45
  and iron absorption, 108
Oxygen, 2
Oyster shell calcium supplements, 50

Paint, lead in, 245, 247, 248–249
Parathormone. *See* Parathyroid
    hormone
Parathyroid gland
  and aluminum, 53, 74
  functions of, 61
Parathyroid hormone
  and aluminum, 282
  and calcium, 32, 41
  and silicon, 218
Parkinson's disease, 74
Patterson, Clair, 245, 251
Pectin
  for lead poisoning, 256
  protection
    against cadmium, 263
    against mercury, 277
Pekarek, R. S., 141
Penicillamine, for Wilson's disease,
    153
Periodontal disease
  and calcium, 37–38, 51, 55–56, 75
  and magnesium, 72, 73, 75
Perl, Daniel, 283
Pestronk, Alan, 232
Peterson, Donald R., 38
Pfeiffer, Carl, 151, 153, 155, 163
Phenothiazines, and manganese, 163
Philpott, William, 191
Phosphate(s)
  and aluminum, 282
  blood level of, 61
  in food additives, 61
  functions of, 60
  and iron absorption, 108
  in soft drinks, 37, 44, 61, 108
  as source for excess phosphorus,
    37, 44
  and subclinical
    hyperparathyroidism, 74
Phospholipids, 60
Phosphorus, 60–63. *See also*
    Calcium-phosphorous ratio
  absorption, 61
  in American diet, 61

blood studies of, as unreliable,
    53
  in body, amount of, 60
  in bone, amount of, 33
  in bone meal, 252
  daily intake of, 44
  deficiency, rarity of, 60, 61
  excessive, and periodontal disease,
    37
  food sources of, 61, 62
  functions of, 60
  and hair analysis, 61, 75
  hair analysis documentation of,
    308
    in animals, 309
    in selected foods, 49
Phosphorous compounds, 60–61
Phytic acid, and zinc absorption, 124,
    138, 139
Plant fibers, silicon in, 216, 218, 219,
    220
Plant foods, iron absorption from,
    108, 114
Pories, Walter, 127
Potassium, 79–91. *See also*
    Sodium-potassium ratio
  absorption, 80
  in Adult Market Baskets, 84, 95
  in American diet, 79
  amount needed, 83–84
  and blood pressure, 81–82
  in body, amount of, 79
  deficiency of, symptoms of, 81
  depletion of, symptoms of, 80–81
  and electrical potential across cell
    membrane, 53
  and energy, 82–83
  excretion, 80
  for fatigue, 67
  food sources of, 84, 86–87, 88, 91
  functions of, 80
  and hair analysis, 85–86, 96–97
  and hair analysis documentation,
    311
  hair analysis interpretation of, 24
  and heart rhythm, 81
  ion, 237
  and muscle strength, 83
  and processed foods, 81, 82, 89,
    90, 93
  supplements, 85

Potassium *(continued)*
  toxicity of, 81
Potassium chloride, 85
Potassium iodide, for radioactive
    fallout, 173
Pregnancy
  and cadmium accumulation, 263
  and copper, 151
  and zinc, 125
Prien, Edwin, 68
Processed foods, 8
  and chromium, 179, 183, 194
  and copper, 153
  and magnesium, 69
  and manganese, 166
  and molybdenum, 209
  and potassium, 81, 82, 89, 90,
    93
  and sodium, 81, 89–90, 93, 96,
    97, 98
  and sodium-potassium ratio, 85
  and zinc, 139
Prostaglandins, and selenium, 202
Prostate gland, and zinc, 133–134, 143
Prostatitis, and zinc, 133
Protein
  in bone, 33
  diet, high in protection against
    cadmium, 263
  in teeth, 34
Protein deficiency, and calcium
    absorption, 41–42
Protein synthesis, and zinc, 122–123
Pulmonary emphysema, and
    cadmium fumes, 264
Pyruvate carboxylase, and
    manganese, 161

Quantities, small, description of, 2

Radioactive fallout, and iodine, 173
Randoin, J., 219
Recker, R., 281
Red-cell protoporphyrin, 110
Rees, Elizabeth, 284, 285
Refined flour, 115–116
  and manganese, 166
  and silicon, 219
  and zinc, 139
Relative chromium response (RCR),
    182, 183

Renin levels, and sodium, 94, 95
Research trace elements. *See* Cobalt;
    Lithium; Nickel; Rubidium;
    Silicon; Strontium; Sulfur; Tin;
    Vanadium
Retinol-binding protein, 134
Rheumatoid arthritis
  and manganese, 164
  and zinc, 136
Riales, Rebecca, 185
Robinson, T., 218
Ronaghy, H., 126
Rubidium, 3, 234–238
  and tumor growth, 234–236

Salt. *See also* Sodium
  and calcium excretion, 45
  diet low in, 94
  iodized, 171
Salt substitute, potassium-based, 85
Sanstead, H. H., 141
Schaffner, Robert, 250
Schizophrenia
  and copper, 151
  and manganese, 151, 163
  and zinc, 151
Schmidt, Alexander, 117
Schrauzer, Gerhard, 201
Schroeder, Henry, 38, 39, 179, 183,
    187, 191
Schultz, R., 204
Schwarz, Klaus, 181, 200, 216, 230,
    257–258
Seafood
  cadmium in, 266
  mercury in, 273–275
Seawater, trace elements in,
    186–187
Sedlacek, Thomas, 128
Seelig, M., 69, 74
Selenium, 6, 200–208
  absorption, 200
  amount needed, 204
  in body, amount of, 3, 200
  and cancer, 172, 201
  excretion, 200
  food sources of, 204, 206
  function of, 200–201
  and hair analysis, 205
  and hair analysis documentation,
    336–338

Selenium *(continued)*
  hair analysis interpretation of, 24
  and heart disease, 201–203, 205
  and immune system, 203–204
  protection
    from cadmium, 202, 263, 265
    from mercury, 277–278
  and soil, 204
  toxicity, 205
Senile dementia, and zinc, 137
Serum ferritin, 19
Sex, and zinc, 133
Sexual impotency, and
    molybdenum, 209
Shamburger, Raymond, 201
Shapiro, Samuel, 264
Sheffy, B., 204
Sickle-cell anemia, and zinc, 137
Silbergold, Ellen K., 246
Silicon, 3, 215–221
  in animal tissues, amount of, 216
  and arthritis, 218
  and atherosclerosis, 216, 217,
    218
  and bone, 216
  and bone fractures, 219
  and cholesterol, 218
  and collagen, 216, 217
  and dietary fiber, 218, 219, 220
  in English diet, amount of, 219
  and exercise, 218
  food sources of, 219
  functions of, 215
  and gastric ulcers, 218
  and growth, 216
  and hair analysis, 220
  and hair analysis documentation,
    339
  and parathyroid hormone, 218
  in plant fibers, 216, 218, 219, 220
  and skin, 216–217
Simkin, Peter, 136
Skin
  and silicon, 216–217
  and zinc, 134–135, 136
Sleep, and magnesium, 67
Slone, Dennis, 264
Sodium, 92–102. *See also* Salt
  in Adult Market Baskets, 84, 85
  amount needed, and potassium, 84
  in body, amount of, 93

and blood pressure, 82, 94–95
in diet, amount of, 79
dietary, 92, 93, 95–96, 99
and electrical potential across cell
    membrane, 53
excretion, 93
and exercise, 93, 96
foods high in, 95–96, 100
food sources of, 97
functions of, 93
and hair analysis, 96–97
and hair analysis documentation,
    312
hair analysis interpretation of, 24
and processed foods, 81, 89–90,
    93, 96, 97, 98
replacement of, 93, 96
in soft water, 38
toxicity, of, 96
Sodium nitrate, 8
Sodium-potassium pump, 79–80, 85
Sodium-potassium ratio, 79
  and blood pressure, 80, 82
  and processed food, 85
Soft drinks, phosphates in, 37, 44,
    61, 108
Soft tissue calcification, 44, 51, 52,
    68
  and calcium-magnesium ratio, 73
  and manganese, 164
Soil
  and cadmium, 264, 266
  and copper, 153, 154
  and iodine, 173
  and loss of trace elements, 9–10
  and manganese, 166
  and molybdenum, 209
  and selenium, 204
  and vanadium, 223
  and zinc, 122, 127, 138, 139
Sorenson, John, 151
Soy protein, and iron absorption,
    108
Spallholz, Julian, 204
Spargo, P., 272
Spencer, Herta, 36, 42, 43, 124
Staub, H. W., 187
Strain, William, 245
Strontium, 3, 239
  and hair analysis documentation,
    344

Sugar, and hair calcium, 52
Sulfite oxidase, 209
Sulfur, 240
  food sources of, 240
Superoxide dismutase, 132
  copper in, 150
  and manganese in, 161, 162, 164
  zinc in, 150
Superoxide radical, 162
Swimming pools, and hair analysis,
  155

Tardive dyskinesia
  lithium for, 163
  and manganese, 163
Taste
  and copper, 137
  and nickel, 137
  and zinc, 137
Teeth
  and calcium, 31, 33–34
  decay of, 209, 210
  fillings, mercury in, 275–276, 277
  and magnesium, 64, 65
  mineral content of, 33–34
  and molybdenum, 209, 210
  phosphorus in, 60
  and strontium, 239
  and zinc, 126
Tension, and magnesium, 67–68
Testosterone, and zinc, 133
Tetany, 34
Thymus gland damage, and zinc, 128
Thyroglobulin, 172
Thyroid gland
  cancer of, and radioactive fallout,
    173
  and copper, 173
  and iodine, 171, 172
Thyroid hormones
  and copper, 152
  and iodine, 171, 172
Thyroxin (T4)
  and copper, 152
  and iodine, 172, 173
Tin, 3, 230
  in diet, amount of, 230
  and hair analysis documentation,
    343
Tipton, Isabel, 179
Tissue biopsy, deficiencies of, 18, 19

Tobacco. See also Cigarette smoke
  nickel in, 228
Topsoil, loss of, 9
Toxic elements, 11–12. See also
  Aluminum; Arsenic; Cadmium;
  Lead; Mercury
Trace element supplements, when to
  take, 20
Trace elements. See also Copper;
  Iodine; Iron; Manganese; Zinc
  in ancient man, 186–187
  and biological amplification, 7, 8
  deficiencies of, 170
  and fertilizers, 138
  in modern man, 186–187
  in seawater, 186–187
  use of word, 3
Trace elements research. See Cobalt;
  Lithium; Nickel; Rubidium;
  Silicon; Strontium; Sulfur; Tin;
  Vanadium
Transferrin, 107
Transferrin saturation, 110
Transmanganin, 162
Tri-iodothyronine (T3)
  and copper, 152
  and iodine, 171, 172
Tumor growth, and rubidium,
  234–236
Turlapaty, Prasad, 65
24-hour urinary copper excretion,
  156

Ulcers
  gastric
    and copper, 151
    and silicon, 218
    and zinc, 136
  leg, and zinc, 135
  skin, and zinc, 135
Ultra-trace elements. See
  Chromium; Molybdenum;
  Selenium
Urine studies, deficiencies of, 18

Vanadium, 3, 222–226
  and acetoacetyl-CoA deacylase,
    223
  in body, amount of, 222
  and cholesterol, 222–223
  deficiency, 222

Vanadium *(continued)*
  in diet, amount of, 223
  food sources of, 224–225
  functions of, 222, 224
  and hair analysis, 224
  and hair analysis documentation,
    340
  and heart disease, 222, 223
  and soil, 223
  toxicity, 224
Viets, Frank, 138
Vitamin A
  deficiency, 1
  with zinc, for acne, 134, 135
Vitamin B1, for lead poisoning,
    254
Vitamin B6, and zinc absorption,
    124
Vitamin B12, cobalt in, 241
Vitamin C
  deficiency, 1
  and iron absorption, 107, 108
  for lead poisoning, 254
  in protection from cadmium, 263
  for vanadium poisoning, 224
Vitamin D
  and calcium absorption, 32, 35
  and zinc absorption, 124
Vitamin E
  and immune system, 203, 204
  and iron absorption, 107,
    118–119
  for leg cramps, 34
Vitamin-mineral supplement, balanced
  taken with meals, 20
  total daily intake of, 20,
    21
Vitamins, 1, 2

Walker, Ray, 149
Warburg, Otto, 235
Water
  and cadmium, 265–266
  and copper, 155–156, 158–159
  "corrosiveness" of, and blood
    pressure, 39
  and heart disease, 38–40
Watson, Robert, 82
Weissman, Robert, 249
Williams, Roger, 47
Wilson's disease, 153, 156–157

Women
  and iron intake, 1
  postmenopausal, and bone
    demineralization, 35, 36, 46–47
  at risk for cadmium toxicity, 263
Wright, Jonathan, 27

Xanthine oxidase, 209

Yokel, Robert, 284

Ziady, F., 67
Zinc, 122–146
  absorption, factors complicating,
    124, 125, 138, 139
  and acne, 134, 135
  in American diet, 140
  and behavior, 126–127
  in body, amount of, 123
  and cadmium, 132, 263, 265
  and calories, 139
  and cancer, 128
  causes of deficiency of, 140
  chelated, 15
  and cholesterol, 130, 131, 132
  and diabetes, 142
  and enzymes, 122, 123, 130,
    137, 150, 172
  excretion, 124–125, 128
  and fertility, 133
  and food preparation, 140
  food sources of, 138–139
  functions of, 122–123
  and gastric ulcers, 136
  and growth, 125, 126, 142–143
  and hair analysis, 141–142
  and hair analysis documentation,
    315–324
  hair analysis interpretation of, 19,
    22
  and healing, 127–128, 132, 135,
    136
  and heart disease, 129–132
  and immunity, 128
  and intelligence, 126–127
  for lead poisoning, 254
  and libido, 133
  and pregnancy, 125
  and processed food, 139
  and prostate gland, 133–134, 143
  and rheumatoid arthritis, 136

Zinc *(continued)*
   and schizophrenia, 151
   and senile dementia, 137
   and sickle-cell anemia, 137
   and skin, 134–135, 136
   and skin ulcers, 135
   and soil, 122, 127, 138, 139
   supplements, when to take, 141
   symptoms of deficiency of, 123
   and taste, 137
   toxicity, 141
   with vitamin A, for acne, 134–135
Zinc-cadmium ratio, and blood
   pressure, 132
Zinc-copper ratio, and heart
   disease, 130–132
Zinc protoporphyrin, in screening
   for lead, 248, 256

ABOUT THE AUTHORS

Richard A. Passwater, Ph.D. is one of the most called-upon authorities for information relating to preventive health care. A noted biochemist, he is credited with popularizing the term "supernutrition" largely as a result of having written two bestsellers on the subject—*Supernutrition: The Megavitamin Revolution* and *Supernutrition for Healthy Hearts*. His other books include *Easy No-Flab Diet, Cancer and Its Nutritional Therapies,* and the recently published *Selenium as Food & Medicine.*

Elmer M. Cranton, M.D., a graduate of Harvard Medical School, is Board Certified as a medical specialist by the American Board of Family Practice and by the American Board of Chelation Therapy. He served as president of the Smyth County Medical Society, Virginia, in 1980 and was president of the American Holistic Medical Association from 1980-1982. He is currently vice president of the American Academy of Medical Preventics. Since 1976, Dr. Cranton has practiced in Trout Dale, Virginia where he specializes in holistic family medicine, preventive medicine, nutrition, EDTA chelation and hyperbolic oxygen therapy.